Parkinson's Disease - Animal Models, Current Therapies and Clinical Trials

Edited by Sarat Chandra Yenisetti, Zevelou Koza, Devendra Kumar, Sushil Kumar Singh and Ankit Ganeshpurkar

Published in London, United Kingdom

Parkinson's Disease - Animal Models, Current Therapies and Clinical Trials
http://dx.doi.org/10.5772/intechopen.100831
Edited by Sarat Chandra Yenisetti, Zevelou Koza, Devendra Kumar, Sushil Kumar Singh and Ankit Ganeshpurkar

Assistant to the Editors: Priyanka Modi and Abhik Das

Contributors
Qing Zhao, Lingjing Jin, Lin Ma, Tingting Sun, Mengdie Zhou, Lama Saad El-Din Mahmoud, Maria Rosa Avila-Costa, José Luis Ordóñez-Librado, Ana Luisa Gutiérrez-Valdez, Enrique Montiel-Flores, Vianey Rodriguez-Lara, Cesar Alfonso Garcia Caballero, Claudia Dorado-Martínez, Leonardo Reynoso-Erazo, Rocío Tron-Alvarez, Javier Sanchez-Betancourt, Ma. Teresa Ibarra-Gutierrez, Veronica Anaya-Martínez, Patricia E. Reyna-Velázquez, Gloria Cruz, Juan Ramírez, Shengdong Nie, Arthur Oscar Schelp, Jéssica Emy Komuro, Daniel Fabiano Barbosa dos Santos, Andreas Batista Schelp, Silvia Justina Papini, Wenming Shi, Changbo Jin, Ahed J. Khatib, Pankaj Singh Dholaniya, Mohammad Ahmad, Neha S, Baby Kumari, MD. Zainul Ali, Bin Song, Jeffrey Schweitzer, Jun Xue, Fangzhou Li, Jiahao Ji, Arturo Solís Herrera, Sarat Chandra Yenisetti, Zevelou Koza, Padmanabhan S. Rajani, Muralidhara, Ajaikumar B. Kunnumakkara, Burak Yaman

First published in London, United Kingdom, 2023 by IntechOpen
IntechOpen is the global imprint of INTECHOPEN LIMITED, registered in England and Wales, registration number: 11086078, 5 Princes Gate Court, London, SW7 2QJ, United Kingdom

British Library Cataloguing-in-Publication Data
A catalogue record for this book is available from the British Library

Additional hard and PDF copies can be obtained from orders@intechopen.com

Parkinson's Disease - Animal Models, Current Therapies and Clinical Trials
Edited by Sarat Chandra Yenisetti, Zevelou Koza, Devendra Kumar, Sushil Kumar Singh and Ankit Ganeshpurkar
p. cm.
Print ISBN 978-1-80356-488-3
Online ISBN 978-1-80356-489-0
eBook (PDF) ISBN 978-1-80356-490-6

For EU product safety concerns:
IN TECH d.o.o., Prolaz Marije Krucifikse Kozulić 3, 51000 Rijeka, Croatia,
info@intechopen.com or visit our website at intechopen.com.

Meet the editors

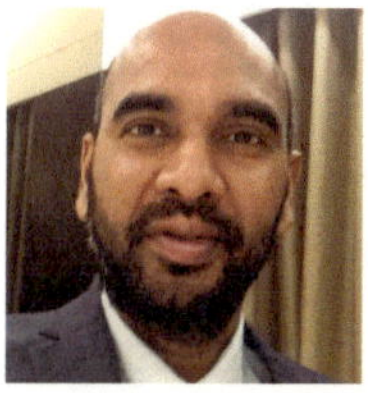

Dr. Sarat Chandra Yenisetti is a professor in the Department of Zoology, Nagaland University (A Central University), India. He received post-doctoral training in neurogenetics from the National Institutes of Neurological Disorders and Stroke (NINDS) of the National Institutes of Health (NIH), USA, and the University of Regensburg, Germany. Dr. Yenisetti's *Drosophila* Neurobiology Laboratory (DNBL) follows *Drosophila* approaches to understand dopaminergic neurodegeneration and identify therapeutic targets for neuroprotection, knowledge of which will help to reduce the burden of Parkinson's disease (PD) in humans. His laboratory developed adult-life, phase-specific *Drosophila* models of PD and demonstrated their importance in understanding the pathophysiology of late-onset neurodegenerative disease (NDD). It also further proved that deciphering the age-mediated regulation of brain-specific molecular networks is essential to screen small molecules/nutraceuticals/drugs with potential neuroprotective efficacy and develop/modulate the therapeutic approaches for late-onset NDDs such as PD.

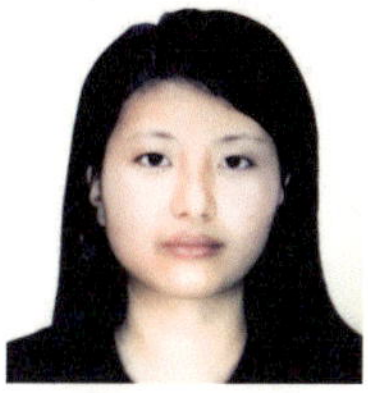

Dr. Zevelou Koza obtained doctoral training from the Drosophila Neurobiology Laboratory (DNBL), Nagaland University, India, and is currently an assistant professor at Patkai Christian College, India. She follows *Drosophila* approaches to understand the sexual dysfunction in Parkinson's disease.

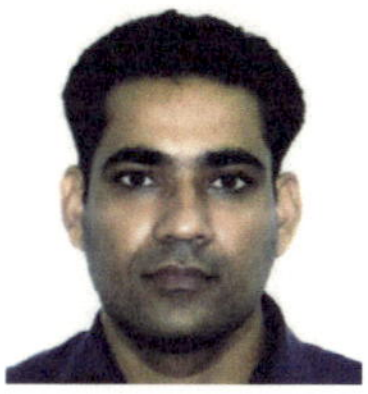

Dr. Devendra Kumar is an assistant professor in the School of Pharmacy and Technology Management. He obtained his Ph.D. in Pharmaceutical Sciences from the Indian Institute of Technology (IIT), Banaras Hindu University (BHU), and completed his postdoctoral research at the University of Texas Health Science Center in San Antonio, USA, in 2021. His research interests include the design, devolvement, and biological screening of small molecules, metal complexes, and peptides for the management of Alzheimer's disease, Fragile X syndrome (FXS), and tuberculosis. Dr. Kumar worked on Alzheimer's disease and developed CNS-active small molecules such as acetylcholine, butylcholinesterase, beta-secretase 1, matrix metalloproteinase-2 and -9 inhibitors, and NMDA receptor antagonists. Along with drug discovery, Dr. Kumar is also working on the pathophysiology of FXS. His work on FXS includes the identification of spine abnormalities and the role of microglia. His focus is the study of microglia–neuron communication in genetically modified animals. He is also working on gene editing tools using clustered regularly interspaced short palindromic repeats (CRISPR) technology and the development of blood–brain barrier-penetrating polymers as the delivery vehicle for CRISPR molecules.

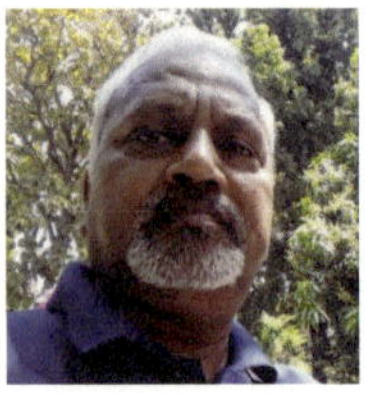

Dr. Kumar Singh is an eminent scientist and teacher in the field of neurodegenerative disorders. He is a fellow of the Royal Society of Chemistry (FRSC) and has authored more than 200 international and national research and review papers. His main research interest is drug development for the treatment of Alzheimer's disease. He was the principal investigator in the development of bioactive molecules as therapeutic agents for Alzheimer's disease and screening their toxicity at the Indian Institute of Technology (IIT) Banaras Hindu University (BHU), as well as the principal investigator in the design and synthesis of matrix metalloproteinase (MMP-2 and -9) inhibitors as therapeutic agents for Alzheimer's disease at the Department of Biotechnology (DBT), Government of India.

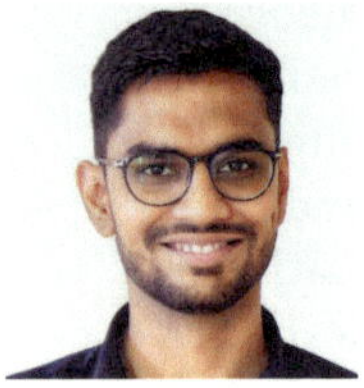

Dr. Ankit Ganeshpurkar's primary goal is to establish a distinct presence in the realm of medicinal chemistry and drug design research, with a specific focus on harnessing computational tools and artificial intelligence to advance the processes of lead discovery and optimization. His research is centered around in silico drug design, lead identification, and optimization. Additionally, his work encompasses the design, synthesis, and thorough biological assessment of novel leads tailored to address diverse pathophysiological conditions, including but not limited to Alzheimer's disease and various neurodegenerative disorders.

Contents

Preface

Parkinson's disease (PD) has been known to humankind since 5000 BC. In ancient Indian civilization, it was known as Kampavata, a condition with symptoms that closely resembled those of modern-day PD, i.e., karpadatale kampa (tremor in the hands and legs), nidrabhanga (sleep disturbances), and kshinmati (slowness of utterance and thought). In modern times, despite being described about 200 years ago, PD is not thoroughly understood due to its complex etiology and heterogeneity in terms of symptoms and progression. Though there are medications and therapies available to manage the symptoms of PD, there is no cure, which provides an opportunity for neurobiologists.

Animal models are precious tools for understanding pathophysiology and unraveling the molecular basis of neuronal degeneration, knowledge of which is immensely useful to screen potential neuroprotective molecules and decipher their mechanism of action. It is important to take advantage of the knowledge generated by biomedical researchers to develop novel therapeutic strategies that should be taken and tested through multiple levels of clinical trials.

The real test lies in connecting all these dots meaningfully and developing a reasonable cure for this neurodegenerative disorder. Thinking in this direction is the genesis for our book, *Parkinson's Disease – Animal Models, Current Therapies and Clinical Trials*. The book examines various topics related to PD, making it a useful resource for basic biomedical researchers, clinicians, technocrats, and science enthusiasts.

I wish to thank all the authors for their valuable contributions. I also wish to acknowledge the staff at IntechOpen, especially Publishing Process Manager Paula Gavran for her support. Thanks go to the publisher for giving me this opportunity to broaden the horizon of my understanding and sharpen my perceptions of PD.

I sincerely believe this book will help move us one step closer to reducing the burden of neurological disease.

Dr. Sarat Chandra Yenisetti, Ph.D.
Professor,
Drosophila Neurobiology Laboratory,
Department of Zoology,
Nagaland University (Central),
Lumami, Nagaland, India

Zevelou Koza
Nagaland University,
Lumami, Nagaland, India

Devendra Kumar
Dehradun Institute of Technology University,
Uttarakhand, India

Sushil Kumar Singh
Banaras Hindu University,
Uttar Pradesh, India

Ankit Ganeshpurkar
Bharati Vidyapeeth Deemed to be University,
Pune, India

Section 1

Parkinson's Disease

Chapter 1

Parkinson's Disease: A Comprehensive Overview of the Disease

Ahed J. Khatib

Abstract

Parkinson's Disease (PD) is the most prevalent neurodegenerative disease following Alzheimer's disease. Its prevalence is increasing over time, and it is expected to reach a peak in 2030. The aim of the present study was to review the literature for various aspects of PD including general characteristics of the disease, its pathology, clinical features, therapeutic clinical trials, and animal models used to study PD. The results of this study showed that no curative therapy for PD has so far been developed. Altogether, PD is still a very hot area in medicine to be studied and to have new therapeutic options.

Keywords: PD, neurodegenerative disease, clinical trials, animal models, pathology of PD

1. Introduction

Parkinson's disease (PD) is a chronic ailment that gradually worsens over time that affects a person's ability to move. It is the second most common cause of neurodegenerative disorders, after Alzheimer's disease [1].

PD is a progressive neurological disorder that is defined by a complicated set of symptoms characterized by tremor, stiffness, and bradykinesia, and as the condition advances, postural instability may appear in certain patients. James Parkinson was the one who originally defined it in 1817, and Jean-Martin Charcot was the one who further characterized it. Our current understanding of the PD is proceeding with its growth. PD is the second most common neurodegenerative disease after Alzheimer's disease (AD), with a prevalence of approximately 0.5–1% among those 65–69 years of age, rising to 1–3% among persons 80 years of age and older [2]. Alzheimer's disease is the most common neurodegenerative disease [3]. It is anticipated that the prevalence and incidence of PD would both rise by more than 30% by the year 2030 because of the aging of the population, which will result in both direct and indirect effects, costs imposed not only on individuals but also on society as a whole and the economy [4].

2. Pathology of PD

PD is pathologically characterized by the loss of nigrostriatal dopaminergic innervation; however, neurodegeneration does not only impact cells located in the nigral dopaminergic neurons; rather, it also involves cells located in other parts of the neural network. Because it affects such a large percentage of the population, Parkinson's disease is a tremendously diverse ailment, for which there is now no reliable diagnostic test [5].

Dopaminergic neuronal death, α-synuclein aggregates, mitochondrial dysfunction, reactive oxygen species, apoptosis, and neuroinflammation are shown to be the pathological hallmarks of PD [6]. α-synuclein is a presynaptic neuronal protein in PD-related genes that ranges in size from 14 to 19 kDa and is responsible for regulating synaptic integrity and cellular activities [7]. α-synuclein is one of the pathogenic markers of PD; throughout the course of PD, α-synuclein accumulates in Lewy bodies and is associated with neuroinflammation [8].

The National Library of Medicine of the United States established the web-based registration known as "ClinicalTrials.gov" in the year 2000. This registry allows users to search for information regarding clinical trials, such as the study design, techniques, outcomes, estimated finish dates, and so on. The data are kept current or maintained by sponsors located all over the world. The list of clinical trials now includes around 2700 PD clinical studies as of this writing. Clinical trial outcomes and endpoints are considered to be comparative effectiveness research [9].

Outcomes can be achieved through the use of a number of different strategies, including cognitive or behavioral scores, magnetic resonance imaging, positron emission tomography, electrophysiological monitoring, or biological biomarkers. Each clinical trial is designed and evaluated for potential treatment advantages in an effort to reduce the occurrence of unfavorable outcomes [9]. In clinical trials, post-approval research is required for comparative research in order to compare clinical trials with accessible standard medicines or therapy. This provides quality of life, safety, and tolerance in order to collect efficient data in the larger patient population [9]. In clinical trials, it is necessary and sufficient to rely on primary endpoints to determine whether a treatment or medication is effective. In light of the primary goals, the secondary endpoints are adequate for claiming or labeling the efficacy of the clinical trial study, and the exploratory and tertiary endpoints provide support for descriptive information [10]. Although levodopa has been used to treat PD for over 50 years, the symptoms of levodopa therapy-induced dyskinesia have not been eliminated completely. As a result, it is of the utmost importance that we investigate the present state of each ongoing clinical study as well as its therapeutic strategy and find novel therapeutic techniques for the treatment of PD [10].

3. Diagnosis of PD

The criteria for a diagnosis require the presence of two of the following clinical features: resting tremor, bradykinesia, rigidity, and/or postural instability. Currently, diagnosis is based on clinical symptoms, and the criteria for a diagnosis require the presence of two of these clinical features [5]. However, clinical criteria may participate in the diagnosis of possible PD [5].

Imaging of the brain, neurological indicators, and clinical symptoms are the three basic components that go into diagnosing PD [11]. The death of dopaminergic neurons in the substantia nigra of the midbrain creates a dopamine shortage in the striatum, which results in motor symptoms of PD [12]. Patients with PD may experience a variety of motor symptoms, such as slowness of movement, rigidity, tremor, freezing, muscle cramps, and dystonia [13]. Patients with idiopathic (typical) PD have an average age of onset between 65 and 70 years old [14]. Early-onset PD is characterized by the development of symptoms in a patient before the age of 50 [14]. The condition is frequently hereditary and has been linked to a number of different genetic alterations [15].

4. Treatment of PD

There is presently no cure for PD, a progressive neurodegenerative disorder; however, treatments are available to relieve PD symptoms and maintain quality of life. PD (PD) affects the nervous system. In the year 2020, approximately 10 million people across the globe were coping with PD. In 1970, the Food and Drug Administration of the United States granted approval for the use of levodopa as a dopamine replacement in the treatment of PD (PD) motor symptoms; the levodopa-carbidopa combination was first made available on the market in 1975. Levodopa has been used to treat PD for more than 50 years, and it is still considered the therapy of choice. Unfortunatcly, thc dyskinesia and OFF symptoms that were produced by levodopa medication have not been alleviated. As a result, it is imperative that we conduct an immediate assessment of the present status of each clinical study and its therapeutic strategy in order to identify new therapeutic approaches for the treatment of PD. From 2008 to June 16, 2021, we analyzed data from 293 clinical trials that were registered on ClinicalTrials.gov. Following the exclusion of levodopa/carbidopa derivative add-on medicines, our search for PD therapy medications or therapies resulted in the identification of 47 trials. Nineteen of them are currently in the phase I stage (41%), 25 are in the phase II stage (53%), and 3 are in the phase III stage (6%). The embryonic dopamine cell implant, the 5-HT1A receptor agonist known as sarizotan, and the adenosine A2A receptor antagonist are all used in the three phase-III clinical trials (caffeine). Each trial's therapeutic method reveals that small compounds are utilized, whereas monoclonal antibodies are utilized in plasma therapy, cell therapy, gene therapy, and herbal extract in the relevant proportions. In addition to this, we talk about the most effective drug or therapy out of all of these trials. We have high hopes that this review can bring novel concepts and fresh perspectives for the further development of PD treatments since it will carefully update the present trial status and conduct an analysis of the therapeutic options [16].

The majority of the treatment's emphasis is placed on providing symptomatic relief with medications that either try to increase the amount of dopamine present in the striatum or work on the region's post-synaptic dopamine receptors. Dopamine is not the sole neurotransmitter implicated in Parkinson's disease (PD), and as a result, several additional medications besides dopamine are also being utilized to target specific symptoms, such as depression and dementia. However, additional research on innovative medicines to slow the rate of neurodegeneration or even to replace dopaminergic cells that have been lost is still being conducted in the research context, and some of these medications are currently in the preliminary stages of clinical trials. The prospect for the development of disease-modifying medicines appears to be encouraging as our understanding of the etiology of PD continues to advance and as more is understood about potential novel therapeutic targets [5].

5. Clinical features of PD

The triad of motor symptoms, which includes tremor, stiffness, and bradykinesia, is the clinical hallmark that has traditionally been linked with PD. As the disease advances, postural instability frequently appears as well. However, PD is also linked to numerous other conditions [17]. Symptoms that are not related to the motor system, and these symptoms may come years or even decades before the motor symptoms. It is possible that the pre-motor or prodromal phase of PD could begin as early as 12–14 years before the actual diagnosis [18]. There is a growing body of evidence that suggests the disease may have its origins in the peripheral autonomic nervous system and/or the olfactory bulb. From there, the pathology may have spread to the central nervous system, where it affected the lower brainstem structures prior to affecting the substantia nigra [19]. The existence of hyposmia, constipation, and rapid eye movement sleep disturbances in people with Parkinson's disease may therefore be explained by this before the onset of motor symptoms. Patients who displayed symptoms of Parkinson's disease 5 years before their diagnosis, including tremor, balance issues, depression, constipation, fatigue, and urinary dysfunction, had a higher risk of developing the disease than patients who did not demonstrate these symptoms [20]. In addition, people who suffer from constipation or tremors are more likely to have a greater likelihood of developing PD during the subsequent 10 years of follow-up [20]. This presymptomatic stage of PD is garnering a growing amount of attention as researchers speculate that it may represent an optimal window of opportunity for treatment intervention. Patients with early PD, defined as those within 2 years of their diagnosis, are included in many clinical studies that investigate prospective therapeutics; nevertheless, even at this point, significant dopaminergic neuron loss has already occurred [21].

6. Etiology of PD

PD is a multifactorial disease, with both genetic and environmental factors playing a role. Age is the biggest risk factor for PD, with the median age of onset being 60 years of age [22]. The incidence of the disease rises with age to 93.1 (per 100,000 person-years) in age groups between 70 and 79 years [23]. Additionally, there are cross-cultural variations, with higher prevalence reported in Europe, North America, and South America compared with African, Asian, and Arabic countries [2].

6.1 Cigarette smoking

Cigarette smoking has been extensively studied with respect to PD, with mostly consistent results. Most of the epidemiological reports are case–control studies showing a reduced risk of developing PD, with larger cohort studies also in agreement [24]. A large meta-analysis including 44 case–control studies and 8 cohort studies from 20 countries showed an inverse correlation between smoking and PD, with a pooled relative risk of 0.39 for current smokers [25]. Two other meta-analyses also reported an inverse correlation between smoking and PD, with a pooled odds ratio ranging from 0.23 to 0.70, indicating a protective mechanism against PD [26, 27]. The reasons underlying this associated reduced risk are not fully understood. Activation of nicotinic acetylcholine receptors on dopaminergic neurons by nicotine or selective agonists has been shown to be neuroprotective in experimental models of PD [28, 29]. Nevertheless, nicotine can also stimulate the release of dopamine, which is involved in the reward mechanisms; it is, therefore, difficult to confirm whether smoking prevents PD or whether PD helps prevent the habitual use of cigarettes [30].

6.2 Caffeine

Several studies have investigated the effect of caffeine on the development of PD and reported a reduced risk of developing PD among coffee drinkers. Caffeine is an adenosine A_{2A} receptor antagonist, which is believed to be protective in PD [31] and has been shown to be neuroprotective in a mouse model of PD [32]. It has been previously reported that there is a 25% risk reduction in developing PD among coffee drinkers [33].

6.3 Genetics

There is a minority of cases (10–15%) that record family history, and approximately 5% exhibit Mendelian inheritance. Although PD is typically an idiopathic condition, there is a minority of cases that report a family history [34]. In addition, an individual's risk of PD is partially the result of polygenic risk factors that have not been adequately characterized as of yet. The genes that have been identified as having the potential to produce PD each receive a "PARK" moniker in the order in which they were discovered. To date, 23 PARK genes have been associated with PD. The PARK genes have been shown to be susceptible to mutations. Either autosomal recessive inheritance (such as in SCNA, LRRK2, and VPS32) or autosomal dominant inheritance (e.g., PRKN, PINK1, and DJ-1). Some of these genes, including PARK5, PARK11, PARK13, PARK18, PARK21, and PARK23, have not been definitively linked to the disease, while others, including PARK3, PARK10, PARK12, PARK16, and PARK22, have been linked to the disease and are considered risk factors [35]. The mutations in GBA1, a gene that codes for glucocerebrosidase, a lysosomal enzyme that is responsible for the hydrolysis of glucocerebrosides are the genetic risk factors that predispose people to PD with the highest relative frequency [36].

7. Treatment

Levodopa treatment is considered the gold standard for improving motor symptoms of PD. Casimir Funk, a scientist from Poland, was the one who first synthesized levodopa in 1911 [37]. According to Abbott [37], a clinical trial of levodopa in 20 PD patients in 1961 was conducted. During the trial, a remarkable improvement in motor function for a few hours was noted. Another clinical study showed that the oral version of levodopa was administered to 28 people with PD, and the results showed positive data for motor improvements [37]. The first combined version of levodopa and carbidopa was employed for the purpose of treating the motor symptoms [38]. Dopamine receptors are activated when levodopa in its combined form is administered. This results in improved motor function across the central nervous system as well as peripheral circulation [39]. Carbidopa functions as a decarboxylase inhibitor to increase the amount of levodopa that is readily available in the brain [39]. Nausea, motor issues, hallucinations, sadness, low blood pressure, irregular sleep, and gambling compulsions are among the most prevalent adverse reactions brought on by the combination of levodopa and carbidopa [40].

7.1 Dopamine receptor agonists

Patients diagnosed with PD often benefit most from a therapeutic class known as dopamine receptor agonists [41]. All dopamine receptors are G protein-coupled receptors, and there are two different types of D1 and D2 dopamine receptors. These dopamine receptors interact with Gs on G proteins, which in turn activate the adenylyl cyclase system and stimulate the production of cAMP [42]. Both the D1 and D5 subtypes are contained within the D1 receptor, while the D2 receptor is made up of the D2, D3, and D4 subtypes [43]. Despite this, once oral dopamine receptor agonists are taken for an extended period of time, treatment stops being effective [44].

In the treatment of PD, we found six clinical trials that utilized four small-molecule medicines that operate as a dopamine receptor agonists. PF-06412562 is a moderately strong, highly selective oral D1/D5 dopamine receptor partial agonist; PF-06412562 has good selectivity than other dopamine receptor subtypes [44]. Oral administration of PF-06412562 demonstrated potential antiparkinsonian efficacy in a phase I trial involving 13 PD patients (NCT03665454) [45]. This was accomplished without the significant acute changes in cardiovascular parameters that were reported with previous D1 agonists. The findings of the trial showed that individuals with advanced PD were able to tolerate PF-06412562 and that the drug fulfilled both the primary and secondary endpoints [46].

7.2 Anti-synuclein aggregation therapy (ASAT)

α-synuclein is an unfolded highly soluble protein that is found in presynaptic neurons throughout the brain [47]. Aggregation of α-synuclein is a pathologic hallmark of synucleinopathies, which can occur in spontaneous or inherited PD. A number of pathological illnesses are brought on by the aggregation of α-synuclein, including synaptic dysfunction, mitochondrial dysfunction, endoplasmic reticulum stress, and oxidative stress [48]. Autophagy and lysosomal disorders are also brought on by this process. All of the pathogenic situations ultimately result in the formation of proteinaceous cytoplasmic inclusions, which are referred to as Lewy bodies and Lewy neurites [48]. The treatment of anti-α-synuclein aggregation primarily works to boost the cellular clearance mechanisms and regulate Lewy bodies [49].

Postuma et al. [18] reported several clinical trials that use anti-α-synuclein aggregation therapy. Five of these clinical trials use monoclonal antibodies (ABVV-0805, BIIB054, and PRX002) or vaccines (AFFITOPE® PD01A). Two of these clinical trials use small molecules (ambroxol and Cu(II)ATSM). (NCT04127695). BIIB054 (cinpanemab) is an IgG1 protein that is produced from the memory B cells of elderly individuals who do not have disorders of the nervous system [18]. The therapy with BIIB054 demonstrated 800 times increased affinity for binding to α-synuclein, which reduced the spread or aggregation of the protein and enhanced motor balances [18].

7.3 Plasma therapy for patients with PD

Antibodies, protein complexes, salts, and chemical molecules are all components that can be found in plasma. As a result, plasma therapy has emerged as an effective treatment option for PD that is also safe and well-tolerated [21].

Plasma therapy may have limited effects since several factors are connected with the disease, including the fact that aggregation of α-synuclein is not the sole factor that contributes to the progression of PD [50]. However, plasma therapy is associated with a number of adverse health effects, including allergic reactions, difficulty breathing, infection with the human immunodeficiency virus (HIV), hepatitis B or hepatitis C virus, or even the possibility of infection with viruses that have not yet been identified [51].

7.4 Based on cells treatment

In cell therapy, dopamine-producing cells are transplanted into the patient's brain in order to produce the desired therapeutic effect. In patients with PD, cell-based therapy is a viable approach that can reduce brain inflammation [52]. Spheramine, also known by its chemical name BAY86–5280, is a human retinal cultured epithelial pigment that is responsible for the production of levodopa [53].

7.5 Gene therapy (GT)

The term "gene therapy" refers to the use of genetically designed therapeutic genes in the treatment of PD. These therapeutic genes actively replace, knockout, or fix the defective genes that are present in PD patients [54]. In gene therapy, numerous serotypes of genetically engineered viral vectors that do not replicate have been utilized [55]. Some examples of these vectors include the adeno-associated virus (AAV) and the lentivirus. Gene therapy has the potential to stop the death of dopaminergic neurons in the brain [56]. In the treatment of PD, gene treatments primarily attempt to restore patients' motor balance by elevating the stimulation of neurotrophic action in the brain [57]. In addition, gene therapy can be used to regulate glucocerebrosidase levels, which is another promising therapeutic method for the treatment of PD [58].

7.6 Agonists or antagonists of the serotonin receptor

The serotonergic neurotransmission system is responsible for the regulation of cognitive and autonomic functions, as well as motor activities and depression [59]. As a result, medications that target serotonergic receptors can influence behavioral aspects and lead to improvements in motor balance [60]. Furthermore, not all of the serotonin receptor agonists are active or controlling in the process of mediating PD. In addition, some of the 5-HT2B receptor agonists were reported to have unwanted side effects. For example, fenfluramine, pergolide, and cabergoline were taken off the market by the pharmaceutical industry because they caused cardiac fibrosis [61].

7.7 Agonists of the muscarinic and nicotinic acetylcholine receptors

Cholinergic receptors are comprised of muscarinic receptors, which are sensitive to muscarine, and nicotinic receptors, which are sensitive to nicotinic, and they are involved in both somatic and autonomic signal transductions in the nervous system [62].

7.8 N-methyl-d-aspartate receptor (NMDAR)

Dysregulation of NMDAR in the cortical-striatal-pallidal-thalmo-cortical network as well as changes in the plasticity of the brain regions are also critical for cognitive function [63]. This is in addition to the loss of dopaminergic neuronal cells that occurs in PD. Synaptic plasticity is increased by NMDAR modulators [63]. NMDAR modulators were shown to have a number of negative side effects including irregular heartbeats, nausea, vomiting, psychosis, catalepsy, constipation, analgesia, and amnesia [64].

7.9 Anti-apoptotic drugs

Apoptosis and necrosis are the two processes that contribute to the destruction of neurons that happens with the course of PD [65]. Two clinical trials involving the use of small molecule anti-apoptotic medicines were identified. These drugs include TCH346 and minocycline. Dibenz[b,f]oxepin-10-ylmethyl-prop-2-ynyl-amine hydrogen maleate salt is another name for TCH346, which is also a name for this compound. Novartis is developing TCH346, which is now in the midst of a phase I/II clinical trial in which 301 early-stage PD patients are participating; the trial status shows that it has been completed, but there are no published data available. According to the findings of the preclinical studies, TCH346 protected dopaminergic neurons against injury [66]. Minocycline is a neuroprotective synthetic tetracycline derivative that primarily targets anti-apoptotic pathways. It modifies microglial cells and lowers oxidative stress and neuroinflammation [67].

7.10 Antioxidants and medications derived from botanical sources

Antioxidants have an action known as free radical scavenging, and this activity is the primary factor that protects dopaminergic neurons and improves mitochondrial function in both sporadic and inherited cases of PD [68]. Mitochondrial malfunction has been linked to the development of PD; free radical scavenging activity can remove damaged mitochondria through the process of mitophagy and provide neuroprotection in PD [69]. One of the pathological characteristics of neuroinflammation is a reduction in the amount of reduced glutathione seen in the brain of PD patients [70].

8. Animal models

Animal models of PD have shown to be extremely useful in the identification of novel treatments for the motor symptoms of PD as well as in the quest for clues as to the underlying cause of the illness. Models that are based on certain disease-causing mechanisms could, in the future, pave the way for the creation of neuroprotective medications for PD that can halt or delay the progression of the disease. There is a wide variety of rodent models that are currently available. These models range from acute pharmacological models, like the rats that were treated with reserpine or haloperidol and displayed one or more parkinsonian signs, to models exhibiting destruction of the dopaminergic nigro-striatal pathway, like the traditional 6-hydroxydopamine (6-OHDA) rats and 1-methyl-4-phenyl-1,2,3,6-tetrahydropyridine (All of these have served as test beds for evaluating potential novel compounds for treating the motor symptoms of PD. In addition, the appearance of abnormal involuntary movements (AIMs) after repeated treatment of 6-OHDA-lesioned rats with L-DOPA has made it possible to investigate the mechanisms that are responsible for treatment-related dyskinesia in PD, as well as the identification of molecules that are able to prevent or reverse the appearance of these symptoms. The systemic administration of the pesticides rotenone and paraquat are examples of other toxin-based models of nigro-striatal tract degeneration. However, despite the fact that these models provide insights into the pathogenesis of the disease, they are not typically utilized in the drug development process. The MPTP-treated primate model of PD is without a doubt the most clinically relevant of all the models that are currently available because it closely resembles the clinical features of PD and because it is the model in which all of the anti-parkinsonian medications that are currently in use have been shown to be effective. When repeatedly exposed to L-DOPA, the MPTP-treated primate develops obvious dyskinesia, and these parkinsonian animals have exhibited reactions to novel dopaminergic drugs that are highly predictive of their effect in man. It is debatable whether or not non-dopaminergic medications demonstrate the same level of response predictability as dopaminergic treatments. New rodent models have been developed in tandem with our growing comprehension of the mechanisms underlying the progression of PD (PD). These agents include proteasome inhibitors such as PSI, lactacystin, and epoximycin, as well as inflammogens such as lipopolysaccharide (LPS). These agents have been shown to produce symptoms in rodents that are similar to those seen in humans. In addition, a new generation of models has emerged with the purpose of imitating the genetic factors that contribute to PD. Even while these more recent models have offered additional insights into the pathophysiology of the disease, researchers have not yet relied heavily on them when developing novel medications. Dopaminergic drug treatment of the illness, as well as the prevention and reversal of drug-related side effects that emerge with disease progression and chronic medication, have been dramatically altered as a result of the availability of experimental animal models of PD. This is something that can be said with a high degree of certainty. However, in terms of expanding into other pharmacological fields for the treatment of PD, we have not made a lot of headway so far. Furthermore, we have not developed models that reflect the progressive nature of the illness and its complexity in terms of the extent of pathology and biochemical change. It is only when this happens that we will have a chance of making progress in the development of medications that can stop or delay the advancement of the disease. In the search for more effective medication treatments for PD, the overriding question that connects all of these models is as follows: how accurately do they recapitulate the human situation, and how predictive are they of the successful translation of pharmaceuticals into the clinic? The purpose of this essay is to provide clarification on the current situation and highlight the strengths and shortcomings of the many models that are available [71].

Akinesia, bradykinesia, rigidity, tremor, and postural abnormalities are the classic motor symptoms of PD. These symptoms are associated with the loss of nigral dopaminergic cells and a decline in caudate-putamen dopamine content, which led to the development of dopamine replacement therapy. Because of this, animal models of PD have played a significant part in the creation of innovative pharmacological approaches to therapy, the development of new treatment methods, and the comprehension of the nature of the pathogenic processes involved in the loss of neuronal function. The discovery that giving rodents and rabbits reserpine or haloperidol led to a temporary parkinsonian-like state was quickly followed by the crucial discovery that giving these animals L-DOPA caused their symptoms to disappear. This was the first evidence that L-DOPA could be used to treat PD [72]. This paved the way for a new era in which animal models of PD were utilized to research the physiological underpinnings of symptomatic treatment. When it was discovered that the injection of 6-hydroxydopamine (6-OHDA) using a unilateral stereotaxic technique into the substantia nigra or the medial forebrain bundle caused the destruction of the nigro-striatal pathway and, as a result, a loss of dopaminergic input to the striatum, this led to further success in the treatment of the condition. Because of this, the "circling" rat model of PD was developed, which went on to dominate research for a good number of years. This also marked the beginning of the era in which toxins were used to produce animal models of PD [73]. These advancements led to the development of novel approaches to treatment, such as the introduction of peripherally acting decarboxylase inhibitors, carbidopa, and benserazide, which limited the peripheral side effects of L-DOPA and allowed for a lowering of dose as more drugs entered the brain. Carbidopa and benserazide are examples of such novel approaches. More recently, the development of selective monoamine oxidase-B (MAO-B) inhibitors, selegiline, and rasagiline, which slow the degradation of dopamine formed from L-DOPA and prolong its duration of effect, as well as the more recent development of catechol-O-methyl-transferase (COMT) inhibitors, entacapone, and tolcapone, which stop either the peripheral or central metabolism of L-DOPA to 3-O-methyldo [22, 74].

Importantly, the chemical and toxin animal-based models of PD ushered in the age of the use of synthetic dopamine agonists, which sparked early interest in the production of anti-parkinsonian action through the stimulation of post-synaptic dopamine receptors in the striatum. A significant number of compounds were put through the available models' screening process, which, of course, resulted in a great number of unsuccessful attempts at both the preclinical and clinical levels. Apomorphine was the very first molecule to be tried out in clinical trials for the treatment of PD after its initial use in research [75]. An early dopamine agonist called piribedil was highly effective, but its clinical application in PD was not properly understood, and rapid dose escalation caused high levels of nausea, vomiting, and gastrointestinal disturbance that tainted its use. This is similar to the situation with many other ground-breaking molecules [76]. However, in the following years, ergot derivatives such as bromocriptine, pergolide, and cabergoline were introduced, which provided effective control of the motor symptoms of PD [77]. Ergots are no longer used because they were found to have valvular effects in the heart, which may represent the broad pharmacology of ergot derivatives and activity on 5-HT2B receptors. As a result, the use of ergots has been phased out [78]. Dopaminergic therapy in PD is presently centered on pramipexole, ropinirole, and rotigotine as oral and transdermal pharmaceuticals. However, non-ergot drugs were previously being used in the treatment of PD. These drugs were discovered by using animal models of the disease [79]. Dopamine receptor subtypes were cloned at the same time that most of the development of dopamine agonists was taking place, and animal models of PD were used as a testing ground to investigate the role that dopamine receptor subtypes play in regulating motor function. In particular, researchers were interested in determining how D1-like and D2-like receptors interact with one another, as well as how this interaction relates to the anti-parkinsonian activity and side effect profile [80].

8.1 Pharmacological models

8.1.1 Reserpine model

One of the initial animal models used in research on PD was a mouse that had been given reserpine. This model was essential in initially proving the therapeutic efficacy of L-DOPA, which is still the treatment of gold standard for PD, despite the fact that it was fairly a primitive pharmacological mimic of the neurochemistry of PD.

Carlsson et al. [81] were the ones who first established that L-DOPA, the endogenous dopamine precursor, has the power to counteract the effects of reserpine pretreatment that were at the time described as having a "tranquilizing" impact on mice. This was done in the late 1950s [81]. This effect was soon replicated in people [82], and the reserpine-treated mouse or, more commonly, the rat became established as a reliable screen for possible symptomatic efficacy of novel medications in PD. The reserpine model has also made substantial contributions to our knowledge of the relationship between monoamine depletion and parkinsonian symptoms from the standpoint of the disease. Reserpine acts by blocking the vesicular monoamine transporter, also known as VMAT2. The typical dose for this medication is four to five milligrams per kilogram subcutaneously. This results in a decrease in storage capacity and, as a consequence, depletion of monoamines in the brain and the peripheral nervous system. These monoamines include noradrenaline, 5-HT, and dopamine. Although the absence of selectivity for dopamine was once thought to be a flaw in the reserpine model's ability to accurately reflect the biochemistry of PD (PD), it was later discovered that the disease also affects the noradrenergic and serotonergic systems [83], which argues in favor of the reserpine model being a relatively good mimic of the disease biochemistry.

8.1.2 MPTP model

Because of its potential to cause persistent Parkinsonism in humans, MPTP is a toxin that is frequently employed for the purpose of producing PD in rodents as well as primates [84]. Subsequent research in non-human primates determined that the pathological basis behind the observed motor deficits was the selective destruction of dopaminergic neurons of the nigro-striatal tract [85]. This led to the development of the most relevant animal model of PD that is still used today. In the study of PD (PD), the MPTP-treated primate model has had an unparalleled influence; nonetheless, we shall begin by concentrating on the application of MPTP in animals that are not primates. It is possible that the relatively rapid clearance of MPP+, which is the poisonous metabolite of MPTP, accounts for the resistance of a great number of animals, including rats, to the toxic effects of MPTP [86]. However, certain strains of mice, most notably black C57 and Swiss Webster, are sensitive to MPTP [86]. Because of this, the MPTP mouse model of PD was able to be developed using these mouse strains. The mechanism that underlies the neurotoxic activity of MPTP has been the focus of extensive research and is now considered to be rather well-known. After receiving a systemic injection often (intraperitoneally or subcutaneously), MPTP is a lipophilic protoxin that quickly penetrates the blood–brain barrier [87]. Once within the brain, MPTP is transformed by MAO-B, which is mostly found in glia and serotonergic neurons, into the intermediate, 1-methyl-4-phenyl-2,3,dihydropyridinium (MPDP+), before its rapid and spontaneous oxidation to the poisonous component, 1-methyl-4-phenylpyridinium (MPP+) [88]. After being released into the extracellular space, MPP+ is taken up by dopaminergic neurons via the DAT. Once inside these neurons, cytoplasmic MPP+ has the ability to stimulate the creation of ROS, which may contribute to the overall neurotoxicity of the compound [89]. On the other hand, the vast majority of MPP+ is finally stored inside mitochondria, which is where the primary harmful process takes place. When MPP+ reaches the mitochondria, it inhibits complex I of the electron transport chain, which in turn reduces the efficiency of mitochondrial respiration. Because of this action, the flow of electrons through the respiratory chain is disrupted, which results in a lower level of ATP synthesis and the creation of reactive oxygen species (ROS), such as superoxide radicals. The combined effects of decreased cellular ATP and elevated ROS production are most likely responsible for the initiation of cell death-related signaling pathways. These pathways include p38 mitogen-activated kinase [90], c-jun N-terminal kinase (JNK) [91], and bax [92]. This model demonstrates a high degree of construct validity due to the fact that many of these mechanisms are also characteristics of the pathophysiology of PD.

8.2 Pesticide-induced models

8.2.1 Rotenone model

The rotenone model of PD is the most well-known of the models that have come out of this, but ever since it was initially presented [93], it has continued to be the subject of much dispute [94]. The pesticide rotenone is extremely lipophilic, just like MPTP, which allows it to easily pass through the blood–brain barrier and diffuse into neurons. Once there, it accumulates within the mitochondria and inhibits complex I in a manner that is very similar to how MPTP does it. However, the subsequent decreases in ATP are not regarded to be the origin of the toxicity; rather, it is believed that glutathione depletion leads to the generation of reactive oxygen species (ROS), which in turn induces oxidative stress [95]. There is no doubt that oxidative damage, in the form of protein carbonyl formation, was discovered in the midbrain, olfactory bulb, striatum, and cortex of rats that were treated with rotenone [95]. This finding is consistent with what is reported in the PD brain after death [96]. The extensive microglial activation that was observed in both the SNpc and striatum following rotenone infusion [97] is consistent with the inflammatory features found in idiopathic PD [98]. This lends support to the construct validity of this model. The recent observation that rotenone suppresses proteasomal activity [99] provides additional support for this theory. Proteasomal activity, which will be discussed further below, is also thought to have a role in PD.

8.3 Paraquat and Maneb model

It is not surprising that attempts have been made to model PD using these agents given that exposure to the herbicide paraquat (1,1′-dimethyl-4,4′-bipyridinium) or the fungicide Maneb (manganese ethylene-bis-dithiocarbamate) has been associated with an increased incidence of PD [100, 101]. Before the Na+-dependent uptake into cells can take place, however, paraquat must first reach the brain through the neutral amino acid transporter [102]. Once it has entered the cell, paraquat causes both indirect mitochondrial toxicity through redox cycling and direct inhibition of complex I (at higher doses). This occurs because paraquat inhibits redox cycling [103]. Following its introduction into the brain, maneb, on the other hand, inhibits complex III of the mitochondrial respiratory chain in a selective manner [104]. It has been demonstrated that the combination of maneb and paraquat results in increased toxicity [105], which may be due to the fact that maneb raises the concentration of paraquat in the brain while simultaneously decreasing its clearance [106]. This provides a clear rationale for combining the administration of these pesticides in order to produce an animal model of PD. This is especially important when considering the fact that human exposure to just one of these pesticides is unlikely because they are used in the same geographical regions.

8.4 Genetic models of PD

The first gene to be unequivocally linked to familial Parkinson's disease (PD) was the alpha-synuclein gene [107]. Researchers were able to zero in on a number of additional familial PD-linked genes after this discovery was made in 1997. These genes were associated with autosomal dominant or recessive forms of Parkinson's disease. These genes are included in this category: parkin [108], DJ-1 [109], PINK1 [110], and LRRK2 [111]. It is essential to note here that despite the fact that mutations in UCHL1 [112] and Omi/HtrA2 [113] have also been proposed to cause parkinsonism, the relevance of these mutations to Parkinson's disease is currently debatable. This is due to the fact that the supposed mutation that causes the disease is either extremely rare in occurrence (e.g., UCHL1 I93M) or present in control population at similar frequencies (e.g., Omi/HtrA2 G399S). Concerning the recently described ATP13A2-linked parkinsonism [114], the clinical phenotype that is associated with it (which is characterized by mild parkinsonism and prominent cognitive defects) is quite different from traditional Parkinson's disease, In general, PD-linked genes are expressed as transgenes in heterologous organisms if their pattern of inheritance in humans indicates that dominant transmission is likely to occur. This is because dominant transmission is the form of inheritance that causes Parkinson's disease. In the event that this cannot be accomplished, orthologous copies of the human gene are removed from animal genomes in order to replicate the recessive loss of gene function. In addition to models based on flies and worms, researchers have had success to this day in developing several mouse models of familial parkinsonism. Despite the fact that non-mammalian models of Parkinson's disease (PD) cannot fully replicate the phenotypic and pathologic characteristics of the human condition, these models are still able to reproduce certain important hallmarks of the disease, such as LB-like inclusions and DA neurodegeneration [115]. Parkinson's disease is a neurodegenerative disorder that affects the brain's dopaminergic neurons. As a consequence of this, these models are beneficial to the investigation of the connection between PD-linked genes and the operation of DA neurons. Noteworthy is the fact that each of the two hemispheres of the adult fly brain contains six clusters of DA neurons, but only one cluster of C neurons. Elegans has a total of eight DA neurons in its brain, and these neurons are split up into three different subsets. Importantly, the well-characterized genetics of these nonmammalian PD models offer a distinct advantage over the mouse model for the rapid identification of modifiers that could shed light on significant pathways involved in the pathogenesis of disease. This advantage cannot be found in any other model. The understanding that one obtains from these pathways might make it easier to create new kinds of therapeutics in the future [116].

8.5 Genetic environmental interactions models of PD

It is generally accepted that the etiology of Parkinson's disease is largely influenced by the interactions that take place between genetic factors and environmental exposures. Even though such interactions are not well defined and are only partially understood, recent epidemiological studies have identified specific interactions that may be of potential importance to human Parkinson's disease (PD). This is despite the fact that such interactions are poorly defined [117].

The specifics of the interactions between genetic predisposition and environmental exposures are not well understood at this time, despite the fact that a large number of researchers believe that the majority of cases are influenced by both genetic predisposition and environmental exposures. Despite this, there is evidence that suggests certain interactions between different factors. The current discussion is limited to those gene–environment interactions that have supporting or suggestive data, despite the fact that the number of gene–environment interactions that could bear pathogenic relevance to PD is extremely large, as is the diversity of those interactions [117].

To be able to have a direct effect on the nigrostriatal dopamine system, a toxicant must first be able to pass through the barrier that separates the blood and the brain (BBB). Due to the BBB's size and polarity requirements, it is highly unlikely that many toxic substances will be able to cross it [118]. It is possible that genetic alterations that change the permeability of the blood–brain barrier (BBB) could either increase the accumulation of toxic substances in the brain or make it possible for toxic substances to enter the brain that are normally kept out. The existence of human data lends credence to the possibility of such an interaction. P-glycoprotein is the product of the multidrug resistance gene (MDR1) and plays a role in the functioning of the blood–brain barrier (BBB). It is interesting to note that the distribution of the 3435 T/T genotype, which has been linked in the past to lower levels of P-glycoprotein expression and function, was highest in early-onset Parkinson's disease patients, second-highest in late-onset Parkinson's disease patients, and lowest in controls [119]. It has been suggested in additional reports that factors such as ethnicity, polymorphisms, and haplotype expression, which are relevant to MDR1, may modulate the risk of Parkinson's disease [120]. Changes in the expression of P-glycoproteins could very well be important to the uptake of toxicants. A positron emission tomography was performed to measure the brain uptake of [(11)C]-verapamil, which is normally expelled from the brain by P-glycoprotein. The results showed that PD patients had increased absorption in the midbrain [121]. According to the findings of this study, Parkinson's disease could be caused by a dysfunctional blood–brain barrier as well as P-glycoprotein. P-glycoprotein dysfunction was not found in early-onset Parkinson's disease patients by a separate imaging study, despite the fact that there was a large amount of variability [122]. Patients with Parkinson's disease had lower levels of MDR1 mRNA in the striatum in their postmortem tissue than controls did [123]. These studies point to a potential pathogenic role for decreased expression or function in Parkinson's disease (PD). It has been demonstrated that mice deficient in the MDR1 gene accumulate anticancer drugs, narcotics, and pesticides [124]. In MDR1/mice, accumulation may take place at much higher levels than in controls, or it may occur in compounds that are normally completely excluded but may gain access. This is dependent on the compound. The direct relevance to dopaminergic toxicants has not yet been established, and it is possible that altered brain entry of normally excluded endogenous factors is significantly more important in modulating PD risk than environmental exposures [117].

9. Pathologic features of PD from our studies

Several studies have been conducted in our laboratories using mouse model. One of the studies aimed to investigate the level of inducible nitric oxide synthase (iNOS) expression in the skeletal muscles of mice with PD and to investigate the influence that training on a treadmill has on the level of iNOS expression in these skeletal muscles. The results showed that the expression of iNOS in the gastrocnemius muscle show a statistically significant increase in the sedentary PD (SPD) group compared to the sedentary control (SC) group ($P = 0.05$). There was an increase in the expression of iNOS in the soleus muscle of those in the SPD group when compared to those in the SC group, although the difference did not reach statistical significance ($P = 0.08$). Additionally, exercise did not result in a significant reduction of the expression of iNOS in the Parkinsonian group (P value 0.13). According to the findings that we have gathered so far, endurance exercise training appears to mitigate the changes in iNOS expression in skeletal muscles that are caused by PD. These findings could be significant when thinking about rehabilitation procedures for Parkinson's disease and the pathophysiology associated with it [125].

Another study was conducted in light of considerations that overexpression of heat shock protein 90 can result in the death of dopaminergic neuronal cells. The study purposed to gain a deeper understanding of the impact that heat shock protein 90 has on the body after it has been subjected to endurance exercise. The results of immunohistochemistry showed that exercise training significantly inhibited heat shock protein 90 overexpression in the soleus and gastrocnemius in rats with Parkinson's disease. This overexpression of heat shock protein 90 is a potential therapeutic target for ameliorating skeletal muscle abnormalities in Parkinson's disease [126].

In another study, Al-Jarrah et al. [127] purposed to analyze the expression of the inducible form of NO (iNOS), and compare it to neuronal nitric oxide (nNOS), in the brain of a chronic mice model of PD, and to investigate the influence that training for endurance will have on the expression of the aforementioned markers. The results showed that nNOS levels were significantly higher in the striatum (ST) of SPD animals in comparison to SC mice ($P > 0.03$). Although there was a lower expression of nNOS in the EC group of mice in comparison to the SC animals, this difference was not statistically significant ($P > 0.8$). When compared to SPD, the amount of nNOS in the EPD showed a substantial decrease as a result of exercise training ($P > 0.04$). Although the expression of iNOS followed a trend that was essentially identical to that of nNOS, the expression of iNOS did not significantly decrease as a result of exercise training in either the EC or EPD groups ($P > 0.2$ and 0.3, respectively). The findings of this research reveal that a period of 4 weeks spent running on a treadmill has a beneficial effect on the expression of nNOS and iNOS in the striatum of a model of Parkinson's disease (PD). It is possible that this could clear up some questions about the pathogenicity of the diseases and the beneficial effects of training on PD [127]. We found other findings from clinical observations in which two patients with PD received certain chemicals including magnesium, chromium, zinc, vitamin D, and tadalafil 5, the results of such an approach showed ameliorating effects of PD symptoms.

10. Conclusions

PD is still a version area of research and clinical trials. There is no curative treatment for PD has been developed so far, a mater that opens the door for continuous inputting efforts to reach a therapeutic goal. In addition to the classical pathological picture of PD, we showed that certain molecular pathways play a major role in the pathogenesis of PD including inducible nitric oxide synthase, HSP90, and in the brain and other tissues of mice with PD. Furthermore, some clinical findings showed that the administration of tadalafil 5, magnesium, zinc, chromium, and vitamin D improves the clinical status of PD.

Author details

Ahed J. Khatib[1,2]

1 Department of Legal Medicine, Toxicology and Forensic Medicine, Jordan University of Science and Technology, Irbid, Jordan

2 International Mariinskaya Academy, Department of Medicine and Critical Care, Department of Philosophy, Academician Secretary of the Department of Sociology, Irbid, Jordan

*Address all correspondence to: ajalkhatib@just.edu.jo

References

[1] Stührenberg M, Berghäuser CS, van Munster M, Pedrosa Carrasco AJ, Pedrosa DJ, on behalf of the iCARE-PD Consortium. Measuring quality of life in Parkinson's disease—A call to rethink conceptualizations and assessments. Journal of Personalized Medicine. 2022;**12**:804. DOI: 10.3390/jpm1205080

[2] Kalia LV, Lang AE. Parkinson's disease. Lancet. 2015;**386**(9996):896-912. DOI: 10.1016/S0140-6736(14)61393-3

[3] Koníˇcková D, Menšíková K, Tuˇcková L, Hényková E, Strnad M, Friedecký D, et al. Biomarkers of neurodegenerative diseases: Biology, taxonomy, clinical relevance, and current research status. Biomedicine. 2022;**10**:1760. DOI: 10.3390/biomedicines10071760

[4] Wanneveich M, Moisan F, Jacqmin-Gadda H, Elbaz A, Joly P. Projections of prevalence, lifetime risk, and life expectancy of Parkinson's disease (2010-2030) in France. Movement Disorders. Sep 2018;**33**(9):1449-1455. DOI: 10.1002/mds.27447. Epub 2018 Aug 25. PMID: 30145805

[5] Kouli A, Torsney KM, Kuan WL. Chapter 1. Parkinson's disease: Etiology, neuropathology, and pathogenesis. In: Stoker TB, Greenland JC, editors. Parkinson's Disease: Pathogenesis and Clinical Aspects [Internet]. Brisbane, AU: Codon Publications; 2018. pp. 3-26. Available from: https://www.ncbi.nlm.nih.gov/books/NBK536722/. DOI: 10.15586/codonpublications.parkinsonsdisease.2018.ch1

[6] Prasad EM, Hung SY. Behavioral tests in neurotoxin-induced animal models of PD. Antioxidants. 2020;**9**:7. DOI: 10.3390/antiox9101007

[7] Maroteaux L, Campanelli JT, Scheller RH. Synuclein: A neuron-specific protein localized to the nucleus and presynaptic nerve terminal. The Journal of Neuroscience. 1988;**8**:2804. DOI: 10.1523/JNEUROSCI.08-08-02804.1988

[8] Maguire-Zeiss KA. α-Synuclein: A therapeutic target for PD? Pharmaceutical Research. 2008;**58**:271-280. DOI: 10.1016/j.phrs.2008.09.006

[9] Velentgas P., Dreyer N.A., Wu A.W. Developing a Protocol for Observational Comparative Effectiveness Research: A User's Guide. Agency for Healthcare Research and Quality (US); Rockville, MD, USA: 2013. Outcome definition and measurement.

[10] Merchant KM, Cedarbaum JM, Brundin P, Dave KD, Eberling J, Espay AJ, et al. A proposed roadmap for PD proof of concept clinical trials investigating compounds targeting alpha-synuclein. Journal of Parkinson's Disease. 2019;**9**:31-61. DOI: 10.3233/JPD-181471

[11] Marino S, Ciurleo R, Di Lorenzo G, Barresi M, De Salvo S, Giacoppo S, et al. Magnetic resonance imaging markers for early diagnosis of PD. Neural Regeneration Research. 2012;**7**:611-619. DOI: 10.3969/j.issn.1673-5374.2012.08.009

[12] Dauer W, Przedborski S. PD: Mechanisms and models. Neuron. 2003;**39**:889-909. DOI: 10.1016/S0896-6273(03)00568-3

[13] Rabinstein AA, Shulman LM. Management of behavioral and psychiatric problems in PD. Parkinsonism & Related Disorders. 2000;**7**:41-50. DOI: 10.1016/S1353-8020(00)00039-0

[14] Horstink DMWIM. PD and parkinsonism in the elderly. Brain. 2000;**123**:2569-2571. DOI: 10.1093/brain/123.12.2569

[15] Foltynie T, Sawcer S, Brayne C, Barker RA. The genetic basis of PD. Journal of Neurology, Neurosurgery, and Psychiatry. 2002;**73**:363-370. DOI: 10.1136/jnnp.73.4.363

[16] Prasad EM, Hung SY. Current therapies in clinical trials of PD: A 2021 update. Pharmaceuticals (Basel, Switzerland). 2021;**14**(8):717. DOI: 10.3390/ph14080717

[17] Maetzler W, Hausdorff JM. Motor signs in the prodromal phase of Parkinson's disease. Movement Disorders. 2012;**27**:627-633

[18] Postuma RB, Anang J, Pelletier A, Joseph L, Moscovich M, Grimes D, et al. Caffeine as symptomatic treatment for Parkinson disease (Café-PD): A randomized trial. Neurology. 2017;**89**:1795-1803. DOI: 10.1212/WNL.0000000000004568

[19] Katzenschlager R, Head J, Schrag A, Ben-Shlomo Y, Evans A, Lees AJ, et al. Fourteen-year final report of the randomized PDRG-UK trial comparing three initial treatments in PD. Neurology. 12 Aug 2008;**71**(7):474-480. DOI: 10.1212/01.wnl.0000310812.43352.66

[20] Schrag A, Horsfall L, Walters K, Noyce A, Petersen I. Prediagnostic presentations of Parkinson's disease in primary care: A case-control study. Lancet Neurology. Jan 2015;**14**(1):57-64. DOI: 10.1016/S1474-4422(14)70287-X

[21] Ma SY, Röyttä M, Rinne JO, Collan Y, Rinne UK. Correlation between neuromorphometry in the substantia nigra and clinical features in Parkinson's disease using disector counts. Journal of the Neurological Sciences. 3 Oct 1997;**151**(1):83-87. DOI: 10.1016/S0022-510X(97)00100-7

[22] Lees AJ. Evidence-based efficacy comparison of tolcapone and entacapone as adjunctive therapy in Parkinson's disease. CNS Neuroscience & Therapeutics. 2008;**14**:83-93

[23] Bower JH, Maraganore DM, McDonnell SK, Rocca WA. Incidence and distribution of parkinsonism in Olmsted County, Minnesota, 1976-1990. Neurology. 12 Apr 1999;**52**(6):1214-1220. DOI: 10.1212/WNL.52.6.1214

[24] Hernán MA, Zhang SM, Rueda-deCastro AM, Colditz GA, Speizer FE, Ascherio A. Cigarette smoking and the incidence of Parkinson's disease in two prospective studies. Annals of Neurology. Dec 2001;**50**(6):780-786. DOI: 10.1002/ana.10028

[25] Hernán MA, Takkouche B, Caamaño-Isorna F, Gestal-Otero JJ. A meta-analysis of coffee drinking, cigarette smoking, and the risk of Parkinson's disease. Annals of Neurology. Sep 2002;**52**(3):276-284. DOI: 10.1002/ana.10277

[26] Ritz B, Ascherio A, Checkoway H, Marder KS, Nelson LM, Rocca WA, et al. Pooled analysis of tobacco use and risk of Parkinson disease. Archives of Neurology. Jul 2007;**64**(7):990-997. DOI: 10.1002/ana.10277

[27] Breckenridge CB, Berry C, Chang ET, Jr RLS, Mandel JS. Association between Parkinson's disease and cigarette smoking, rural living, well-water consumption, farming and pesticide use: Systematic review and meta-analysis. PLoS One. 7 Apr 2016;**11**(4):e0151841. DOI: 10.1371/journal.pone.0151841

[28] Bordia T, McGregor M, Papke RL, Decker MW, McIntosh JM, Quik M. The α7 nicotinic receptor agonist ABT-107 protects against nigrostriatal damage in rats with unilateral 6-hydroxydopamine lesions. Experimental Neurology. Jan 2015;**263**:277-284. DOI: 10.1016/j.expneurol.2014.09.015

[29] Srinivasan R, Henley BM, Henderson BJ, Indersmitten T, Cohen BN, Kim CH, et al. Smoking-relevant nicotine concentration attenuates the unfolded protein response in dopaminergic neurons. The Journal of Neuroscience. 6 Jan 2016;**36**(1):65-79. DOI: 10.1523/JNEUROSCI.2126-15.2016

[30] Ritz B, Lee P-C, Lassen CF, Arah OA. Parkinson disease and smoking revisited: Ease of quitting is an early sign of the disease. Neurology. 14 Oct 2014;**83**(16):1396-1402. DOI: 10.1212/WNL.0000000000000879

[31] Ross GW, Abbott RD, Petrovitch H, Morens DM, Grandinetti A, Tung KH, et al. Association of coffee and caffeine intake with the risk of Parkinson disease. Journal of the American Medical Association. 24 May 2000;**283**(20):2674-2679. DOI: 10.1001/jama.283.20.2674

[32] Chen JF, Xu K, Petzer JP, Staal R, Xu YH, Beilstein M, et al. Neuroprotection by caffeine and A(2A) adenosine receptor inactivation in a model of Parkinson's disease. The Journal of Neuroscience. 15 May 2001;**21**(10):RC143. DOI: 10.1523/JNEUROSCI.21-10-j0001.2001

[33] Noyce AJ, Bestwick JP, Silveira-Moriyama L, Hawkes CH, Giovannoni G, Lees AJ, et al. Meta-analysis of early nonmotor features and risk factors for Parkinson disease. Annals of Neurology. Dec 2012;**72**(6):893-901. DOI: 10.1002/ana.23687

[34] Deng H, Wang P, Jankovic J. The genetics of Parkinson disease. Ageing Research Reviews. 1 Mar 2018;**42**:72-85. DOI: 10.1016/j.arr.2017.12.007

[35] Schulte C, Gasser T. Genetic basis of Parkinson's disease: Inheritance, penetrance, and expression. The Application of Clinical Genetics. 1 Jun 2011;**4**:67-80

[36] Nichols WC, Pankratz N, Marek DK, Pauciulo MW, Elsaesser VE, Halter CA, et al. Mutations in GBA are associated with familial Parkinson disease susceptibility and age at onset. Neurology. 27 Jan 2009;**72**(4):310-316. DOI: 10.1212/01.wnl.0000327823.81237.d1

[37] Abbott A. Levodopa: The story so far. Nature. 2010;**466**:S6-S7. DOI: 10.1038/466S6a

[38] Lesser RP, Fahn S, Snider SR, Cote LJ, Isgreen WP, Barrett RE. Analysis of the clinical problems in parkinsonism and the complications of long-term levodopa therapy. Neurology. 1979;**29**:1253-1260. DOI: 10.1212/WNL.29.9_Part_1.1253

[39] Guebila MB, Thiele I. Model-based dietary optimization for late-stage, levodopa-treated, PD patients. NPJ Systems Biology and Applications. 2016;**2**:16013. DOI: 10.1038/npjsba.2016.13

[40] Dodd ML, Klos KJ, Bower JH, Geda YE, Josephs KA, Ahlskog JE. Pathological gambling caused by drugs used to treat parkinson disease. Archives of Neurology. 2005;**62**:1377-1381. DOI: 10.1001/archneur.62.9.noc50009

[41] Annus Á, Vécsei L. Spotlight on opicapone as an adjunct to levodopa in PD: Design, development and potential place in therapy. Drug Design, Development and Therapy.

2017;**11**:143-151. DOI: 10.2147/DDDT.S104227

[42] Gurevich EV, Gainetdinov RR, Gurevich VV. G protein-coupled receptor kinases as regulators of dopamine receptor functions. Pharmaceutical Research. 2016;**111**:1-16. DOI: 10.1016/j.phrs.2016.05.010

[43] Beaulieu JM, Gainetdinov RR. The physiology, signaling and pharmacology of dopamine receptors. Pharmacy Review. 2011;**63**:182-217. DOI: 10.1124/pr.110.002642

[44] Ghiglieri V, Bagetta V, Pendolino V, Picconi B, Calabresi P. Corticostriatal plastic changes in experimental L-DOPA-induced dyskinesia. Parkinson's Disease. 2012;**2012**:358176. DOI: 10.1155/2012/358176

[45] Papapetropoulos S, Liu W, Duvvuri S, Thayer K, Gray DL. Evaluation of D1/D5 partial agonist PF-06412562 in PD following oral administration. Neurodegenerative Diseases. 2018;**18**:262-269. DOI: 10.1159/000492498

[46] Huang X, Lewis MM, Van Scoy LJ, De Jesus S, Eslinger PJ, Arnold AC, et al. The D1/D5 dopamine partial agonist PF-06412562 in advanced-stage PD: A feasibility study. Journal of Parkinson's Disease. 2020;**10**:1515-1527. DOI: 10.3233/JPD-202188

[47] Silveira CRA, MacKinley J, Coleman K, Li Z, Finger E, Bartha R, et al. Ambroxol as a novel disease-modifying treatment for PD dementia: Protocol for a single-centre, randomized, double-blind, placebo-controlled trial. BMC Neurology. 2019;**19**:20. DOI: 10.1186/s12883-019-1252-3

[48] Parashos SA, Luo S, Biglan KM, Bodis-Wollner I, He B, Liang GS, et al. Measuring disease progression in early Parkinson disease: The national institutes of health exploratory trials in Parkinson disease (NET-PD) experience. JAMA Neurology. 2014;**71**:710-716. DOI: 10.1001/jamaneurol.2014.391

[49] Schwarzschild MA, Schwid SR, Marek K, Watts A, Lang AE, Oakes D, et al. Serum urate as a predictor of clinical and radiographic progression in Parkinson disease. Archives of Neurology. 2008;**65**:716-723. DOI: 10.1001/archneur.2008.65.6.nct70003

[50] Kaplitt MG, Feigin A, Tang C, Fitzsimons HL, Mattis P, Lawlor PA, et al. Safety and tolerability of gene therapy with an adeno-associated virus (AAV) borne GAD gene for PD: An open label, phase I trial. Lancet. 2007;**369**:2097-2105. DOI: 10.1016/S0140-6736(07)60982-9

[51] Bartus RT, Baumann TL, Siffert J, Herzog CD, Alterman R, Boulis N, et al. Safety/feasibility of targeting the substantia nigra with AAV2-neurturin in Parkinson patients. Neurology. 2013;**80**:1698-1701. DOI: 10.1212/WNL.0b013e3182904faa

[52] Marks WJ Jr, Bartus RT, Siffert J, Davis CS, Lozano A, Boulis N, et al. Gene delivery of AAV2-neurturin for PD: A double-blind, randomised, controlled trial. Lancet Neurology. 2010;**9**:1164-1172. DOI: 10.1016/S1474-4422(10)70254-4

[53] Ghosh S, Won SJ, Wang J, Fong R, Butler NJM, Moss A, et al. α-Synuclein aggregates induce c-Abl activation and dopaminergic neuronal loss by a feed-forward redox stress mechanism. Progress in Neurobiology. 2021;**202**:102070. DOI: 10.1016/j.pneurobio.2021.102070

[54] Gordon PH, Yu Q, Qualls C, Winfield H, Dillon S, Greene PE, et al.

Reaction time and movement time after embryonic cell implantation in Parkinson disease. Archives of Neurology. 2004;**61**:858-861. DOI: 10.1001/archneur.61.6.858

[55] McRae C, Cherin E, Yamazaki TG, Diem G, Vo AH, Russell D, et al. Effects of perceived treatment on quality of life and medical outcomes in a double-blind placebo surgery trial. Archives of General Psychiatry. 2004;**61**:412-420. DOI: 10.1001/archpsyc.61.4.412

[56] Politis M, Lindvall O. Clinical application of stem cell therapy in PD. BMC Medicine. 2012;**10**:1. DOI: 10.1186/1741-7015-10-1

[57] Axelsen TM, Woldbye DPD. Gene therapy for PD, an update. Journal of Parkinson's Disease. 2018;**8**:195-215. DOI: 10.3233/JPD-181331

[58] Lang AE, Gill S, Patel NK, Lozano A, Nutt JG, Penn R, et al. Randomized controlled trial of intraputamenal glial cell line-derived neurotrophic factor infusion in Parkinson disease. Annals of Neurology. 2006;**59**:459-466. DOI: 10.1002/ana.20737

[59] Sangkuhl K, Klein TE, Altman RB. Selective serotonin reuptake inhibitors pathway. Pharmacogenetics and Genomics. 2009;**19**:907-909. DOI: 10.1097/FPC.0b013e32833132cb

[60] Baumgarten HG, Grozdanovic Z. Psychopharmacology of central serotonergic systems. Pharmacopsychiatry. 1995;**28**:73-79

[61] Brea J, Castro-Palomino J, Yeste S, Cubero E, Párraga A, Domínguez E, et al. Emerging opportunities and concerns for drug discovery at serotonin 5-HT2B receptors. Current Topics in Medicinal Chemistry. 2010;**10**:493-503. DOI: 10.2174/156802610791111524

[62] Carlson AB, Kraus GP. StatPearls. Treasure Island, FL: StatPearls Publishing LLC.; 2020. Physiology, cholinergic receptors

[63] Barth AL, Schneider JS, Johnston TH, Hill MP, Brotchie JM, Moskal JR, et al. NYX-458 improves cognitive performance in a primate PD model. Movement Disorders. 2020;**35**:640-649. DOI: 10.1002/mds.27962

[64] Olivares D, Deshpande VK, Shi Y, Lahiri DK, Greig NH, Rogers JT, et al. N-methyl D-aspartate (NMDA) receptor antagonists and memantine treatment for Alzheimer's disease, vascular dementia and PD. Current Alzheimer Research. 2012;**9**:746-758. DOI: 10.2174/156720512801322564

[65] Ribeiro H, Sarmento-Ribeiro AB, Andrade JP, Dourado M. Apoptosis and (in) pain—potential clinical implications. Biomedicine. 2022;**10**:1255. DOI: 10.3390/biomedicines10061255

[66] Andringa G, Eshuis S, Perentes E, Maguire RP, Roth D, Ibrahim M, et al. TCH346 prevents motor symptoms and loss of striatal FDOPA uptake in bilaterally MPTP-treated primates. Neurobiology of Disease. 2003;**14**:205-217. DOI: 10.1016/S0969-9961(03)00125-6

[67] Grotegut P, Perumal N, Kuehn S, Smit A, Dick HB, Grus FH, et al. Minocycline reduces inflammatory response and cell death in a S100B retina degeneration model. Journal of Neuroinflammation. 2020;**17**:375. DOI: 10.1186/s12974-020-02012-y

[68] Kumar H, Lim H-W, More SV, Kim B-W, Koppula S, Kim IS, et al. The role of free radicals in the aging brain and PD: Convergence and parallelism. International Journal of Molecular

Sciences. 2012;**13**:10478-10504. DOI: 10.3390/ijms130810478

[69] Lin M-W, Lin CC, Chen Y-H, Yang H-B, Hung S-Y. Celastrol inhibits dopaminergic neuronal death of PD through activating mitophagy. Antioxidants. 2020;**9**:37. DOI: 10.3390/antiox9010037

[70] Sechi G, Deledda MG, Bua G, Satta WM, Deiana GA, Pes GM, et al. Reduced intravenous glutathione in the treatment of early PD. Progress in Neuro-Psychopharmacology & Biological Psychiatry. 1996;**20**: 1159-1170. DOI: 10.1016/S0278-5846 (96)00103-0

[71] Duty S, Jenner P. Animal models of PD: A source of novel treatments and clues to the cause of the disease. British Journal of Pharmacology. 2011;**164**(4):1357-1391. DOI: 10.1111/j. 1476-5381.2011.01426.x

[72] Lees AJ, Tolosa E, Olanow CW. Four pioneers of L-dopa treatment: Arvid Carlsson, Oleh Hornykiewicz, George Cotzias, and Melvin Yahr. Movement Disorders. 2015;*30*(1):19-36. DOI: 10.1002/mds.26120

[73] Ungerstedt U. 6-Hydroxy-dopamine induced degeneration of central monoamine neurons. European Journal of Pharmacology. 1968;**5**:107-110

[74] Fernandez HH, Chen JJ. Monoamine oxidase-B inhibition in the treatment of Parkinson's disease. Pharmacotherapy. 2007;**27**:174S-185S

[75] Lees AJ. Dopamine agonists in Parkinson's disease: A look at apomorphine. Fundamental & Clinical Pharmacology. 1993;**7**:121-128

[76] Rondot P, Ziegler M. Activity and acceptability of piribedil in Parkinson's disease: A multicentre study. Journal of Neurology. 1992;**239**(Suppl. 1):S28-S34

[77] Montastruc JL, Rascol O, Senard JM. Current status of dopamine agonists in Parkinson's disease management. Drugs. 1993;**46**:384-393

[78] Elangbam CS. Drug-induced valvulopathy: An update. Toxicologic Pathology. 2010;**38**:837-848

[79] Bonuccelli U, Del DP, Rascol O. Role of dopamine receptor agonists in the treatment of early Parkinson's disease. Parkinsonism & Related Disorders. 2009;**15**(Suppl. 4):S44-S53

[80] Jenner P. The rationale for the use of dopamine agonists in Parkinson's disease. *Neurology*. 1995;**45**:S6-S12

[81] Carlsson A, Lindqvist M, MagnussonT.3,4-Dihydroxyphenylalanine and 5-hydroxytryptophan as reserpine antagonists. Nature. 1957;**180**:1200

[82] Degkwitz R, Frowein R, Kulenkampff C, et al. Uber die Wirkungen von L-DOPA beim Menschen und deren Beeinflussung durch Reserpin, Chlorpromazin, Ipronazid und Vitamin B6. Klinische Wochenschrift. 1960;**38**:120-123

[83] Jellinger KA. Pathology of Parkinson's disease. Changes other than the nigrostriatal pathway. Molecular and Chemical Neuropathology. 1991;**14**:153-197

[84] Langston JW, Ballard P, Tetrud JW, Irwin I. Chronic parkinsonism in humans due to a product of meperidine-analog synthesis. Science. 1983;**219**:979-980

[85] Jenner P, Rupniak NM, Rose S, Kelly E, Kilpatrick G, Lees A, et al. 1-Methyl-4-phenyl-1,2,3,6-tetrahydropyridine-induced parkinsonism in the common

marmoset. Neuroscience Letters. 1984;**50**:85-90

[86] Johannessen JN, Chiueh CC, Burns RS, Markey SP. Differences in the metabolism of MPTP in the rodent and primate parallel differences in sensitivity to its neurotoxic effects. Life Sciences. 1985;**36**:219-224

[87] Riachi NJ, LaManna JC, Harik SI. Entry of 1-methyl-4-phenyl-1,2,3,6-tetrahydropyridine into the rat brain. Journal of Pharmacology and Experimental Therapeutics. 1989;**249**:744-748. [PubMed] [Google Scholar]

[88] Chiba K, Trevor A, Castagnoli N Jr. Metabolism of the neurotoxic tertiary amine, MPTP, by brain monoamine oxidase. Biochemical and Biophysical Research Communications. 1984;**120**:574-578

[89] Javitch JA, D'Amato RJ, Strittmatter SM, Snyder SH. Parkinsonism-inducing neurotoxin, *N*-methyl-4-phenyl-1,2,3,6-tetrahydropyridine: Uptake of the metabolite *N*-methyl-4-phenylpyridine by dopamine neurons explains selective toxicity. Proceedings of the National Academy of Sciences of the United States of America. 1985;**82**:2173-2177

[90] Karunakaran S, Saeed U, Mishra M, Valli RK, Joshi SD, Meka DP, et al. Selective activation of p38 mitogen-activated protein kinase in dopaminergic neurons of substantia nigra leads to nuclear translocation of p53 in 1-methyl-4-phenyl-1,2,3,6-tetrahydropyridine-treated mice. The Journal of Neuroscience. 2008;**28**:12500-12509

[91] Saporito MS, Thomas BA, Scott RW. MPTP activates c-Jun NH(2)-terminal kinase (JNK) and its upstream regulatory kinase MKK4 in nigrostriatal neurons in vivo. Journal of Neurochemistry. 2000;**75**:1200-1208

[92] Tatton NA, Kish SJ. In situ detection of apoptotic nuclei in the substantia nigra compacta of 1-methyl-4-phenyl-1,2,3,6-tetrahydropyridine-treated mice using terminal deoxynucleotidyl transferase labelling and acridine orange staining. Neuroscience. 1997;**77**:1037-1048

[93] Betarbet R, Sherer TB, MacKenzie G, Garcia-Osuna M, Panov AV, Greenamyre JT. Chronic systemic pesticide exposure reproduces features of Parkinson's disease. Nature Neuroscience. 2000;**3**:1301-1306

[94] Greenamyre JT, Cannon JR, Drolet R, Mastroberardino PG. Lessons from the rotenone model of Parkinson's disease. Trends in Pharmacological Sciences. 2010;**31**:141-142. author reply 142-143

[95] Sherer TB, Betarbet R, Testa CM, Seo BB, Richardson JR, Kim JH, et al. Mechanism of toxicity in rotenone models of Parkinson's disease. The Journal of Neuroscience. 2003;**23**:10756-10764

[96] Alam ZI, Daniel SE, Lees AJ, Marsden DC, Jenner P, Halliwell B. A generalised increase in protein carbonyls in the brain in Parkinson's but not incidental Lewy body disease. Journal of Neurochemistry. 1997;**69**:1326-1329. DOI: 10.1046/j.1471-4159.1997.69031326.x

[97] Sherer TB, Betarbet R, Kim JH, Greenamyre JT. Selective microglial activation in the rat rotenone model of Parkinson's disease. Neuroscience Letters. 2003;**341**:87-90

[98] Tansey MG, Goldberg MS. Neuroinflammation in Parkinson's disease: Its role in neuronal death and implications for therapeutic intervention. Neurobiology of Disease. 2010;**37**:510-518

[99] Wang XF, Li S, Chou AP, Bronstein JM. Inhibitory effects of pesticides on proteasome activity: Implication in Parkinson's disease. Neurobiology of Disease. 2006;**23**:198-205

[100] Ascherio A, Chen H, Weisskopf MG, O'Reilly E, McCullough ML, Calle EE, et al. Pesticide exposure and risk for Parkinson's disease. Annals of Neurology. 2006;**60**:197-203

[101] Costello S, Cockburn M, Bronstein J, Zhang X, Ritz B. Parkinson's disease and residential exposure to maneb and paraquat from agricultural applications in the central valley of California. American Journal of Epidemiology. 2009;**169**:919-926

[102] Shimizu K, Ohtaki K, Matsubara K, Aoyama K, Uezono T, Saito O, et al. Carrier-mediated processes in blood–brain barrier penetration and neural uptake of paraquat. Brain Research. 2001;**906**:135-142

[103] Miller GW. Paraquat: The red herring of Parkinson's disease research. Toxicological Sciences. 2007;**100**:1-2

[104] Zhang J, Fitsanakis VA, Gu G, Jing D, Ao M, Amarnath V, et al. Manganese ethylene-bis-dithiocarbamate and selective dopaminergic neurodegeneration in rat: A link through mitochondrial dysfunction. Journal of Neurochemistry. 2003;**84**:336-346

[105] Thiruchelvam M, Brockel BJ, Richfield EK, Baggs RB, Cory-Slechta DA. Potentiated and preferential effects of combined paraquat and maneb on nigrostriatal dopamine systems: Environmental risk factors for Parkinson's disease? Brain Research. 2000;**873**:225-234

[106] Barlow BK, Thiruchelvam MJ, Bennice L, Cory-Slechta DA, Ballatori N, Richfield EK. Increased synaptosomal dopamine content and brain concentration of paraquat produced by selective dithiocarbamates. Journal of Neurochemistry. 2003;**85**:1075-1086

[107] Polymeropoulos MH, Lavedan C, Leroy E, Ide SE, Dehejia A, Dutra A, et al. Mutation in the alphasynuclein gene identified in families with Parkinson's disease. Science. 1997;**276**:2045-2047

[108] Kitada T, Asakawa S, Hattori N, Matsumine H, Yamamura Y, Minoshima S, et al. Mutations in the parkin gene cause autosomal recessive juvenile parkinsonism. Nature. 1998;**392**:605-608

[109] Bonifati V, Rizzu P, Van Baren MJ, Schaap O, Breedveld GJ, Krieger E, et al. Mutations in the DJ-1 gene associated with autosomal recessive early-onset Parkinsonism. Science. 2002;**299**:256-259

[110] Valente EM, Abou-Sleiman PM, Caputo V, Muqit MM, Harvey K, Gispert S, et al. Hereditary early-onset Parkinson's disease caused by mutations in PINK1. Science. 2004;**304**:1158-1160

[111] Zimprich A, Biskup S, Leitner P, Lichtner P, Farrer M, Lincoln S, et al. Mutations in LRRK2 cause autosomal-dominant parkinsonism with pleomorphic pathology. Neuron. 2004;**44**:601-607

[112] Leroy E, Boyer R, Auburger G, Leube B, Ulm G, Mezey E, et al. The ubiquitin pathway in Parkinson's disease. Nature. 1998;**395**:451-452

[113] Strauss KM, Martins LM, Plun-Favreau H, Marx FP, Kautzmann S, Berg D, et al. Loss of function mutations in the gene encoding Omi/HtrA2 in Parkinson's disease. Human Molecular Genetics. 2005;**14**:2099-2111

[114] Ramirez A, Heimbach A, Grundemann J, Stiller B, Hampshire D, Cid LP, et al. Hereditary parkinsonism with dementia is caused by mutations in ATP13A2, encoding a lysosomal

type 5 P-type ATPase. Nature Genetics. 2006;**38**:1184-1191

[115] Lakso M, Vartiainen S, Moilanen AM, Sirvio J, Thomas JH, Nass R, et al. Dopaminergic neuronal loss and motor deficits in *Caenorhabditis elegans* overexpressing human alpha-synuclein. Journal of Neurochemistry. 2003;**86**:165-172

[116] Lim K-L, Ng C-H. Genetic models of Parkinson disease. Biochimica et Biophysica Acta. 2009;**1792**:604-615

[117] Cannon JR, Greenamyre JT. Gene-environment interactions in Parkinson's disease: Specific evidence in humans and mammalian models. Neurobiology of Disease. 2013;**57**:38-46. DOI: 10.1016/j.nbd.2012.06.025

[118] Pardridge WM. The blood-brain barrier: Bottleneck in brain drug development. NeuroRx. 2005;**2**:3-14

[119] Furuno T, Landi MT, Ceroni M, Caporaso N, Bernucci I, Nappi G, et al. Expression polymorphism of the blood-brain barrier component P-glycoprotein (MDR1) in relation to Parkinson's disease. Pharmacogenetics. 2002;**12**(7):529-534. DOI: 10.1097/00008571-200210000-00004 PMID: 12360103

[120] Tan EK, Chan DK, Ng PW, Woo J, Teo YY, Tang K, et al. Effect of MDR1 haplotype on risk of Parkinson disease. Archives of Neurology. 2005;**62**(3):460-464. DOI: 10.1001/archneur.62.3.460 PMID: 15767512

[121] Kortekaas R, Leenders KL, van Oostrom JC, Vaalburg W, Bart J, Willemsen AT, et al. Blood-brain barrier dysfunction in parkinsonian midbrain in vivo. Annals of Neurology. 2005;**57**(2):176-179. DOI: 10.1002/ana.20369 PMID: 15668963

[122] Bartels AL, van Berckel BN, Lubberink M, Luurtsema G, Lammertsma AA, Leenders KL. Blood-brain barrier P-glycoprotein function is not impaired in early Parkinson's disease. Parkinsonism & Related Disorders. 2008;**14**(6):505-508. DOI: 10.1016/j.parkreldis.2007.11.007. Epub 2008 Mar 5. PMID: 18325822

[123] Westerlund M, Belin AC, Olson L, Galter D. Expression of multi-drug resistance 1 mRNA in human and rodent tissues: Reduced levels in Parkinson patients. Cell and Tissue Research Nov 2008;**334**(2):179-185. DOI: 10.1007/s00441-008-0686-5. Epub 2008 Oct 15. PMID: 18855017

[124] Schinkel AH, Wagenaar E, Mol CA, van Deemter L. P-glycoprotein in the blood-brain barrier of mice influences the brain penetration and pharmacological activity of many drugs. The Journal of Clinical Investigation. 1996;**1;97**(11):2517-2524. DOI: 10.1172/JCI118699. PMID: 8647944; PMCID: PMC507337

[125] Erekat N, Al Khatib A, Al-Jarrah M. Endurance exercise training attenuates the up regulation of iNOS in the skeletal muscles of chronic/progressive mouse model of Parkinson's disease. Journal of Neurology Research. 2013;**3**(3-4):108-113

[126] Erekat N, Al-Khatib A, Al-Jarrah M. Heat shock protein 90 is a potential therapeutic target for ameliorating skeletal muscle abnormalities in Parkinson's disease. Neural Regeneration Research. 2014;**9**(6):616-621

[127] Al-Jarrah M, Obaidat H, Bataineh Z, Walton L, Al-Khateeb A. Endurance exercise training protects against the upregulation of nitric oxide in the striatum of MPTP/probenecid mouse model of Parkinson's disease. NeuroRehabilitation. 2013;**32**(1):141-147. DOI: 10.3233/NRE-130831. PMID: 23422467

Chapter 2

Air Pollution and Parkinson's Disease

Changbo Jin and Wenming Shi

Abstract

Parkinson's disease (PD) is the second most common neurodegenerative disease of unclear etiology that is thought to be caused by a combination of genetic and environmental factors. Air pollution, the largest environmental health risk globally, has been suggested to be associated with PD risk, while not all results are uniform. In this chapter, we summarize the recent advances in the epidemiology of six criteria air pollutants-fine particulate matter ($PM_{2.5}$), inhalable particles (PM_{10}), nitrogen dioxide (NO_2), sulfur dioxide (SO_2), carbon monoxide(CO), and ozone exposure with PD risk, and provided an overview of the potential mechanisms of air pollution on PD. Based on the current evidence from the human's studies and animal models, this chapter provides a novel insight for the understanding of how environmental exposure influences the pathogenesis of neurodegeneration and prevents the occurrence or development of PD.

Keywords: Parkinson's disease, air pollution, $PM_{2.5}$, inflammation, neurotoxicity

1. Introduction

Air pollution, a major cause of premature death and disease, is the largest environmental health risk globally [1, 2]. According to the Global Burden of Disease (GBD) study in 2019, air pollution has been ranked as the fourth death cause in the world [3], which poses a heavy threat to both individuals and society. With rapid urbanization and industrialization, air pollution levels have continuously increased over the past decades. Parkinson's disease (PD), the second most common neurodegenerative disease, is characterized by the pathological accumulation of proteins, inflammation, and neuron loss [4]. It is reported that the global prevalence of PD doubled over the next 30 years [4]. Recent epidemiological studies have found that air pollutants exposure is significantly associated with the increased risk of PD, while not all results are uniform [5–8]. The variability among these studies is likely attributed to the measurement of air pollutants, exposure assessment and duration, and correction for other confounding. In this chapter, we summarize the recent advances in the epidemiology of air pollution exposure and PD, including the evidence of the effects of six criteria air pollutants-fine particulate matter ($PM_{2.5}$), inhalable particles (PM_{10}), nitrogen dioxide (NO_2), sulfur dioxide (SO_2), carbon monoxide (CO), and ozone with PD, and provided a narrative review of the potential mechanisms of air pollution on PD risk. This chapter serves to provide a novel insight for the understanding of how environmental exposure influences the pathogenesis of neurodegeneration and reduces the risk of PD.

2. Air pollution: sources, composition, and monitoring

Air pollution is a heterogeneous mixture composed of particulate matter (PM) and gaseous components that are released directly into the atmosphere (primary pollutants) but also generated by reacting with other components (secondary pollutants) that vary both temporally and spatially [9]. Expansion of industry and vehicle traffic had a major impact on the overall air quality in urban areas over the past decades. In addition, indoor solid fuels burning, agricultural production, and waste incineration also contribute to negative effects on air quality.

Urban airborne PM typically can be described by four modes (**Figure 1**), which primarily composed of PM_{10} (particles <10 μm in diameter), $PM_{2.5}$ (particles <2.5 μm in diameter), and ultrafine particles (UFP, $PM_{0.1}$, particles <0.1 μm in diameter). However, only $PM_{2.5}$ and PM_{10} are monitored by regulatory agencies in different countries (i.e., the Environmental Protection Agency in the USA) due to the "mass-based" estimation approach [10]. The sources of PM are diverse and mainly include anthropogenic causes (e.g., traffic gas emissions and fossil fuel burning) and natural sources such as dust storms, wildfires, and volcanic eruptions, which are related to climate change.

Nitrogen oxides (NOx), SO_2, CO, and ozone are the critical gaseous components in the atmosphere. NOx is a mixture of gases that consists of nitrogen and oxygen, such as NO_2 and nitric oxide (NO) that can be produced by traffic or indoor cooking stoves or the burning of coal, oil, or natural gas. The sources of SO_2 are primarily from burning fossil fuels, non-ferrous metal smelting, steel, and industry production process. CO is produced by motor vehicle emissions, industrial boilers, and waste incineration. Ozone, a secondary pollutant, is formed when NOx reacts with volatile organic carbons (VOCs) and oxygen in the presence of heat and light. Its main sources include

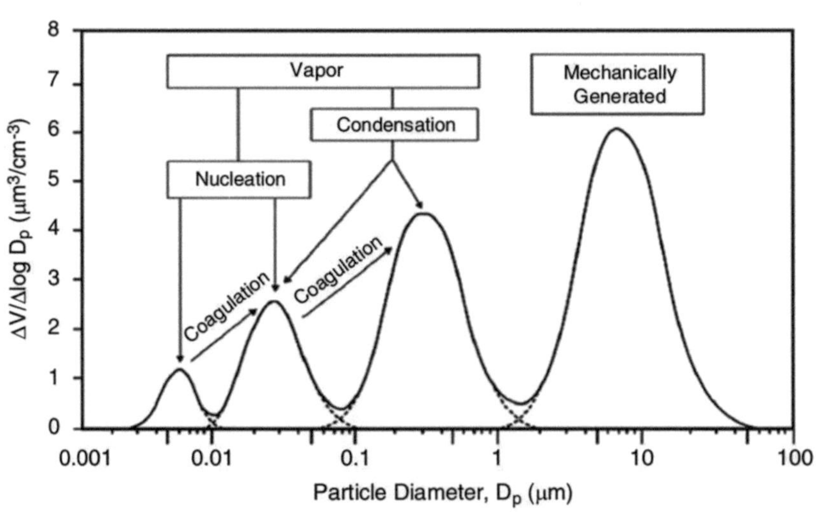

Figure 1.
The size distribution of airborne particulate matter (Adapted from USA. EPA 2004).

Pollutants	Averaging period	USA	E.U.	China
Sulfur dioxide	1 hour	75 ppb	350 μg/m^3	150 μg/m^3
Carbon monoxide	8 hour	10 mg/m^3	10 μg/m^3	10 mg/m^{3a}
Nitrogen dioxide	1 hour	100 ppb	200 μg/m^3	200 μg/m^3
Ozone	8 hour	0.07 ppm	120 μg/m^3	100 μg/m^3
$PM_{2.5}$	1 year	15 μg/m^3	25 μg/m^3	15 μg/m^3
PM_{10}	1 day	150 μg/m^3	50 μg/m^3	50 μg/m^3
Lead	1 year	0.15 μg/m^3	0.5 μg/m^3	0.5 μg/m^3

[a]*The averaging period for carbon monoxide is 1 hour.*

Table 1.
Air quality standards in the USA, EU, and in China.

traffic gas, factories, and electric utilities. To accelerate the control of air pollution, a series of air quality standards for the primary air pollutants have been established in the USA, EU, and China (**Table 1**).

In general, ambient air pollutants are monitored by traditional monitoring methods with fixed air stations, while they are expensive, sparsely distributed, and require high maintenance. To overcome the limitations in the traditional methods, a growing body of relatively new approaches including land-use regression (LUR) models, satellite remote sensing, and disperse models have been developed to estimate the air pollution levels with high spatial resolution. In the LUR modeling approach, levels of vehicle exhaust markers, such as NOx and PM, are measured simultaneously at many locations throughout an urban area using relatively inexpensive passive monitors. Various geographic information system (GIS) parameters (such as traffic and roadway density, land use, and population density) are used to predict the measured concentrations. For satellite-based models, Shi et al. used the V4.CH.02 product of the Dalhousie University Atmospheric Composition Analysis Group to simulate the annual average $PM_{2.5}$ and its chemical constituents at approximately 0.01° × 0.01° resolution [11]. This dataset combines satellite retrievals and simulation of aerosol optical depth (AOD) from multiple sources (MISR, MODIS Dark Target, MODIS, and SeaWiFS Deep Blue, MODIS MAIAC, and GEOS-Chem), chemical transported models, and near-surface $PM_{2.5}$ concentrations [11, 12]. Additionally, to measure an individual's exposure of air pollution, low-cost sensors with real-time monitoring are becoming popular in the field of environmental epidemiology.

3. Epidemiological findings of air pollution with PD risk

3.1 Particulate matter and PD risk

PM has been suggested to be related to the risk of PD, while the evidence from different study designs is inconsistent. Among others, $PM_{2.5}$ is the most consistent and robust indicator of air pollution [11]. A prospective cohort study of 2.19 million participants in Ontario showed that long-term exposure to $PM_{2.5}$ was associated with a 4% increase in incident PD (95%CI:1.01, 1.08) [7]. Another nationwide cohort study among 63.03 million individuals aged ≥65 years in the USA found that annual $PM_{2.5}$ exposure was positively associated with an increased risk of first hospital admission for PD (hazard ratio, HR = 1.13, 95%CI:1.12, 1.14) [13]. Regarding the short-term effects of $PM_{2.5}$, Zanobetti et al. found that each 10 μg/m^3 increase in lag 2-day average $PM_{2.5}$ was positively associated with the hospitalization risk of PD (3.23%, 95%CI:1.08, 5.43) [14]. Moreover, a study performed in New York State to explore the chemical constituents of $PM_{2.5}$ with PD hospitalization by using a satellite-based model at 1 km × 1 km spatial resolution and the results showed that organic matter (OM) and nitrate exposure significantly increased the risk of PD aggravation [15]. However, the associations of PM exposure are not uniform in some studies [6, 16]. A large cohort from the Health Professionals Follow-up Study (HPFS) showed that exposure to ambient PM_{10} or PM_{coarse} was not significantly associated with PD risk among US men [16]. A recent meta-analysis conducted in 2020 involving 10,077,029 participants presented no significant relationship between long-term PM_{10} exposure and PD incidence. With every 10 μg/m^3 increment, the relative risks (RRs) and 95% CIs were 1.01 (0.97, 1.05) for PM_{10} exposure [17].

3.2 Nitrogen oxides with PD risk

Nitrogen oxides (NOx) are recognized as traffic-related air pollutants, which are released during any high-temperature combustion and then rapidly converted to NO_2. The associations found between NO_2 exposure and PD risk are mixed. In a Denmark study, Ritz et al. used a dispersion model to estimate the NO_2 exposure and the results showed positive relationships with PD risk, with a 9% higher risk (95% CI:3, 16.0%) [18]. Similar associations were also observed in a nationally representative cohort of 78,830 individuals [19], the findings indicated that long-term exposure to ambient NO_2 was related to an increased risk of PD in Korea (HR for highest vs. lowest quartile, 1.41; 95% CI: 1.02, 1.95; $P_{trend} = 0.045$). However, a matched case-control study in the Netherlands reported no significant association between 16 years of residential exposure to ambient NO_2 and the development of PD (aOR = 0.87, 95% CI: 0.54, 1.41) [6]. Moreover, a nested case–control study in Taiwan investigated multiple chemical compounds exposure with the incidence of PD, and no significant associations for NO_2, NO, and NO_X exposure were observed [8]. A recent meta-analysis summarized the studies of ambient air pollution with PD risk, the pooled odds ratio (OR) for the effect of NO_2 (per 1 μg/m^3) on PD was 1.01 (95%CI,1.00, 1.02, $I^2 = 69\%$) [20].

3.3 Sulfur dioxide with PD risk

Studies of the association between SO_2 exposure and PD risk are relatively fewer. Most studies reported no significant effects of ambient SO_2 exposure on the risk of PD. A nested case-control study performed in Taiwan using the National Health Insurance Research Dataset (NHIRD) explored the multiple air pollutants exposure with incident PD, and the findings showed no significant relationship for SO_2 exposure. Jo et al. [19] used the data from the Korea National Health Insurance Service and estimated the pollutants levels based on the nearest air monitoring stations to examine such association. The results found no statistically significant relationship between long-term exposure to ambient SO_2 and incident PD (HR = 1.02, 95%CI: 0.74, 1.41). Another population-based cohort study was also conducted in Korea, which examined the short-term effects of air pollutants exposure on PD aggravation, with a positive association. Each unit increase in the 8-day moving average of SO_2

level was significantly related to PD aggravation (OR = 1.54, 95%CI:1.11, 2.14 per 1 ppb) [21]. As reported in a recent meta-analysis in 2022, the pooled association was not statistically significant for SO_2 exposure [20].

3.4 Carbon monoxide with PD risk

Overall, the research on CO has demonstrated an effect on the risk of PD, but there are inconsistencies across studies. A population-based case-control study in Taiwan suggested that traffic-related pollutants exposure such as NOx and CO increased PD risk in Taiwanese population. The multi-pollutant models showed that the OR was 1.17 (1.07, 1.27) for ambient CO above the 75th percentile exposure compared with the lowest percentile [22]. A case-crossover study in Seoul found that short-term exposure to ambient CO significantly related to the risk of PD aggravation. The OR was 1.46 (95%CI, 1.05, 2.04) for each 0.1 ppm increment in the 8-day moving average of CO concentrations [21]. Conversely, some studies found no significant effects of ambient CO exposure on PD risk [8, 19]. Given the inconsistencies of studies, a systematic review and meta-analysis were conducted in 2019 to summarize the results from 10 studies. The pooled association indicated that the risk of PD was 1.65 (1.10, 2.48) for each 1 ppm increment of ambient CO exposure [23].

3.5 Ozone with PD risk

Studies of ambient ozone exposure with the risk of PD have been reported but remain inconclusive. Several studies found significant associations between exposure to ozone and PD risk [7, 24]. Zhao et al. [24] estimated the ambient average level of ozone by a combination of chemical transport models and ground measurement. The association analysis indicated that long-term exposure to ozone was significantly related to the increased risk of mortality due to PD in Canada (HR = 1.09, 95%CI:1.04, 1.14). A systematic review and meta-analysis included 21 studies with 222,051 individuals who found that ozone exposure might contribute to a higher risk of PD. The pooled results presented that with each 10 $\mu g/m^3$ increase in the concentration of ozone, the adjusted RR was 1.01 (95%CI: 1.00, 1.02) [25]. Furthermore, a most up-to-date meta-analysis by Dhiman et al. further confirms the positive association of ozone exposure [20].

4. Major study design in air pollution epidemiology

4.1 Studies on acute health effects

In the field of air pollution epidemiology, time-series study, case-crossover study, and panel study are often used to assess the acute health effects of pollutants. A time-series design by controlling for confounders that do not vary temporally but can only address short-term acute effects [26]. In recent years, time-series study has been widely applied to investigate the short-term exposure to air pollution on various health endpoints. Similar findings have been documented in different areas with different air pollution backgrounds, as well as in different study populations around the world [27–29]. This method is particularly advantageous where the catchment area is unclear, for hospital-based studies in densely populated areas where not all hospitals can be included, counts of admissions or outpatients might be comparable for high-polluted versus low-polluted days. Therefore, time-based comparisons within a population are useful for assessing acute health effects from community-wide exposures and may provide more valid estimates than comparisons between communities. The statistic methods of the generalized additive model (GAM) or Poisson regression models are often applied to analyze in these studies, whereas temperature and relative humidity are controlled for potential meteorological effects [30].

Case cross-over study is another typical design used for examining the acute effects of air pollution. The concept of "case-crossover study" is firstly named by Dr. Maclure at the Harvard University in 1991. The key feature of this study design is that each case serves its own control. The method is analogous to a crossover experiment viewed retrospectively, except that researcher does not control when a patient starts and stops being exposed to the possible trigger. Furthermore, the exposure frequency is measured in only a sample of the total period when the patient was at risk of the onset of disease [31]. Confounding from individual time-invariant characteristics is completely controlled, as the individual supplies his/her own referent periods. Compared with the time-series study, the strength of case-crossover study not only can control many potential confounding by its novel design rather than statistical models but also can help avoid many ethical issues.

Panel study, sample a set of fixed individuals on whom observations are made at regular time intervals, is usually completed in time. In recent decades, a growing number of epidemiological studies have applied the panel design to investigate the association of individual-level air pollutants exposure with health outcomes. Panel studies are usually performed over a short period, require intensive observation within this period, and have a relatively narrow focus. Thus, it may be difficult for recruitment and retention as they are demanding on participants, leading to issues with completeness and sample size [32]. Linear mixed models, mixed-effect models, or generalized estimating equations (GEEs) are usually used in this study design to examine the health effects of air pollutants.

4.2 Studies on long-term health effects

Compared with acute health effects, studies on long-term exposure of air pollutants are more common in the field of environmental epidemiology. Cohort studies, case-control studies, or cross-sectional studies are often used to analyze the relationship. The ecological study, a type of cross-sectional design, can be used to determine the regional characteristics of air pollution. Ecologic studies utilize group-level data on outcomes (i.e., rates of disease, prevalence proportions, or mean measurements) in relation to group-level data on exposures. With the emergence of some new technologies such as LUR model or satellite-based models, the estimation of the temporal and spatial changes of ambient concentrations of air pollutants has been improved [11, 24]. As reported in a recent model study, satellite-retrieved AOD provides a unique opportunity to characterize the long-term trends of ground-level $PM_{2.5}$ at high spatial resolution [33]. Given the ecological study is easily subject to ecological fallacy and confounding, results from ecological studies should be viewed critically.

Cohort study is widely recognized as an ideal approach to investigating the long-term effects of air pollutants exposure on health outcomes. However, due to the high expense and time-consuming nature, it brings many challenges to the practices of scientific research.

5. Potential mechanisms of air pollution on Parkinson's disease

The primary pathology in PD involves dopaminergic neuron loss, particularly in the substantia nigra (SN), and systematic inflammation. In the context of air pollution, studies have indicated that diesel exhaust can increase α-synuclein (α-syn) levels and lead to neuroinflammation, which is associated with the development of PD. It is suggested that several pathways by which air pollutants can affect the central nervous system (CNS) and contribute to the pathogenesis of PD. The direct neurotoxicity and neuroinflammation, air pollutants-lung-brain connection, and changes of gut and microbiome play important roles in the occurrence and development of PD. The details of the possible mechanisms are summarized in **Figure 2**.

5.1 Direct neurotoxicity and neuroinflammation

It is believed that many components of air pollution can reach the brain and thus contribute to the pathogenesis of PD by direct neurotoxicity and/or neuroinflammation. The two fractions of PM-$PM_{2.5}$ and UFP are predominantly implicated in CNS effects. Both of them are acutely toxic to cardiovascular and lung tissue. Given the small particle size and high activity, these particles can cross the blood-air barrier of the lungs, gaining access to peripheral circulation and the brain. The nasal olfactory pathway is suggested to be a critical portal of entry, where inhaled UFP reaches trigeminal nerves, brainstem, and hippocampus [34, 35]. Furthermore, a growing number of studies have indicated these PMs can enter the brain and may be related to neurodegenerative pathology in vivo [36–38]. Additionally, evidence has shown that the concentrations of some polycyclic aromatic hydrocarbons (PAHs) in human brains are very high. This can help support the concept that specific components of air pollution can bioaccumulate in the nervous system, poses significant risks through direct neurotoxicity [39].

Oxidative stress and inflammation have been associated with the neurodegenerative process including PD. In vitro studies have reported that PM exposure can induce inflammation in airway epithelial cells mediated by oxidative stress [40]. It is believed that oxidative stress plays a role in PD pathogenesis and can cause α-syn aggregation [41]. Pathological α-syn aggregates appear to spread throughout the CNS in a predictable manner, which determines the clinical symptom of PD. Mitochondrial damage has also been implicated in the development of PD and can lead to oxidative stress and neuronal loss. Dysfunction of mitochondria promotes the formation of reactive oxygen species (ROS), which can induce α-syn aggregation [42]. In addition, animal models showed that systematic inflammation could result in neuroinflammation and loss of dopaminergic neurons, especially in combination with increased α-syn levels, which posed an elevated risk for incident PD.

5.2 Lung-brain connection

Exposure to air pollution also leads to peripheral or systematic inflammation, which, in turn, can contribute to CNS inflammation. Epithelial cells lining the airway can physically block larger size PM and secrete cytokines including tumor necrosis factor-α (TNF-α) and interleukin-1 beta (IL-1β), which promote the synthesis of other cytokines and lead to immune cell activation. Just as an example, chronic low-level inflammation

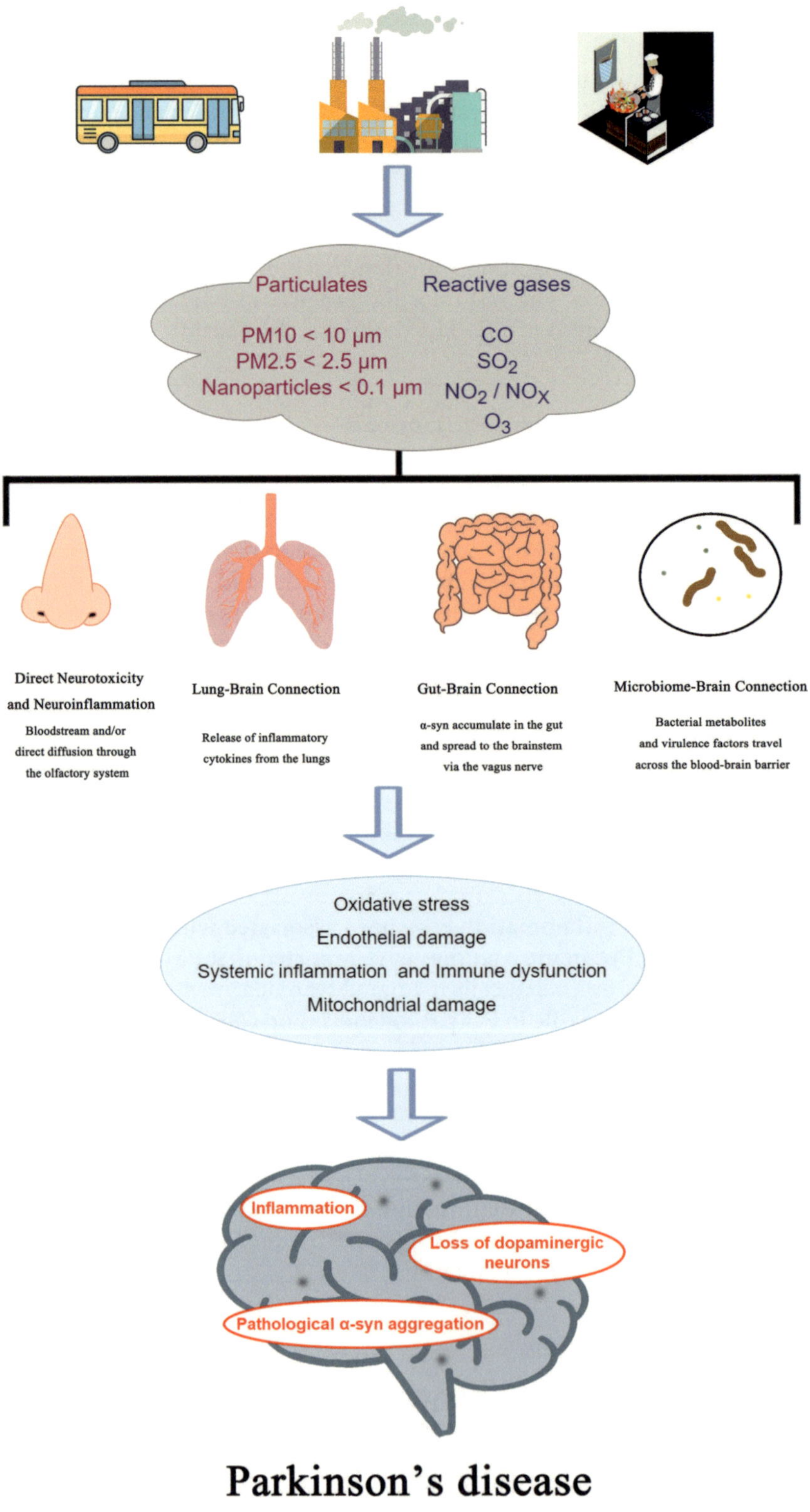

Figure 2.
The potential mechanisms of air pollutants exposure on risk of PD.

is linked to multiple systemic injections of low lipopolysaccharide (LPS), a cell wall component of Gram-negative bacteria that is a potent pro-inflammatory stimulus, rendering animals more vulnerable to further pro-inflammatory insult [43]. The blood-brain barrier (BBB) is weakened by systemic inflammation-derived proinflammatory cytokines and chemokines, which can allow proinflammatory cytokines and inflammatory cells to enter the brain. Once passing to the brain, these factors from the periphery, along with brain-derived cytokines, chemokines, α-syn, and amyloid precursor proteins, can activate CNS immune cells and induce downstream effects [44, 45]. In brief, air pollutants exposure induces a systemic inflammatory response, which may lead to neuroinflammation and an elevated risk of PD.

5.3 Gut-brain connection

Studies from both animal experiments and humans have supported the hypothesis that pathological α-syn can accumulate in the gut, spread to the brainstem by the vagus nerve, and eventually induce neuronal loss in the SN. To our knowledge, there is little direct evidence of air pollutants can induce α-syn aggregates in the gut, which spreads to the CNS, while there is an increasing body of publications demonstrating that air pollutants can change the gut mucosa, which is thought to promote α-syn pathology. In animal studies, α-syn preformed fibrils injected into the duodenum induces α-syn spread into brainstem nuclei and then to the SN [46]. Moreover, it is reported that air pollution exposure can induce inflammation and leakiness in the gut. It may be a trigger for α-syn aggregates and alter the risk of inflammatory bowel disease (IBD) [44]. To date, it remains unclear how air pollutants exert these changes in the gut, while they may act or partly affect by altering the microbiome.

5.4 Microbiome-brain connection

Microbiome has recently encountered the interest of neuroscience, which may be associated with the risk of PD. Air pollutants exposure has been linked to alterations in the microbiome, while primarily in animals. The imbalances in the microbiome can lead to disruption of the epithelial barrier of the gut and allow various bacterial metabolites and virulence factors to pass through the intestinal lining, enter the bloodstream and subsequently across the BBB. Metabolites of gut microbes, such as short-chain fatty acids (SCFA, i.e., acetate, propionate, and butyrate), have also been suggested to activate microglia and increase neuroinflammation [47]. In addition, some molecules including synaptogenic proteins, SCFA, levodopa (L-dopa), γ-aminobutyric acid, and serotonin can be produced, suppressed, and overused by strains of microbiota. These changes can have a direct effect on neurological function. As reported in a mice model, PD-derived gut microbiota may exacerbate α-syn-mediated motor impairments and neuronal disease, whereas germ-free mice displayed milder α-syn pathology [48]. An experimental study in mice found that ambient $PM_{2.5}$ exposure exhibited significant changes in gut microbial diversity [49]. A significant increment was observed in Bacteroidales, which probably involved degradation of the mucous layer and elevated gut permeability [44]. Though the mice microbiome is different from that in humans, these studies may help provide implications for air pollution affecting the PD risk by changing the microbiome. Future studies are warranted to validate these findings.

6. Summary and future perspectives

The etiology of PD is complex but undoubtedly involves a combination of gene and environmental factors. To our knowledge, epidemiological investigations of air pollution exposure and PD risk have covered a wide variety of sizes and types of pollutants, populations, geographical locations, and related factors. Air pollution has been suggested to contribute to a significant percentage of PD cases worldwide. Several potential mechanisms include direct neural toxicity, CNS inflammation, and alternations in the microbiome may promote neurodegeneration and increase the risk of PD. However, this field is still in its early stage, some important questions remain unanswered, and some challenges are listed below.

1. $PM_{2.5}$ constituents with PD risk

   Since $PM_{2.5}$ is a complex mixture of more than 50 chemical constituents (such as black carbon, OM, water-soluble ions, and metals), different chemical constituents of $PM_{2.5}$ on PD risk as well as the possible mechanisms may be varied. It is meaningful for identifying the roles of various constituents of $PM_{2.5}$ played in the development of PD.

2. Critical exposure windows

   Given the development of PD is a chronic condition with a latency of about a decade [50], the critical windows of air pollutants exposure on PD risk needed to be identified in the future. With the rapid development of wearable personal monitoring sensors, we may foresee future possibilities for more precise and accurate personal exposure to pollutants, which can greatly benefit studies of air pollution and PD.

3. Interaction of gut microbiome and air pollutants

   The involvement of human gut microbe with PD risk is an exciting emergent field of research. Besides the inhalation pathway, the PMs can also be swallowed and end up in the gut. The particles can then induce systematic inflammation, or interact with the gut microbiome in other ways, thus potentially impacting PD risk. Future investigations are needed to explore the interaction between air pollutants and gut-microbiome concerning the risk of PD.

4. Gene modifications and vulnerable population

   As reported that the PD risk increased threefold when joint exposure to the AA genotype of the IL-1β gene and ambient NO_2 [22]. It would be interesting to explore the interactions of the gene (such as APOEε4) with air pollutants on PD risk. Additionally, it is significant to identify the vulnerable characteristics of the population in future studies.

We believe that the understanding of the relationship between air pollution and PD will improve in the coming years as more investigations are conducted and more reproducible findings are reported.

Conflict of interests

None declared.

Abbreviations

PD	Parkinson's disease
$PM_{2.5}$	fine particulate matter
PM_{10}	inhalable particles
NO_2	nitrogen dioxide
SO_2	sulfur dioxide
CO	carbon monoxide
UFP	ultrafine particles
RR	relative risk
OR	odds ratio
HR	hazard risk
95%CI	95% confidence interval
α-syn	α-synuclein
CNS	central nervous system
BBB	blood-brain barrier
SN	substantia nigra
OM	organic matter
AOD	aerosol optical depth

Author details

Changbo Jin[1] and Wenming Shi[2*]

1 Tongji University School of Medicine, Shanghai, China

2 School of Public Health, Li Ka Shing Faculty of Medicine, The University of Hong Kong, Hong Kong, Hong Kong, SAR, China

*Address all correspondence to: shiwmfd@126.com

References

[1] Cohen AJ, Brauer M, Burnett R, et al. Estimates and 25-year trends of the global burden of disease attributable to ambient air pollution: An analysis of data from the Global Burden of Diseases Study 2015. Lancet. 2017;**389**(10082):1907-1918

[2] Lelieveld J, Evans JS, Fnais M, Giannadaki D, Pozzer A. The contribution of outdoor air pollution sources to premature mortality on a global scale. Nature. 2015;**525**(7569):367-371

[3] Collaborators GRF. Global burden of 87 risk factors in 204 countries and territories, 1990-2019: A systematic analysis for the Global Burden of Disease Study 2019. Lancet. 2020;**396**(10258):1223-1249

[4] Tolosa E, Garrido A, Scholz SW, Poewe W. Challenges in the diagnosis of Parkinson's disease. Lancet Neurology. 2021;**20**(5):385-397

[5] Lee H, Kim OJ, Jung J, Myung W, Kim SY. Long-term exposure to particulate air pollution and incidence of Parkinson's disease: A nationwide population-based cohort study in South Korea. Environmental Research. 2022;**212**(Pt A):113165

[6] Toro R, Downward GS, van der Mark M, et al. Parkinson's disease and long-term exposure to outdoor air pollution: A matched case-control study in the Netherlands. Environment International. 2019;**129**:28-34

[7] Shin S, Burnett RT, Kwong JC, et al. Effects of ambient air pollution on incident Parkinson's disease in Ontario, 2001 to 2013: A population-based cohort study. International Journal of Epidemiology. 2018;**47**(6):2038-2048

[8] Chen CY, Hung HJ, Chang KH, et al. Long-term exposure to air pollution and the incidence of Parkinson's disease: A nested case-control study. PLoS One. 2017;**12**(8):e0182834

[9] Brook RD, Rajagopalan S, Pope CR, et al. Particulate matter air pollution and cardiovascular disease: An update to the scientific statement from the American Heart Association. Circulation. 2010;**121**(21):2331-2378

[10] Costa LG, Cole TB, Dao K, Chang YC, Coburn J, Garrick JM. Effects of air pollution on the nervous system and its possible role in neurodevelopmental and neurodegenerative disorders. Pharmacology & Therapeutics. 2020;**210**:107523

[11] Shi W, Liu C, Annesi-Maesano I, et al. Ambient PM2.5 and its chemical constituents on lifetime-ever pneumonia in Chinese children: A multi-center study. Environment International. 2021;**146**:106176

[12] van Donkelaar A, Martin RV, Li C, Burnett RT. Regional estimates of chemical composition of fine particulate matter using a combined geoscience-statistical method with information from satellites, models, and monitors. Environmental Science & Technology. 2019;**53**(5):2595-2611

[13] Shi L, Wu X, Danesh YM, et al. Long-term effects of PM2.5 on neurological disorders in the American Medicare population: A longitudinal cohort study. Lancet Planet Health. 2020;**4**(12):e557-e565

[14] Zanobetti A, Dominici F, Wang Y, Schwartz JD. A national case-crossover analysis of the short-term effect of PM2.5

on hospitalizations and mortality in subjects with diabetes and neurological disorders. Environmental Health. 2014;**13**(1):38

[15] Nunez Y, Boehme AK, Li M, et al. Parkinson's disease aggravation in association with fine particle components in New York State. Environmental Research. 2021;**201**:111554

[16] Palacios N, Fitzgerald KC, Hart JE, et al. Air pollution and risk of Parkinson's disease in a large prospective study of men. Environmental Health Perspectives. 2017;**125**(8):087011

[17] Wang Y, Liu Y, Yan H. Effect of long-term particulate matter exposure on Parkinson's risk. Environmental Geochemistry and Health. 2020;**42**(7):2265-2275

[18] Ritz B, Lee PC, Hansen J, et al. Traffic-related air pollution and Parkinson's disease in denmark: A case-control study. Environmental Health Perspectives. 2016;**124**(3):351-356

[19] Jo S, Kim YJ, Park KW, et al. Association of NO2 and other air pollution exposures with the risk of Parkinson disease. JAMA Neurology. 2021;**78**(7):800-808

[20] Dhiman V, Trushna T, Raj D, Tiwari RR. Is ambient air pollution a risk factor for Parkinson's disease? A meta-analysis of epidemiological evidence. International Journal of Environmental Health Research. 2022:1-18 [Online ahead of print]

[21] Lee H, Myung W, Kim DK, Kim SE, Kim CT, Kim H. Short-term air pollution exposure aggravates Parkinson's disease in a population-based cohort. Scientific Reports. 2017;**7**:44741

[22] Lee PC, Raaschou-Nielsen O, Lill CM, et al. Gene-environment interactions linking air pollution and inflammation in Parkinson's disease. Environmental Research. 2016;**151**:713-720

[23] Hu CY, Fang Y, Li FL, et al. Association between ambient air pollution and Parkinson's disease: Systematic review and meta-analysis. Environmental Research. 2019;**168**:448-459

[24] Zhao N, Pinault L, Toyib O, Vanos J, Tjepkema M, Cakmak S. Long-term ozone exposure and mortality from neurological diseases in Canada. Environment International. 2021;**157**:106817

[25] Han C, Lu Y, Cheng H, Wang C, Chan P. The impact of long-term exposure to ambient air pollution and second-hand smoke on the onset of Parkinson disease: A review and meta-analysis. Public Health. 2020;**179**:100-110

[26] Ritz B, Wilhelm M. Ambient air pollution and adverse birth outcomes: methodologic issues in an emerging field. Basic & Clinical Pharmacology & Toxicology. 2008;**102**(2):182-190

[27] Ma Y, Wang W, Li Z, et al. Short-term exposure to ambient air pollution and risk of daily hospital admissions for anxiety in China: A multicity study. Journal of Hazardous Materials. 2022;**424**(Pt B):127535

[28] Thuong D, Dang TN, Phosri A, et al. Fine particulate matter and daily hospitalizations for mental and behavioral disorders: A time-series study in Ho Chi Minh City, Vietnam. Environmental Research. 2022;**213**:113707

[29] Vicedo-Cabrera AM, Sera F, Liu C, et al. Short term association between ozone and mortality: Global two stage

time series study in 406 locations in 20 countries. BMJ. 2020;**368**:m108

[30] Shang Y, Sun Z, Cao J, et al. Systematic review of Chinese studies of short-term exposure to air pollution and daily mortality. Environment International. 2013;**54**:100-111

[31] Maclure M, Mittleman MA. Should we use a case-crossover design? Annual Review of Public Health. 2000;**21**:193-221

[32] Li S, Williams G, Jalaludin B, Baker P. Panel studies of air pollution on children's lung function and respiratory symptoms: A literature review. The Journal of Asthma. 2012;**49**(9):895-910

[33] Meng X, Liu C, Zhang L, et al. Estimating PM2.5 concentrations in Northeastern China with full spatiotemporal coverage, 2005-2016. Remote Sensing of Environment. 2021;**253**:112203

[34] Wang J, Liu Y, Jiao F, et al. Time-dependent translocation and potential impairment on central nervous system by intranasally instilled TiO(2) nanoparticles. Toxicology. 2008;**254**(1-2):82-90

[35] Wang B, Feng WY, Wang M, et al. Transport of intranasally instilled fine Fe2O3 particles into the brain: Micro-distribution, chemical states, and histopathological observation. Biological Trace Element Research. 2007;**118**(3):233-243

[36] Peters A, Veronesi B, Calderon-Garciduenas L, et al. Translocation and potential neurological effects of fine and ultrafine particles a critical update. Particle and Fibre Toxicology. 2006;**3**:13

[37] Calderon-Garciduenas L, Reed W, Maronpot RR, et al. Brain inflammation and Alzheimer's-like pathology in individuals exposed to severe air pollution. Toxicologic Pathology. 2004;**32**(6):650-658

[38] Calderon-Garciduenas L, Maronpot RR, Torres-Jardon R, et al. DNA damage in nasal and brain tissues of canines exposed to air pollutants is associated with evidence of chronic brain inflammation and neurodegeneration. Toxicologic Pathology. 2003;**31**(5):524-538

[39] Pastor-Belda M, Campillo N, Arroyo-Manzanares N, et al. Bioaccumulation of polycyclic aromatic hydrocarbons for forensic assessment using gas chromatography-mass spectrometry. Chemical Research in Toxicology. 2019;**32**(8):1680-1688

[40] Edwards RD, Liu Y, He G, et al. Household CO and PM measured as part of a review of China's National improved stove program. Indoor Air. 2007;**17**(3):189-203

[41] Takahashi M, Ko LW, Kulathingal J, Jiang P, Sevlever D, Yen SH. Oxidative stress-induced phosphorylation, degradation and aggregation of alpha-synuclein are linked to upregulated CK2 and cathepsin D. The European Journal of Neuroscience. 2007;**26**(4):863-874

[42] Musgrove RE, Helwig M, Bae EJ, et al. Oxidative stress in vagal neurons promotes parkinsonian pathology and intercellular alpha-synuclein transfer. The Journal of Clinical Investigation. 2019;**129**(9):3738-3753

[43] Perry VH, Cunningham C, Holmes C. Systemic infections and inflammation affect chronic neurodegeneration. Nature Reviews. Immunology. 2007;7(2):161-167

[44] Murata H, Barnhill LM, Bronstein JM. Air pollution and

the risk of Parkinson's disease: A review. Movement Disorders. 2022;**37**(5):894-904

[45] Kempuraj D, Thangavel R, Selvakumar GP, et al. Brain and peripheral atypical inflammatory mediators potentiate neuroinflammation and neurodegeneration. Frontiers in Cellular Neuroscience. 2017;**11**:216

[46] Kim S, Kwon SH, Kam TI, et al. Transneuronal propagation of pathologic alpha-synuclein from the gut to the brain models Parkinson's disease. Neuron. 2019;**103**(4):627-641.e7

[47] Warner BB. The contribution of the gut microbiome to neurodevelopment and neuropsychiatric disorders. Pediatric Research. 2019;**85**(2):216-224

[48] Sampson TR, Debelius JW, Thron T, et al. Gut microbiota regulate motor deficits and neuroinflammation in a model of Parkinson's disease. Cell. 2016;**167**(6):1469-1480.e12

[49] Mutlu EA, Comba IY, Cho T, et al. Inhalational exposure to particulate matter air pollution alters the composition of the gut microbiome. Environmental Pollution. 2018;**240**:817-830

[50] Shi W, Kan L, Li Y. Concerns remain regarding ambient NO2 exposure and the risk of Parkinson disease. JAMA Neurology. 2022;**79**(1):89

Section 2

Animal Models of Parkinson's Disease

Chapter 3

Behavioral and Cytological Differences between Two Parkinson's Disease Experimental Models

Maria Rosa Avila-Costa, José Luis Ordoñez-Librado, Ana Luisa Gutierréz-Valdez, Javier Sanchez-Betancourt, Ma Teresa Ibarra-Gutiérrez, Patricia E. Reyna-Velázquez, Verónica Anaya-Martínez, Cesar Alfonso Garcia Caballero, Enrique Montiel-Flores, Claudia Dorado-Martínez, Leonardo Reynoso-Erazo, Vianey Rodríguez-Lara and Rocío Tron-Alvarez

Abstract

The knowledge about the biochemical and behavioral changes in humans with PD has allowed proposing animal models for its study; however, the results obtained so far have been heterogeneous. Recently, we established a novel PD model in rodents by manganese chloride ($MnCl_2$) and manganese acetate ($Mn(OAc)_3$) mixture inhalation. After inhaling, the rodents presented bilateral loss of SNc dopaminergic neurons. Later, we conclude that the alterations are of dopamine origin since L-DOPA reverted the alterations. After six months, SNc significantly reduced the number of cells, and striatal dopamine content decreased by 71%. The animals had postural instability, action tremor, and akinesia; these symptoms improved with L-DOPA, providing evidence that Mn mixture inhalation induces comparable alterations that those in PD patients. Thus, this study aimed to compare the alterations in two different PD experimental models: 6-OHDA unilateral lesion and Mn mixture inhalation through open field test, rotarod performance and the number of SNc dopaminergic neurons. The results show that the Mn-exposed animals have motor alterations and bilateral and progressive SNc neurons degeneration; in contrast, in the 6-OHDA model, the neuronal loss is unilateral and acute, demonstrating that the Mn exposure model better recreates the characteristics observed in PD patients.

Keywords: Mn inhalation, Parkinson's disease experimental models, motor behavior, TH immunohistochemistry, rotarod performance

1. Introduction

Parkinson's disease (PD) is a neurodegenerative disorder with movement abnormalities, which include tremor, rigidity, akinesia, bradykinesia, masked face, and postural and gait abnormalities [1] involving the continued dopaminergic cell loss projecting from the substantia nigra compacta (SNc) to the striatum. Within neurodegenerative diseases, it is the second most frequent, resulting in motor disorders, abnormal dopamine signaling, and dopamine cell death [2, 3].

While its causes are still not fully understood, experimental models have postulated essential evidence. Based on clinical and experimental findings, PD was the first neurodegenerative disorder to be modeled and treated by neurotransmitter replacement therapy [4].

When selecting an animal PD model, one has to be considering the differences and similarities between humans and animals' behavior, physiology, and anatomy. The prevailing models have helped understand the disease's causes and compromised resources for new treatment approaches [5]. Nevertheless, the dopamine deafferentation simulated in animals, by the wide variety of neurotoxins or genetic manipulations, some PD models destroy the dopaminergic neurons rapidly and not progressively. In genetic PD models, the dopaminergic loss, while more progressive, is limited in amount or may not occur at all [5, 6].

The typical PD models (**Table 1**) induce nigrostriatal dopaminergic cell loss, frequently with 1-methyl-4-phenyl-1,2,3,6-tetrahydropyridine (MPTP), 6-hydroxydopamine (6-OHDA), rotenone or paraquat [4, 6–9]. It is known that these models induce mitochondrial dysfunction and/or reactive oxygen species, but none completely simulate the pathology and symptoms seen in humans [7, 9]. 6-OHDA and MPTP are neurotoxins that rapidly and selectively destroy the dopaminergic neurons (within 1–3 days), while PD pathogenesis obeys a progressive progression over decades [4, 10].

The consequences of manganese (Mn) as a PD model have been investigated since its toxicity (known as manganism) is related to extrapyramidal motor system symptoms [11–14].

For a long time, there has been some controversy about Mn-induced dopaminergic alterations; whereas some researchers reported that Mn alters dopaminergic innervation, particularly in the basal ganglia, and produces Parkinson-like disorder [14–18],

Model	Characteristics	Disadvantages
6-OHDA	First established model, neuronal degeneration in 24 hours. Enters via Dopamine transporter (DAT) and inhibits the mitochondrial respiratory chain	Unilateral injection, acute model. Unilateral damage, measurable by ipsi or contralateral rotation
MPTP	Humans and monkeys produces the same symptoms/histopathology and response to L-DOPA. It is transformed to MPP+ in the glia and enters through the DAT.	Lower susceptibility in rodents, the administration is acute or subacute. In rodents there is recovery
Rotenone	Damage to the SNc and cytoplasmic inclusions is similar to Lewy bodies. Inhibition of mitochondrial respiratory chain.	In neuronal selectivity, not all animals are affected.

Table 1.
Some PD experimental models.

many authors suggested that Mn neurotoxicity is unlike from PD in symptoms, pathology, and etiology [18, 19], particularly in the evident preservation of SNc dopaminergic somas [20–24].

We recently established an innovative PD model in mice [25, 26] and rats [27] by the inhalation of the mixture of two Mn compounds, Manganese chloride ($MnCl_2$) and Manganese acetate ($Mn(OAc)_3$). After Mn mixture inhalation, the rodents presented a significant loss of SNc dopaminergic neurons (67.58%) [26]. Later, we determine whether L-DOPA treatment improves the behavior to ensure that the alterations are of dopamine origin [27, 28]. Consequently, after six months of Mn compounds inhalation, striatal dopamine concentration decreased by 71%, and SNc showed a significant reduction in the number of TH^+ neurons. The animals presented action tremor and postural instability, which were improved with L-DOPA—suggesting that $MnCl_2$/Mn $(OAc)_3$ mixture inhalation induces comparable symptoms and neurochemical and cellular alterations to those observed in PD patients, providing a valuable model for the study of this disease [25–28]. Additionally, Mn inhalation is progressive and bilateral, making it more reliable. Thus, this study aimed to compare motor alterations in two different PD experimental models: 6-OHDA unilateral lesion (the most common used PD-experimental model [29] and $MnCl_2/Mn(OAc)_3$ mixture inhalation through open field test determining: walking distance (ambulation), rearing and walking speed, freezing time, rotarod performance and bradykinesia and counting the number of TH neurons in the SNc.

2. Methods

Male adult Wistar rats (starting weight 180–200 g) were placed during the recovery from the 6-OHDA surgery; two weeks after the surgery or Mn mixture inhalation, they were accommodated in groups of four with an inverted dark-light cycle (12:12 h) and fed with Purina Rat Chow and water *ad libitum*. Body weight was recorded daily. The experimental protocol follows the National Institute of Health Guide for the Care and Use of Laboratory Animals (NIH Publications No. 80-23) revised in 1996 and the Rules for Research in Health Matters (Mexico). We strive to limit the animals' amount and their distress. Rotarod performance and open field were tested before the lesion or Mn inhalations as preliminary parameters (average condition) of each rat's motor coordination, postural balance, and muscle rigidity to follow up on their performance throughout the experiment. The rats were first tested in the rotarod and trained to remain on the rod at 5 rpm and 10 rpm for 2 min, discarding those that, after three consecutive days, were unable to stay on the rod [30].

2.1 Stereotactic surgery

The rats were anesthetized with sodium pentobarbitone (35 mg/kg, intraperitoneal) and placed in a stereotaxic apparatus (David Kopf Instruments, Tujunga, CA). They were injected with 4 ml of saline solution containing 8 mg of 6-OHDA (Sigma Chemical Company, Mexico) and 0.2 mg of ascorbic acid (n = 6) into the left medial forebrain bundle (MFB). For the unilateral lesion, the stereotaxic coordinates were as follows: AP=–6.1 mm anterior to the interaural line; L = 1.6 mm lateral to bregma; and V = – 8.1 mm vertical from dura according to Paxinos and Watson [31]. A sham lesion was made with the vehicle using the exact coordinates (n = 6, control group). The injections were administered over a 4-min period using a Hamilton syringe attached to a glass micropipette with a 20–50 mm tip diameter.

2.2 Manganese inhalation

Inhalations were performed as described by [25, 32]. Six rats were placed in an acrylic chamber inhaling 0.04 M $MnCl_2$ and 0.02 M Mn $(OAc)_3$ one hour thrice a week for six months. Six control rats inhaled only the vehicle—deionized water—for the same period. Inhalations were performed in closed acrylic boxes (40 cm wide/70 cm long and 25 cm high) connected to an ultra-nebulizer (Shinmed, Taiwan) with 10 l/min continuous flux. The ultra-nebulizer produces droplets in a 0.5–5 mm range. A trap for the vapor was on the contrary side with a sodium bicarbonate solution to precipitate the remaining metal. During exposures, animals were constantly monitored for respiration rate, depth, and regularity. The exposure system was continuously monitored for temperature, oxygen level, and Mn concentration [25, 32].

2.3 Motor behavior

2.3.1 Rotarod performance

The rotarod consists of a four-lane rotating rod (diameter 7.5 cm) and infrared beams to detect the moment of fall. The rat's body was placed perpendicular to the rotating axis and the head against the direction of the rotation; the animal must move forward to stay on the rod. Each rat was tested for about 15 min between the different testing speeds, thus reducing stress and fatigue. The rats were trained twice on the rotarod at the constant rate of 5 and 10 rpm for two min during three consecutive days before the performance evaluation. In the evaluating session, the rats were placed on the rod, and their performance was tested at different constant speeds (5, 10, 15, 20, and 25 rpm) for a maximum of two min at each rate. All rats were video recorded while on the rod to assess their motor coordination and posture [30]. Control, 6-OHDA-lesioned and Mn-inhaled groups were evaluated before the experimental procedures and after three and six months.

2.3.2 Open field test

The rats' behavior in the open field was evaluated before the experimental procedures and after three and six months. The rat was placed in the center of a square arena (80 × 80 cm) with 40 cm high, opaque black walls in a quiet, red-light-illuminated room. The motor behavior was video recorded for 20 min. The geometrical coordinates of the rat position in the arena were measured from the recorded videos to obtain the spatiotemporal sequence of the movements. The following behavioral parameters were measured: walking distance (ambulation), rearing, and walking speed. Bradykinesia was estimated by the reduction in walking speed assessed by the time taken by the rat to move from one corner of the open field to the next with relative speed. The arena was cleaned with a water/alcohol (70%) solution before every behavioral testing to avoid a possible bias due to odors and residues left by rats tested earlier [30]. All experiments were carried out from 11:00 a.m. to 3:00 p.m.

The times the rat passed through the center of the arena (central lines; **Figure 1**) of the open field were counted and multiplied by the distance (115 cm).

2.4 Tyrosine hydroxylase (TH) immunocytochemistry

After six months, for the immunohistochemical study, the rats were deeply anesthetized under pentobarbitone anesthesia (35 mg/kg, i.p.) after the last behavioral

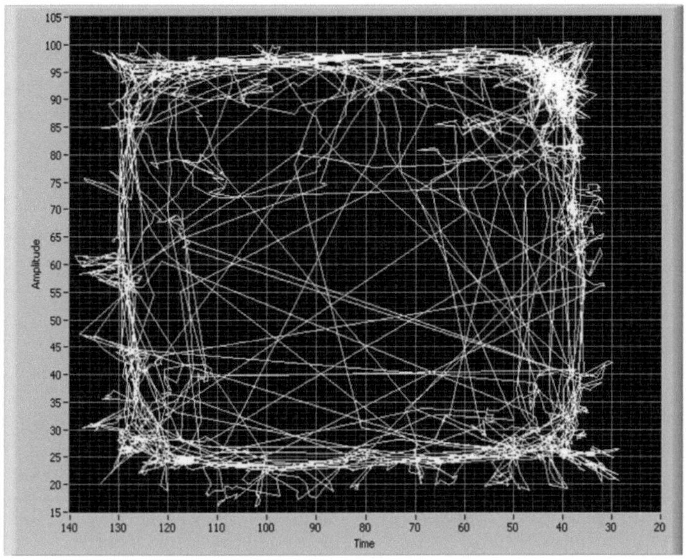

Figure 1.
Open field test. Rat trace in the center of the arena.

test and perfused transcardially with 120 ml of 0.9% saline, followed by 300 ml of 4% paraformaldehyde.

Coronal sections (50 μm) were acquired on a vibrating microtome containing the mesencephalon for immunocytochemistry. TH (Chemicon International Inc., Temecula, California, USA; 1: 1000) immunostaining with the ABC detection method (Vector Lab MI, USA) was performed for light microscope analysis. The analysis was carried out using a computer-assisted system (Image-Pro Plus; Media Cybernetics, Del Mar, California, USA) connected by a CCD camera to an Optiphot 2 Microscope (Nikon, Mexico). The number of TH^+ neurons was counted in 1500 mm^2 from each animal's seven SNc sections per hemisphere [25–28, 32].

3. Statistical analysis

An unpaired t-test was used to analyze the number of cells. Motor performances were analyzed using repeated-measures ANOVA on mean values of motor activity per certain period, and *post hoc* comparisons were made with Tukey's test. Group differences were considered statistically significant at $p < 0.05$. All analyses were conducted with GraphPad Prism Software Inc., Version 9 for Mac [25–28].

4. Results

4.1 Rotarod performance

This test estimates motor coordination and balance. Both features are under the dorsal striatum control [33, 34].

First, we explored the deficit degree in motor coordination and balance produced by the unilateral MFB lesion six months after; we found that the fall latency (or permanence on the roll) decreased significantly from 15 rpm ($p < 0.05$), as seen in **Figure 2**.

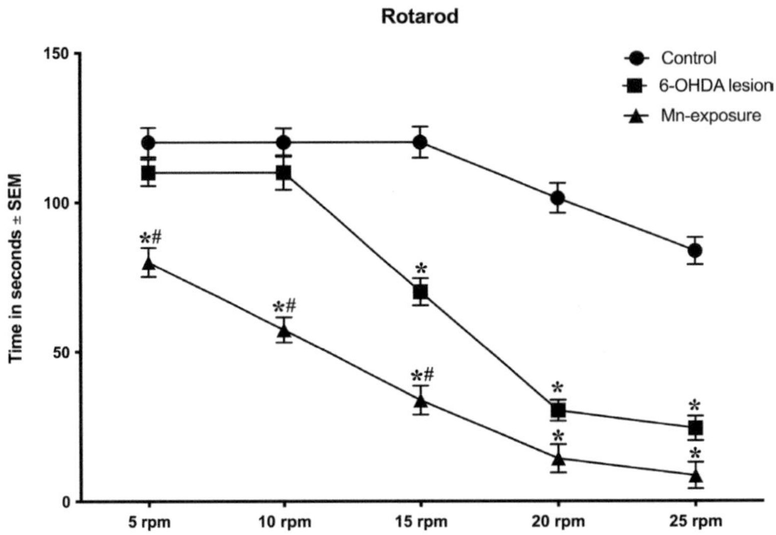

Figure 2.
Rotarod Permanence time at (5, 10, 15, 20, 25 rpm) of the control, 6-OHDA-lesioned, and Mn-exposed groups after six months. It is observed that the higher the rod speed, the performance in this test was more deficient. Performance in the pre-exposure test was considered 100%. (= P < 0.005 6-OHDA-lesion and Mn-exposure versus control group; # = P < 0.005 Mn-exposure versus 6-OHDA-lesion; repeated-measures ANOVA followed by Tukey post hoc test).*

Figure 2 also shows the Mn mixture-exposed rats' results, observing a progressive decrease in rod permanence directly proportional to the months of exposure. Between the pre-exposure stage vs. three months, an evident reduction is kept in the permanence time at revolutions 20 and 25, decreasing by 46% and 8%, respectively. However, after six months, the decrease in the rode permanence time was evident in the five evaluated revolutions (5, 10, 15, 20, and 25 rpm) due to the significant falls between 70 to 90%. **Figure 2** shows the performance in the test after six months of experimental performances. The pre-groups are not shown because they were considered 100%.

4.2 Open-field test

In addition to assessing gross motor deficit, we decided to explore the effect of the lesion and Mn-inhalation on the animals' overall spontaneous motor behavior. Open-field testing after the 6-OHDA lesion revealed that voluntary movement and exploration decreased significantly to 44.87 ± 29.50% on average (**Figure 3**). As seen in the representative traces of the route (**Figure 4A**), the animal in its intact condition moved profusely through the open field, exploring the entire perimeter of the arena and sometimes the center, with few periods of inactivity. After three months of the unilateral MFB 6-OHDA lesion, the same animal made a much smaller movement (which is reflected in the low density of lines in the x-y axes), almost did not cross the center of the arena, and presented prolonged periods in which it stopped staying in expectation, or simply immobile in the corners (akinesia), this is observed in the route as a space between the movements on the t-axis (see the middle trace of **Figure 4A**). The Mn-exposed group also decreased the exploratory activity compared to the pre-exposure stage (**Figure 5**). The animals, before Mn inhalation, traveled the average maximum distance of 5875 cm in 20 min (this value was taken as 100%); after three months of exposure, a significant decrease was observed; on average, each animal traveled a distance of 3250 cm which is equivalent to

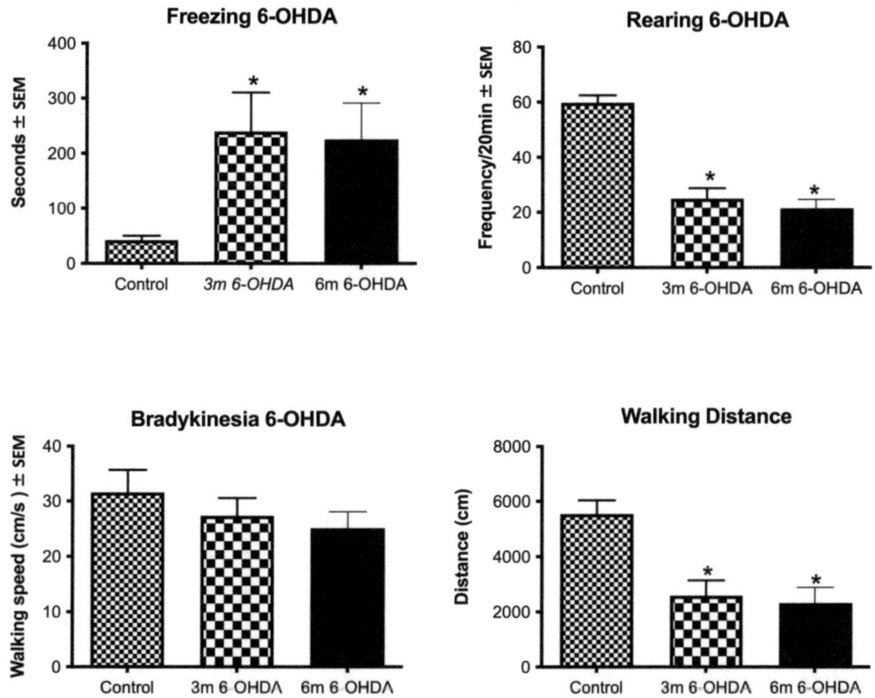

Figure 3.
*The 6-OHDA lesion altered the ambulatory performance assessed by the distance traveled, the walking distance, and the rearing frequency, inducing bradykinesia and freezing in the first ten minutes. (One-way repeated-measures ANOVA) but it did not significantly affect bradykinesia. *P < 0.001 compared with control. The data are given as the mean ± SEM).*

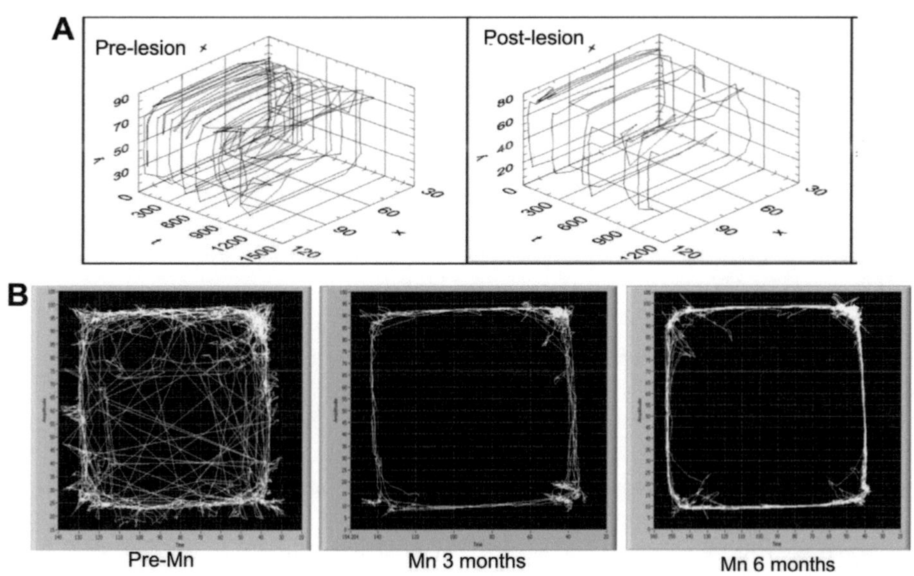

Figure 4.
(A) The representative traces are shown in a three-dimensional form of a rat's path (x-y in time) in the two stages of the protocol after the 6-OHDA lesion. The number of lines is proportional to the total distance traveled. (B) Images showing the path of a rat in the pre-and after Mn exposure stages. It is evident that after Mn inhalation, and presumably by the loss of dopaminergic innervation, the animals did so attached to the walls when they wandered.

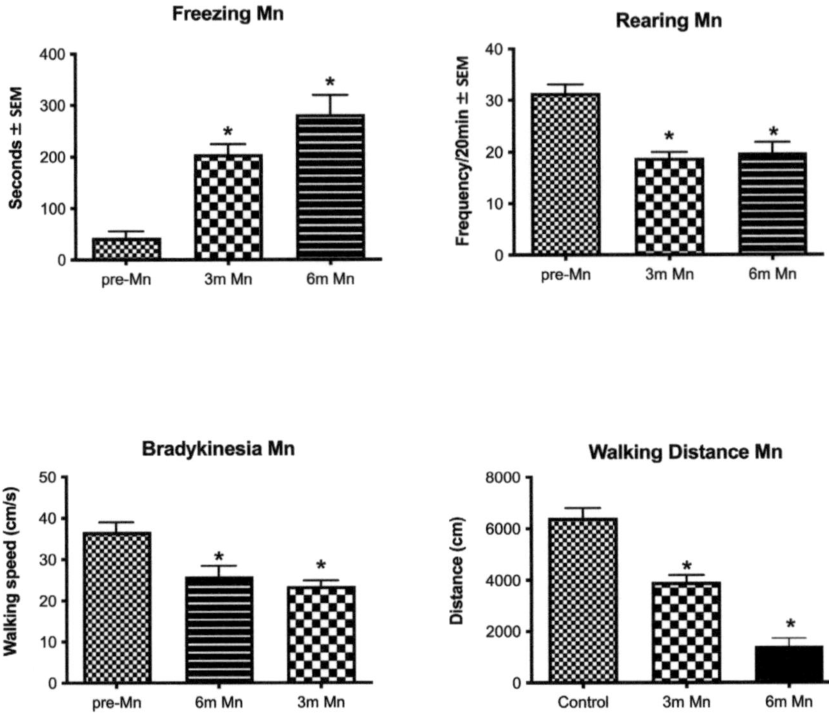

Figure 5.
*$MnCl_2/Mn(OAc)_3$ inhalation decreased ambulatory activity measured by distance traveled, rearing frequency, and walking distance, and induced significant bradykinesia and freezing during the first ten minutes in the open field (one-way repeated-measures ANOVA). * $P < 0.001$ compared with control (the data are given as the mean ± SEM).*

45% decrease (**Figure 5**); however, at six months the decline was more evident, corresponding to 66% covering a distance of 1985.83 cm in 20 min (**Figures 4B** and 5).

As can be seen, the inhalation of Mn, by producing bilateral dopaminergic damage, accentuates the alterations in a time-dependent manner (in both rotarod and open field tests) more clearly compared to the unilateral 6-OHDA-lesioned group. Moreover, the qualitative evaluation showed that Mn-exposed animals exhibit hindlimb weakness, poverty of spontaneous movement (akinesia), slowness of movement (bradykinesia), action tremor, and postural instability.

4.3 Tyrosine hydroxylase immunocytochemistry

TH^+ neurons counting found that in the 6-OHDA unilaterally lesioned rats, SNc had 95.4% of dopaminergic neurons lost on the ipsilateral side than the contralateral (**Figures 6** and 7). The number of TH^+ neurons in the control group, both contra and ipsilateral SNc, remained unaffected (94 ± 1.9 and 93 ± 1.7, respectively) (**Figure 6**). In contrast, we found a substantial loss of TH-positive neurons in the SNc of 6-OHDA lesioned animals in both contralateral (73 ± 1.9) and ipsilateral (5 ± 1.6) SNc compared to controls as shown in **Figures 6** and 7.

Also, after six months of $MnCl_2/Mn(OAc)_3$ inhalation, a significant loss of the TH^+ neurons in the SNc was observed (70.58%) compared to the control group (**Figures 6** and 7).

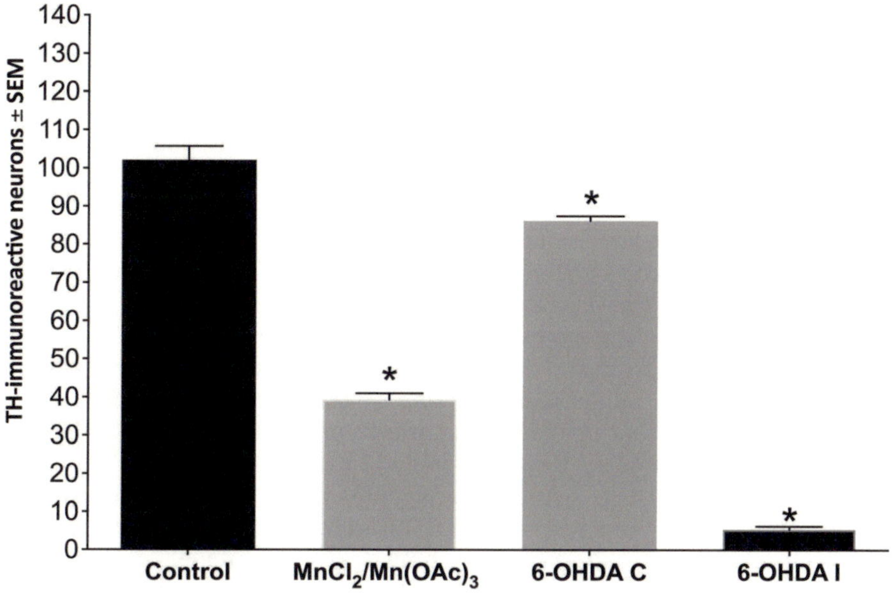

Figure 6.
SNc TH^+ cell number. The data are presented as the mean ± SEM. A statistically significant decrease in TH-immunoreactive cells was detected in $MnCl_2/Mn(OAc)_3$-exposed group and both 6-OHDA-lesioned contralateral and ipsilateral SNc; being more drastic in the 6-OHDA ipsilateral SNc (= $P < 0.05$ versus control group; ANOVA test).*

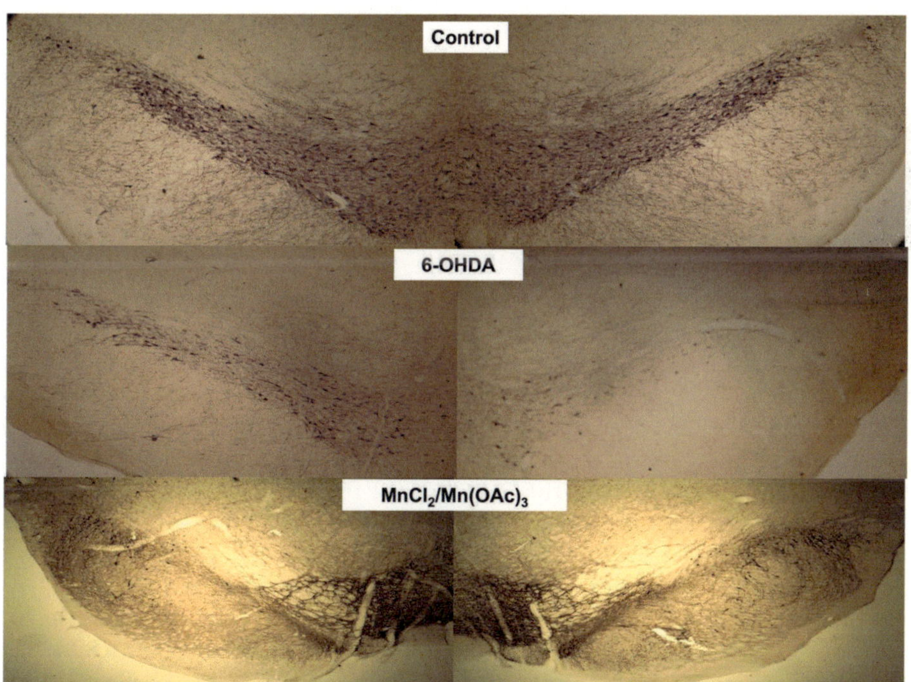

Figure 7.
Illustrative TH^+ from coronal sections containing the SNc of control, 6-OHDA, and $MnCl_2/Mn(OAc)_3$-exposed rats; it is evident the loss of dopaminergic neurons in both experimental groups is more drastic in the 6-OHDA ipsilateral SNc (magnification 10×).

Figures 6 and 7 clearly show the laterality of the neural loss in the unilaterally 6-OHDA-lesioned animals, unlike the rats that inhaled Mn, who presented significant bilateral cell loss.

5. Discussion

A reliable PD experimental model must gradually mimic the physiological and behavioral symptoms such as bradykinesia, akinesia, tremor, and muscle rigidity, allowing intervention in the early stages of the disease [5, 35, 36].

There are currently several experimental models that reproduce PD. These models were aimed to induce nigrostriatal dopaminergic depletion. Selective neurotoxins such as 6-OHDA, MPTP, paraquat, or rotenone are generally used [4, 7, 9]. These models induce neuronal death by inhibiting mitochondrial function and producing ROS. Still, none fully reproduce the symptoms and pathology seen in PD patients, in part because the activity of the neurotoxins is acute, fast, unilateral, and nonprogressive, and the response to these neurotoxins is different between species [4].

Our results evidence that the alterations between the two models are similar; however, the animals exposed to the Mn mixture had time-dependent behavioral alterations, while the animals lesioned with 6-OHDA presented alterations almost immediately, the neuronal loss is massive and mainly unilateral, so it is complicated to prove a treatment with 5% remaining dopaminergic neurons.

5.1 Rotarod performance

The rotarod is commonly used to behaviorally assess the degree of dopaminergic depletion (maximum or partial) in PD models [37]; this test also assesses akinesia and postural instability symptoms.

The exact mechanism underlying this test is the failure of the dopamine-depleted rats to remain on the rod; these deficits become increasingly apparent as the speed of rotation increases and the rats are obligated to move faster. There is also evidence of loss in the ability to apply force with the affected extremities; therefore, there is fatigue [38], and they tend to fall (fall latency). It has recently been shown that PD patients present instability and movement inaccuracy which becomes more prominent when they are asked to move faster [39]. The motor alterations became more evident at 20 and 25 rpm; after six months of dopamine depletion, motor coordination decreased significantly in the five evaluated revolutions. The dopamine-depleted animals tended to remain static before starting the test, so when the rotarod was turned on, it was easy for them to lose their balance and fall or not coordinate their steps with the movement of the rod when the revolutions increased. Similar results have also been reported by Rozas et al. [37] using the rotarod test in mice that received injections of MPTP, the animals showed a reduction in the time spent on the rod, related to the SNc dopamine loss. Subsequently, Razgado-Hernandez et al. [30] report the association between the degree of motor coordination deficit and the balance produced by 6-OHDA unilateral lesion in the MFB, where there is an 89.4% loss of TH^+ neurons in the lesioned SNc.

Our data demonstrate that the Mn-exposed rats had more trouble staying on the rod since the dopaminergic denervation is bilateral, just like the PD patients.

5.2 Open field performance

The open field is a reliable test in rodents to assess motor activity as it measures (spontaneous motor behavior) that is an analog in PD patients when they present hypokinesia (decreased ambulation) and bradykinesia (reduced speed of movement).

Among the cardinal PD symptoms are akinesia and postural instability. Akinesia can be the most disabling symptom (along with tremors). It can be subdivided into different components such as delayed initiation of movement (prolonged reaction time (bradykinesia), inability to reach an object with continuous movement, rapid fatigue with repetitive motions, and balance disorders [35, 39]. The locomotion decrease is indicative of an altered state of motor behavior typical of parkinsonism, and the reduction obtained is similar to that reported by [40] for a unilateral 6-OHDA MFB lesion. In the 6-OHDA-lesioned rats, the walking distance appears unaffected, so there is no bradykinesia; we found some akinesia probably associated with a lack of motivation to move and explore the environment.

In contrast, regarding the animals exposed to Mn, before the inhalation, the rats maintained spontaneous exploration activity; however, when Mn-exposed, the spontaneous activity significantly decreased; this decrease was progressive; after three months, the decline was 45%, but after six months it was 76%, this response indicates that the model reproduces the symptoms of hypokinesia (decreased ambulation) which causes them to walk less distance and bradykinesia since their walking speed was altered, alterations reported previously by our group [41]. We also observed tremors, a symptom the 6-OHDA-lesioned rats did not present. Qualitative inspection indicated that Mn-exposed rats display hind-limb weakness, poverty of spontaneous movement (akinesia), slowness of movement (bradykinesia), action tremor, postural instability, and freezing behavior. About these alterations, Harischandra et al. [15] stated that mice exposed subchronically to Mn by intragastric gavage displayed hypoactivity; this alteration was associated with 50% striatal dopamine depletion; Eriksson et al. [42] found that after five months of Mn exposure the animals developed unsteady gait, subsequently action tremor and were hypoactive. The animals lost strength in both upper and lower extremities, and their paw movements were clumsy [42].

It is well known that rats with both MFB 6-OHDA lesions have postural instability and little ability to preserve equilibrium after tasks with destabilizing forces. Similarly, spontaneous movements are significantly altered [43]; this has not been reported after the unilateral 6-OHDA lesion.

Parkinsonian-like tremors have been scarce in unilaterally 6-OHDA-lesioned rats [44, 45]; nevertheless, Schallert et al. [46] have reported infrequent tremors in the paw and the wrist of rats with almost complete dopamine denervation (either bilateral or unilateral). This tremor is observed when the paw is placed off the floor in a non-weight-bearing posture [46]. It is also known that bilaterally 6-OHDA- lesioned rats show most of the PD motor symptoms. However, 6-OHDA bilateral lesion is not a typical PD model since the lesioned animals need intensive care since they present adipsia and aphagia and die a few days after the lesion [47]. Therefore, the MFB unilateral 6-OHDA lesion is the most commonly used PD model, even though it does not replicate all the PD symptoms and pathological characteristics. Likewise, the acute kind of the experimental models contrasts with the dopaminergic nigral neuron's progressive degeneration in PD [41].

5.3 Tyrosine hydroxylase immunocytochemistry

We observed a severe decrease (95%) of TH^+ cells after the unilateral 6-OHDA lesion in the ipsilateral SNc. The MFB 6-OHDA unilateral lesion produces a severe SNc degeneration, mainly in the ipsilateral side, within the first hours after the lesion, corroborated by apomorphine-induced circling behavior [48] and TH^+ cell count (see **Figures 6** and 7). Our results concur with Surmeier [49], who reported that PD patients have up to 95% of dopaminergic neuron reduction in the advanced stages of the disease. Similarly, it has been confirmed that the MFB unilateral lesion decreases 95–98% of the SNc ipsilateral number of TH^+ neurons [50, 51]. We also found a significant cell loss in the contralateral SNc, as reported previously by our group [52, 53]; however, the cell loss in the contralateral SNc is not enough to simulate PD symptoms. Similarly, it has been described that the reserpine rat PD model is known to induce a substantial dopamine depletion with a rapid development of striatal dopaminergic receptors supersensitivity (within 12–24 h after reserpine) [54]. Other authors have shown that most severely lesioned parkinsonian primates subjected to chronic MPTP regimens present 70–80% nigral TH^+ cell loss and >95% striatal dopamine depletion [55].

According to previous reports [25–28, 41], we found a substantial loss of TH^+ neurons, as shown in **Figures 6** and 7, displaying a very similar pattern to that reported in the middle to advanced stages of the PD; it has been described neurochemical variations in humans and animals Mn-intoxicated involving the decrease in dopamine concentration and TH^+ immunoreactivity in the SNc and striatum [13, 15, 16, 56–59]. Hence, it has been supposed that Mn interacts with catechols specific to dopaminergic neurons to diminish them promptly, causing these cells to no longer be viable [60, 61]. However, there has been controversy about Mn-inducing SNc dopaminergic damage [18, 20, 22, 24, 62–65]. According to these authors, Mn exposure leads mainly to Globus Pallidus and striatal alterations without affecting the SNc dopaminergic neurons. Our results are probably because we exposed the animals to a mixture of divalent and trivalent Mn. Divalent Mn pro-oxidant activity seems to depend on trivalent Mn trace amounts, which may enable Mn^{2+} small portion to oxidize to Mn^{3+}. This relationship between both Mn compounds results in a continuous redox cycle [66]. It seems that divalent Mn does not have oxidative effects; nevertheless, the transition of Mn^{2+} to Mn^{3+} accelerates its oxidant capability, which might consequence in the production of reactive oxygen species, cell membrane damage, and lipid peroxidation [61], which, in turn, could affect catecholamines [67, 68]; therefore, the inherent transformation of divalent Mn to trivalent Mn and the existence of more trivalent Mn might provoke mitochondrial dysfunction and more reactive oxygen species [68, 69] manifested as the evident motor alterations and the dopaminergic neuronal death, reported here.

Numerous reasons have been suggested to explain the SNc dopaminergic cell's susceptibility to Mn. First, the lack of cellular antioxidant defenses, and second, the mitochondrial oxidative energy metabolism disruption [69]. This has led to the assumption that extreme brain Mn levels provoke oxidative stress leading to neurodegeneration [66]. However, the main reason for the specificity of Mn for the SNc dopaminergic neurons is related to the dopamine transporter (DAT); it has been reported that Mn arrives in the neurons via DAT [70–73]; DAT is related to the MPTP [74], and 6-OHDA neurotoxicity [75], where SNc is more vulnerable than other dopaminergic areas, such as the ventral tegmental area (VTA). It seems that the VTA and SNc dopaminergic cells exhibit topography, biochemistry, and susceptibility to pathological processes differences [76]; the middle and medial SNc express higher levels of DAT than the VTA [74, 77]; thus, Mn possibly get SNc dopaminergic cells through the greater amounts of DAT reported on those neurons. Moreover, in PD, the most vulnerable neurons are the SNc dopaminergic ones and not those of the VTA [76, 77].

Currently, available PD experimental models have contributed significantly to our knowledge of the disease's neurotransmitter changes, potential neuroprotective therapeutics, and pathophysiology [6, 7]. However, so far, we do not have the most suitable model. MPTP experimental model is the best available one for some reasons, and it has been essential for testing neurorestorative and neuroprotective approaches [4]. Nevertheless, the MPTP model disadvantages are acute damage to the dopaminergic system and infrequent generation of inclusion bodies, different susceptibility among species, and recovery after exposure ceased [78]. Both MPTP and 6-OHDA models differ from the slowly progressive pathology of human PD [4]. In addition, PD genetic models seem to simulate some features of the disease without extensive SNc neuronal loss [79]. Transgenic mice overexpressing wild-type and mutant alfa-synuclein demonstrate motor deficits without loss of dopaminergic neurons [4, 80].

The substantial reduction (72 %) in the number of SNc dopaminergic cells after divalent/trivalent Mn inhalation observed here establishes an evident reduction of this catecholamine content. Therefore, we suppose the motor PD symptoms are due to dopaminergic denervation since L-DOPA-treated animals almost entirely improved their motor performance [27, 28].

6. Conclusion

For some years, PD has shown a significant increase in its prevalence, which is why it has been the focus of multiple investigations worldwide. All these investigations strive to explain the pathophysiological mechanisms of the disease and the best therapeutic alternatives. To accomplish this, we have resorted to the design and use of various animal models, representing an opportunity to study aspects of the disease from different perspectives.

When choosing an animal PD model, the stated objective, scope of the research, and the similarities or discrepancies between the anatomy, physiology, and behavior of humans and animals should be considered. In this chapter, we compared the motor alterations of the model due to unilateral 6-OHDA lesions and inhalation of the $MnCl_2/Mn(OAc)_3$ mixture.

Our results showed that 6-OHDA unilateral lesion produces acute loss of dopaminergic neurons. These animals did not appear to present bradykinesia and tremor, both clinical aspects that are considered cardinal in PD patients. Unlike 6-OHDA or MPTP PD models, where all symptoms happen in a few days or weeks, or even hours, while in PD patients progress over decades [81]; our Mn mixture-inhaled model seems to be adequate because the symptoms and cell death are bilateral and, and the variances between species are insignificant [25–28]. According to Schober [78], an ideal PD model must develop the following characteristics: (1) an average number of SNc dopaminergic neurons at birth followed by the gradual and selective loss of these cells beginning in adulthood; (2) easily detectable and quantifiable motor deficits; (3) Lewy bodies; (4) the model, ideally must have a reasonably short time course to simulate the PD pathogenesis (about 3–6 months), which would grant a prompt assessment of therapeutic schemes [78]. Therefore, we replicate at least three of those features with our model [25–28]. However, additional studies are required to clarify whether Mn-mixture inhalation produces Lewy bodies, reduces striatal dopamine concentrations, and determine if the animals recover after the inhalation.

Finally, our data and the findings of the Mn-model apport crucial knowledge concerning a better understanding of the mechanisms related to the PD nigrostriatal degeneration since it adequately simulates the neurochemical, neuroanatomical, and some behavioral characteristics of PD.

Acknowledgements

This work was supported by COMECyT FICDTEM-2021-066 and PAPIIT-DGAPA IN216821 grants. We are very grateful to Patricia Aley-Medina, Jesús Espinosa-Villanueva and Veronica Rodriguez Mata for their excellent photographic and technical assistance.

Conflict of interest

Authors have declared that no competing interests exist.

Author details

Maria Rosa Avila-Costa[1*], José Luis Ordoñez-Librado[1], Ana Luisa Gutierréz-Valdez[1], Javier Sanchez-Betancourt[1], Ma Teresa Ibarra-Gutiérrez[2], Patricia E. Reyna-Velázquez[3], Verónica Anaya-Martínez[3,4], Cesar Alfonso Garcia Caballero[1], Enrique Montiel-Flores[1], Claudia Dorado-Martínez[1], Leonardo Reynoso-Erazo[5], Vianey Rodríguez-Lara[6] and Rocío Tron-Alvarez[5]

1 Facultad de Estudios Superiores Iztacala, Neuromorphology Lab, UNAM, Tlalnepantla, Mexico

2 Molecular and Cellular Neurobiology Lab, National Institute of Neurology and Neurosurgery, Mexico

3 Department of Physiology, Biophysics and Neurosciences, Cinvestav, Mexico City, Mexico

4 Faculty of Health Sciences, Center for Research in Health Sciences, Anahuac University, Huixquilucan, Mexico

5 Facultad de Estudios Superiores Iztacala, Health Education Project, UNAM, Tlalnepantla, Mexico

6 Facultad de Medicina, Department of Cell Biology, Nacional University of Mexico (UNAM), Mexico City, Mexico

*Address all correspondence to: nigraizo@unam.mx

References

[1] Naskar A, Manivasagam T, Chakraborty J, Singh R, Thomas B, Dhanasekaran M, et al. Melatonin synergizes with low doses of L-DOPA to improve dendritic spine density in the mouse striatum in experimental Parkinsonism. Journal of Pineal Research. 2013;**55**:304-301

[2] Rangel-Barajas C, Coronel I, Florán B. Dopamine receptors and neurodegeneration. Aging and Disease. 2015;**6**:349-368

[3] Michel PP, Hirsch EC, Hunot S. Understanding dopaminergic cell death pathways in parkinson disease. Neuron. 2016;**90**:675-691

[4] Betarbet R, Sherer TB, Greenamyre JT. Animal models of Parkinson's disease. BioEssays. 2002;**24**:308-318

[5] Gubellini P, Kachidian P. Animal models of Parkinson's disease: An updated overview. Revue Neurologique (Paris). 2015;**171**:750-761

[6] Emborg ME. Evaluation of animal models of Parkinson's disease for neuroprotective strategies. Journal of Neuroscience Methods. 2004;**139**:121-143

[7] Bove J, Prou D, Perier C, Przedborski S. Toxin-induced models of Parkinson's disease. NeuroRx. 2005;**2**:484-494

[8] Greenamyre JT, Betarbet R, Sherer TB. The rotenone model of Parkinson's disease: Genes, environment, and mitochondria. Parkinsonism & Related Disorders. 2003;**9**(Suppl. 2):S59-S64

[9] Konnova EA, Swanberg M. Animal models of Parkinson's disease. In: Stoker TB, Greenland JC, editors. Parkinson's Disease: Pathogenesis and Clinical Aspects. Brisbane (AU): Codon Publications; 2018

[10] von Bohlen und Halbach O, Schober A, Krieglstein K. Genes, proteins, and neurotoxins involved in Parkinson's disease. Progress in Neurobiology. 2004;**73**:151-177

[11] Cook DG, Fahn S, Brait KA. Chronic manganese intoxication. Archives of Neurology. 1974;**30**:59-64

[12] Calne DB, Chu NS, Huang CC, Lu CS, Olanow W. Manganism and idiopathic parkinsonism: Similarities and differences. Neurology. 1994;**44**:1583-1586

[13] Pal PK, Samii A, Calne DB. Manganese neurotoxicity: A review of clinical features, imaging and pathology. Neurotoxicology. 1999;**20**:227-238

[14] Kwakye GF, Paoliello MM, Mukhopadhyay S, Bowman AB, Aschner M. Manganese-induced Parkinsonism and Parkinson's disease: Shared and distinguishable features. International Journal of Environmental Research and Public Health. 2015;**12**:7519-7540

[15] Harischandra DS, Ghaisas S, Zenitsky G, et al. Manganese-induced neurotoxicity: New insights into the triad of protein misfolding, mitochondrial impairment, and neuroinflammation. Frontiers in Neuroscience. 2019;**13**:654

[16] Guilarte TR, Gonzales KK. Manganese-induced Parkinsonism is not idiopathic Parkinson's disease: Environmental and genetic evidence. Toxicological Sciences. 2015;**146**:204-212

[17] Kulshreshtha D, Ganguly J, Jog M. Manganese and movement disorders:

A review. The Journal of Movement Disorders. 2021;**14**:93-102

[18] Kissani N, Naji Y, Mebrouk Y, Chraa M, Ghanima A. Parkinsonism and chronic manganese exposure: Pilot study with clinical, environmental and experimental evidence. Clinical Parkinsonism & Related Disorders. 2020;**3**:100057

[19] Lee EY, Flynn MR, Du G, et al. Nigral MRI features of asymptomatic welders. Parkinsonism & Related Disorders. 2021;**85**:37-43

[20] Calabresi P, Ammassari-Teule M, Gubellini P, Sancesario G, Morello M, Centonze D, et al. A synaptic mechanism underlying the behavioral abnormalities induced by manganese intoxication. Neurobiology of Disease. 2001;**8**:419-432

[21] Salari M, Etemadifar M, Dargahi L, Valian N, Rezaee M. Manganese-induced parkinsonism responsive to intranasal insulin: A case report. Clinical Case Reports. 2022;**10**:e05562

[22] Olanow CW. Manganese-induced parkinsonism and Parkinson's disease. Annals of the New York Academy of Sciences. 2004;**1012**:209-223

[23] Lin M, Colon-Perez LM, Sambo DO, et al. Mechanism of manganese dysregulation of dopamine neuronal activity. The Journal of Neuroscience. 2020;**40**:5871-5891

[24] Perl DP, Olanow CW. The neuropathology of manganese-induced parkinsonism. Journal of Neuropathology and Experimental Neurology. 2007;**66**:675-682

[25] Ordonez-Librado JL, Anaya-Martinez V, Gutierrez-Valdez AL, Colin-Barenque L, Montiel-Flores E, Avila-Costa MR. Manganese inhalation as a Parkinson disease model. Parkinson's Disease. 2010;**2011**:612989

[26] Ordonez-Librado JL, Gutierrez-Valdez AL, Colin-Barenque L, Anaya-Martinez V, Diaz-Bech P, Avila-Costa MR. Inhalation of divalent and trivalent manganese mixture induces a Parkinson's disease model: Immunocytochemical and behavioral evidences. Neuroscience. 2008;**155**:7-16

[27] Sanchez-Betancourt J, Anaya-Martinez V, Gutierrez-Valdez AL, Ordonez-Librado JL, Montiel-Flores E, Espinosa-Villanueva J, et al. Manganese mixture inhalation is a reliable Parkinson disease model in rats. Neurotoxicology. 2012;**33**:1346-1355

[28] Ordonez-Librado JL, Anaya-Martinez V, Gutierrez-Valdez AL, Montiel-Flores E, Corona DR, Martinez-Fong D, et al. L-DOPA treatment reverses the motor alterations induced by manganese exposure as a Parkinson disease experimental model. Neuroscience Letters. 2010;**47**:79-82

[29] Ungerstedt U. 6-Hydroxy-dopamine induced degeneration of central monoamine neurons. European Journal of Pharmacology. 1968;**5**:107

[30] Razgado-Hernandez LF, Espadas-Alvarez AJ, Reyna-Velazquez P, Sierra-Sanchez A, Anaya-Martínez V, Jimenez-Estrada I, et al. The transfection of BDNF to dopamine neurons potentiates the effect of dopamine D3 receptor agonist recovering the striatal innervation, dendritic spines and motor behavior in an aged rat model of Parkinson's disease. PLoS One. 2015;**10**:e0117391

[31] Paxinos G, Watson C. The Rat Brain in Stereotaxic Coordinates. London: Academic Press, Elsevier; 2005

[32] Avila-Costa MR, Montiel Flores E, Colin-Barenque L, Ordoñez JL, Gutiérrez AL, Niño-Cabrera HG, et al. Nigrostriatal modifications after vanadium inhalation: An immunocytochemical and cytological approach. Neurochemical Research. 2004;**29**:1365-1369

[33] Robbe D. To move or to sense? Incorporating somatosensory representation into striatal functions. Current Opinion in Neurobiology. 2018;**52**:123-130

[34] Durieux PF, Schiffmann SN, de Kerchove d'Exaerde A. Differential regulation of motor control and response to dopaminergic drugs by D1R and D2R neurons in distinct dorsal striatum subregions. The EMBO Journal. 2012;**31**:640-653

[35] Raza C, Anjum R, Shakeel NUA. Parkinson's disease: Mechanisms, translational models and management strategies. Life Sciences. 2019;**226**:77-90

[36] Zeng XS, Geng WS, Jia JJ. Neurotoxin-induced animal models of parkinson disease: Pathogenic mechanism and assessment. ASN Neuro. 2018;**10**:1759091418777438

[37] Rozas G, López-Martín E, Guerra MJ, Labandeira-García JL. The overall rod performance test in the MPTP-treated-mouse model of Parkinsonism. Journal of Neuroscience Methods. 1998;**83**:165-175

[38] Boix J, Padel T, Paul G. A partial lesion model of Parkinson's disease in mice--characterization of a 6-OHDA-induced medial forebrain bundle lesion. Behavioural Brain Research. 2015;**284**:196-206

[39] Freed WJ, Fernandez L, Huys R, Issartel J, Azulay JP, Eusebio A. Movement speed-accuracy trade-off in Parkinson's disease. Frontiers in Neurology. 2018;**9**:897

[40] Eskow Jaunarajs KL, George JA, Bishop C. L-DOPA-induced dysregulation of extrastriatal dopamine and serotonin and affective symptoms in a bilateral rat model of Parkinson's disease. Neuroscience. 2012;**218**:243-256

[41] Ordoñez-Librado JL, Gutierrez-Valdez AL, Montiel-Flores E, Rodríguez-Lara V, Reynoso-Erazo L, Tron-Alvarez R, Avila-Costa M. R. Divalent and trivalent manganese mixture inhalation as a Parkinson disease model. Challenges in Disease and Health Research Vol. 6. BP International; 2021. 102-125.

[42] Eriksson H, Mägiste K, Plantin L-O, Fonnum F, Hedström K-G, Theodorsson-Norheim E, et al. Effects of manganese oxide on monkeys as revealed by a combined neurochemical, histological and neurophysiological evaluation. Archives of Toxicology. 1987;**61**:46-52

[43] Wang Z, Flores I, Donahue EK, et al. Cognitive flexibility deficits in rats with dorsomedial striatal 6-hydroxydopamine lesions tested using a three-choice serial reaction time task with reversal learning. Neuroreport. 2020;**31**:1055-1064

[44] Lindner MD, Cain CK, Plone MA, Frydel BR, Blaney TJ, Emerich DF, et al. Incomplete nigrostriatal dopaminergic cell loss and partial reductions in striatal dopamine produce akinesia, rigidity, tremor and cognitive deficits in middle-aged rats. Behavioural Brain Research. 1999;**102**:1-16

[45] Cenci MA, Whishaw IQ, Schallert T. Animal models of neurological deficits: How relevant is the rat? Nature Reviews. Neuroscience. 2002;**3**:574-579

[46] Schallert T, Petrie BF, Whishaw IQ. Neonatal dopamine depletion: Spared and unspared sensorimotor and attentional disorders and effects of further depletion in adulthood. Psychobiology. 1989:386-396

[47] Ungerstedt U. Adipsia and aphagia after 6-hydroxydopamine induced degeneration of the nigro-striatal dopamine system. Acta Physiologica Scandinavica. Supplementum. 1971;**367**:95-122

[48] Ungerstedt U, Arbuthnott GW. Quantitative recording of rotational behavior in rats after 6-hydroxy-dopamine lesions of the nigrostriatal dopamine system. Brain Research. 1970;**24**:485-493

[49] Surmeier DJ. Determinants of dopaminergic neuron loss in Parkinson's disease. The FEBS Journal. 2018;**285**:3657-3668

[50] Allbutt HN, Henderson JM. Use of the narrow beam test in the rat, 6-hydroxydopamine model of Parkinson's disease. Journal of Neuroscience Methods. 2007;**159**:195-202

[51] Dowd E, Dunnett SB. Comparison of 6-hydroxydopamine-induced medial forebrain bundle and nigrostriatal terminal lesions in a lateralised nose-poking task in rats. Behavioural Brain Research. 2005;**159**:153-161

[52] Avila-Costa M, Gutierrez-Valdez A, Ordonez-Librado J, Martinez V, Colin-Barenque L, Espinosa-Villanueva J, et al. Time course changes of the striatum neuropil after unilateral dopamine depletion and the usefulness of the contralateral striatum as a control structure. Neurological Research. 2008;**30**:1068-1074

[53] Anaya-Martinez V, Gutierrez-Valdez AL, Ordonez-Librado JL, Montiel-Flores E, Sanchez-Betancourt J, Sanchez Vazquez del Mercado C, et al. The presence of perforated synapses in the striatum after dopamine depletion, is this a sign of maladaptive brain plasticity? Microscopy (Oxf). 2014;**63**:427-435

[54] Trugman JM, James CL. Rapid development of dopaminergic supersensitivity in reserpine-treated rats demonstrated with 14C-2-deoxyglucose autoradiography. The Journal of Neuroscience. 1992;**12**:2875-2879

[55] Di Monte DA, McCormack A, Petzinger G, Janson AM, Quik M, Langston WJ. Relationship among nigrostriatal denervation, parkinsonism, and dyskinesias in the MPTP primate model. Movement Disorders. 2000;**15**:459-466

[56] Ellingsen DG, Shvartsman G, Bast-Pettersen R, Chashchin M, Thomassen Y, Chashchin V. Neurobehavioral performance of patients diagnosed with manganism and idiopathic Parkinson disease. International Archives of Occupational and Environmental Health. 2019;**92**:383-394

[57] Thiruchelvam M, Richfield EK, Baggs RB, Tank AW, Cory-Slechta DA. The nigrostriatal dopaminergic system as a preferential target of repeated exposures to combined paraquat and maneb: Implications for Parkinson's disease. The Journal of Neuroscience. 2000;**20**:9207-9214

[58] Sistrunk SC, Ross MK, Filipov NM. Direct effects of manganese compounds on dopamine and its metabolite Dopac: An in vitro study. Environmental Toxicology and Pharmacology. 2007;**23**:286-296

[59] Sriram K, Lin GX, Jefferson AM, Roberts JR, Chapman RS, Chen BT, et al.

Dopaminergic neurotoxicity following pulmonary exposure to manganese-containing welding fumes. Archives of Toxicology. 2010;**84**:521-540

[60] Peres TV, Schettinger MR, Chen P, et al. Manganese-induced neurotoxicity: A review of its behavioral consequences and neuroprotective strategies. BMC Pharmacology and Toxicology. 2016;**17**:57

[61] Archibald FS, Tyree C. Manganese poisoning and the attack of trivalent manganese upon catecholamines. Archives of Biochemistry and Biophysics. 1987;**256**:638-650

[62] Aschner M, Erikson KM, Herrero Hernandez E, Tjalkens R. Manganese and its role in Parkinson's disease: From transport to neuropathology. Neuromolecular Medicine. 2009;**11**:252-266

[63] Erikson KM, Dobson AW, Dorman DC, Aschner M. Manganese exposure and induced oxidative stress in the rat brain. Science of the Total Environment. 2004;**334-335**:409-416

[64] Struve MF, McManus BE, Wong BA, Dorman DC. Basal ganglia neurotransmitter concentrations in rhesus monkeys following subchronic manganese sulfate inhalation. American Journal of Industrial Medicine. 2007;**50**:772-778

[65] Gwiazda RH, Lee D, Sheridan J, Smith DR. Low cumulative manganese exposure affects striatal GABA but not dopamine. Neurotoxicology. 2002;**23**:69-76

[66] HaMai D, Bondy SC. Oxidative basis of manganese neurotoxicity. Annals of the New York Academy of Sciences. 2004;**1012**:129-141

[67] Ali SF, Duhart HM, Newport GD, Lipe GW, Slikker W. Manganese-induced reactive oxygen species: Comparison between Mn+2 and Mn+3. Neurodegeneration. 1995;**4**:329-334

[68] Díaz-Véliz G, Mora S, Gómez P, Dossi MT, Montiel J, Arriagada C, et al. Behavioral effects of manganese injected in the rat substantia nigra are potentiated by dicumarol, a DT-diaphorase inhibitor. Pharmacology, Biochemistry, and Behavior. 2004;**77**:245-251

[69] Morello M, Canini A, Mattioli P, Sorge RP, Alimonti A, Bocca B, et al. Sub-cellular localization of manganese in the basal ganglia of normal and manganese-treated rats: An electron spectroscopy imaging and electron energy-loss spectroscopy study. Neurotoxicology. 2008;**29**:60-72

[70] Gunter TE, Gavin CE, Aschner M, Gunter KK. Speciation of manganese in cells and mitochondria: A search for the proximal cause of manganese neurotoxicity. Neurotoxicology. 2006;**27**:765-776

[71] Ingersoll RT, Montgomery EB, Aposhian HV. Central nervous system toxicity of manganese. II: Cocaine or reserpine inhibit manganese concentration in the rat brain. Neurotoxicology. 1999;**20**:467-476

[72] Erikson KM, John CE, Jones SR, Aschner M. Manganese accumulation in striatum of mice exposed to toxic doses is dependent upon a functional dopamine transporter. Environmental Toxicology and Pharmacology. 2005;**20**:390-394

[73] Anderson JG, Cooney PT, Erikson KM. Inhibition of DAT function attenuates manganese accumulation in the globus pallidus. Environmental Toxicology and Pharmacology. 2007;**23**:179-184

[74] Masoud ST, Vecchio LM, Bergeron Y, et al. Increased expression

of the dopamine transporter leads to loss of dopamine neurons, oxidative stress and l-DOPA reversible motor deficits. Neurobiology of Disease. 2015;**74**:66-75

[75] Lehmensiek V, Tan EM, Liebau S, et al. Dopamine transporter-mediated cytotoxicity of 6-hydroxydopamine in vitro depends on expression of mutant alpha-synucleins related to Parkinson's disease. Neurochemistry International. 2006;**48**:329-340

[76] Brichta L, Greengard P. Molecular determinants of selective dopaminergic vulnerability in Parkinson's disease: An update. Frontiers in Neuroanatomy. 2014;**8**:152

[77] Bhaskar S, Gowda J, Prasanna J, Kumar A. Does altering proteasomal activity and trafficking reduce the arborization mediated specific vulnerability of SNpc dopaminergic neurons of Parkinson's disease? Medical Hypotheses. 2020;**143**:110062

[78] Schober A. Classic toxin-induced animal models of Parkinson's disease: 6-OHDA and MPTP. Cell and Tissue Research. 2004;**318**:215-224

[79] Goldberg MS, Fleming SM, Palacino JJ, Cepeda C, Lam HA, Bhatnagar A, et al. Parkin-deficient mice exhibit nigrostriatal deficits but not loss of dopaminergic neurons. The Journal of Biological Chemistry. 2003;**278**:43628-43635

[80] Giasson BI, Duda JE, Quinn SM, Zhang B, Trojanowski JQ, Lee VMY. Neuronal α-Synucleinopathy with severe movement disorder in mice expressing A53T Human α-Synuclein. Neuron. 2002;**34**:521-533

[81] Bloem BR, Okun MS, Klein C. Parkinson's disease. Lancet. 2021;**397**: 2284-2303

Chapter 4

Early Diagnosis of Parkinson's Disease: Utility of Animal Models

Neha S, Mohammad Ahmad, Baby Kumari, MD. Zainul Ali and Pankaj Singh Dholaniya

Abstract

The effectiveness of the treatment strategies for Parkinson's disease (PD) is highly dependent on the time of therapeutic intervention. This makes early diagnosis of PD an essential factor for its treatment; however, the complexities of the symptoms make it difficult to diagnose at an early stage. Moreover, by the time the symptoms start to appear, the disease has already been propagated in the patients. Even for the researchers, it is difficult to understand the important early diagnostic biomarkers due to the unavailability of the patients at the early stage, that is, before the manifestation of visible symptoms. The solution to this problem appears to develop animal models and monitor them from the early days to discover the diagnostic biomarkers. In this chapter, we shall discuss the use of animal models in the research intended to discover early diagnostic biomarkers for PD and why it is important to use animal models.

Keywords: alpha-synuclein, animal models, biomarkers, dopaminergic neurons, early diagnosis, neurodegeneration, Parkinson's disease, prodromal stage, rotenone, substantia nigra, transgenic models

1. Introduction

The number of Parkinson's disease (PD) cases per year is rising worldwide. In the coming two decades, it is estimated to outpace Alzheimer's disease in terms of casualties [1]. The economic burden of PD is also very high, as it can be understood by the fact that the US alone spends more than $50 billion annually on PD [2]. The disease goes unnoticed in the earlier stages as neurons are highly arborized and redundant; therefore, when degeneration of dopaminergic neurons starts, other neurons compensate for this loss. Consequently, motor symptoms appear when nearly half of the dopaminergic neurons have degenerated [2, 3]. PD's effects on the central nervous system are prolonged, and the neuronal damage cannot be reversed, making the disease's symptoms and progression inexorable. By the time PD is diagnosed, individuals have difficulty coordinating their bodies due to tremors, bradykinesia, stiffened limbs or trunk, and poor balance. Also, moving, speaking, swallowing, and other ordinary functions can become problematic as the symptoms progress. Apart from obvious motor-related symptoms, there are a few non-motor symptoms such as behavioral changes, sleep-related disorders, cognitive impairment, constipation etc.

that severely impact the healthy well-being of the individuals. Interestingly, some non-motor symptoms such as hyposmia, REM sleep behavior disorder (RBD), constipation, etc., follow motor symptoms over many years [4–8]. The multifactorial nature of PD makes it difficult for clinical diagnosis as the symptoms and causes are not universal among all patients. Particularly early diagnosis of PD is challenging because the symptoms at an early stage overlap with other diseases and normal aging. There is a need to identify biomarkers that can be helpful in early and accurate diagnosis, which must be aimed to prevent PD progression. In this chapter, we first discuss the different aspects of PD diagnosis, followed by challenges in early diagnosis. We also discuss the existing animal models used in PD research. Later we shall focus on various diagnostic markers and the utility of animal models. We conclude by stating the importance of animal models in PD research intended to discover early diagnostic biomarkers.

2. Different aspects of PD diagnosis

There are different aspects to diagnose PD, such as (1) Non-motor symptom assessment, (2) Brain imaging, and (3) Molecular markers-based diagnosis—e.g., metabolome analysis, miRNA-based analysis, genome sequencing.

2.1 Non-motor symptoms assessment

It has been shown that a few non-motor symptoms appear before the inception of the motor symptoms, e.g., Smell loss or hyposmia is a common phenomenon in PD (75–95%), however, a study reports ~25% of the normal population faces smell loss at later stages of life [9–11]. Constipation associated problems have been reported in PD, but only 15–20% of patients suffer from this problem [6, 7]. RBD is often reported in PD patients. It has been reported that ~67% of patients with RBD complaints whose nigrostriatal dopaminergic system is damaged, develop PD within 4 years [4, 5]. Although these non-motor symptoms help in PD diagnosis, their accuracy is very low. As these symptoms are not exclusive to PD, there is a need to identify a set of important non-motor symptoms that can accurately predict PD condition.

2.2 Brain imaging

With advancements in radiology, one could think of having non-invasive imaging (MRI, PET etc.) techniques to identify degenerated regions in the brain, such as substantia nigra, but the depletion is gradual which will go undetected in the early stages. Moreover, performing MRIs are too expensive to be carried out for a healthy population. Despite that, if someone wants to deploy imaging for early diagnosis, then it is necessitated to build some machine learning models (e.g., Deep learning methods such as Convolution Neural Networks etc.) for analyzing the whole brain regions that can be used for early diagnosis and predict the disease condition better than the existing models [12].

2.3 Molecular markers-based diagnosis

Metabolome-based analysis has been thriving in the last decade, and it is now extensively used for diagnosing PD using various sample matrices, such as

Cerebrospinal fluid metabolome, Blood metabolome, Tissue metabolome, Fecal metabolome, Urine metabolome. Although the initial metabolome results seem promising, it has some serious impediments to deal with, as the metabolome varies demographically and individually. Moreover, differences in genotype, presence of other diseases, lifestyle, diet, past medical records, and use of dissimilar tools and techniques for analysis enormously impact the results and conclusions. The reproducibility and validity of the results can be improved by standardizing the protocols, taking large samples, including various demographic populations in one study, and joint analysis with other methods. Among all, blood biomarkers are the most straightforward and cost-effective way of diagnosing a disease, but it does not seem to keep up to the mark in the case of PD. Heretofore, not a single biomarker has been found that can be employed universally in diagnosing the disease at the early stages. Many laboratories have conducted experiments relating to identification of circulating miRNAs, and they have come with a few novel miRNAs that are beneficial for early diagnosis of PD, but the results vary among the laboratories. This might be because of the difference in genotyping, symptoms, small sample size, demographic constraints, implementation of different protocols etc. Since miRNA can be collected aptly, if we improvise our approach, we can expect beneficial results. There is a dearth of rigorous standardization of the techniques, and one must address the above-mentioned challenges to improve the outcome. Nevertheless, different body fluids biomarkers such as α-synuclein aggregation or the formation of toxic tau isoforms are also considered hallmarks in PD. But they are deposited at the later stages of PD; therefore, they cannot be detected in the early stages and hence are not helpful for early diagnosis. There is a need to identify a biomarker that can be detected in the early stages of the disease. Scientists also contemplate a few miRNAs found in CSF as potential biomarkers, but sampling CSF is cumbersome and costly, and it also may lead to some untoward circumstances. Apart from CSF, it is required to identify miRNA from other body fluids, which can be collected easily and help diagnose the disease early [13, 14].

Few researchers have come up with machine learning (ML) models using various features to predict the disease condition. Several models focused on pre-motor symptoms of the disease and can predict the disease condition with acceptable accuracy. There is a need to tune the models with more data and play with other parameters and features, deploy other ML algorithms to improve the accuracy of the disease early diagnosis [15].

3. Challenges in early diagnosis

PD begins much before the motor symptoms occur, also known as the Preclinical phase of the disease that may last several years. Symptoms of this phase include hyposmia, depression, anxiety, and sleep difficulties along with autonomic nervous system disorders such as digestion, breathing, salivation, bladder malfunction, excessive sweating, and sexual dysfunction [16]. Clinical PD begins with onset of motor symptoms such as resting tremors, bradykinesia, limb rigidity, and coordination issues. Symptoms usually proceed gradually, often starting on one side of the body, such as reduced one-sided arm swing and intermittent tremors. Cognitive impairment (a non-motor symptom) appears often after the motor symptoms [17]. Many patients with PD develop dementia, however the time frame varies significantly from one individual to another. Dementia is a primary reason for PD patients to enter long-term care facilities [18]. However, it has been observed that the onset of motor symptoms i.e. clinical PD starts much earlier than it can be diagnosed with current diagnostic criteria. Hitherto, no biomarkers have been found which will assist accurate diagnosis of these conceptual phases of pre-diagnostic PD with high sensitivity and specificity [19].

Furthermore, it should be noted that perception of a PD case on early diagnosis may be significantly influenced by their demographics, their family history, or a genetically identical state [20]. However, there is also the possibility of entering in disease-modifying therapy trials associated with gene targeting. Along with the fact that different mutations for PD have been reported, exhibiting a varying degree of penetrance in various populations. As a result, while some populations are susceptible to one mutation, the same mutation may not be active as a risk factor for the development or progression of the disease in other populations. Genetic testing of unselected PD cohorts revealed that up to 10% of cases with Glucocerebrosidase gene A (GBA) mutations had type 1 GD (Gaucher's disease), which is known to dramatically enhance the risk of acquiring PD (and is considerably high in few populations, like Ashkenazi Jewish demography) [21, 22]. Leucine-rich repeat kinase 2 (LRRK2) gene mutations are present in a substantial number of PD patients in several groups, including Ashkenazi Jewish and Berber Arab communities [23–25]. Similarly, it has been discovered that Han Chinese people have a substantial association with GAK gene mutation [26].

Despite various studies, PD diagnosis and misclassification in routine clinical practice are frequent, with error rates between 15–24% [27–29]. Approximately 10% of cases that were diagnosed with PD by neurologists had alternate pathologies (like multiple system atrophy, tauopathies and progressive supranuclear palsy), despite the adoption of strict clinical diagnostic criteria [30]. A recent meta-analysis of 11 clinicopathological investigations revealed a shared accuracy in clinical diagnosis of PD cases of only 81% which is a reason why various forms of secondary parkinsonism and tremor diseases such as essential tremor, are frequently misdiagnosed as PD [31]. Early diagnostic separation of PD from atypical parkinsonian disorders presents the toughest challenge even for qualified professionals. Diseased defined by neuronal deposition of phosphorylated tau aggregates like tauopathies and progressive supranuclear palsy are among the parkinsonism disorders including multiple system atrophy which are pathologically characterized by presence of cytoplasmic glial inclusions formed due to aggregation of *α-synuclein* in oligodendrocytes. All these conditions can be exceedingly difficult to identify from one another and from PD in the early stages of the disease [32, 33]. According to clinicopathological research clinical diagnostic mistakes account for 7 to 35% of cases [34–36]. It is important to optimize the clinical biomarkers that can be used to differentiate between PD and these main subtypes of atypical degenerative parkinsonism.

To address this need, various cross-sectional case-control studies have strived to define the prognostic value of non-genetic, genetic risk and prodromal clinical factors (biomarkers identified from studies on animal models) to establish the probability of translation to clinically identified PD. Some of the studies which have been initiated to better characterize this using a variety of risk factors or markers and prodromal features are:

- The Parkinson's Associated Risk Study (PARS) is a multicentre study in the United States that compares older individuals with and without hyposmia and involves annual physical exams and twice-yearly dopamine transporter SPECT scans [37].

- The Prospective Validation of Risk Factors for the Development of Parkinsonian Syndromes (PRIPS) study focused on early diagnosis of PD by analyzing risk factors such as age, male gender, family history, hyposmia, subtle motor impairment and enlarged substantia nigra hyperechogenicity. The study was performed on 1847 individuals from three European nations aged over 50 years [38].

- The Tübingen Evaluation of Risk Factors for Early Detection of Neurodegeneration (TREND) study highlight the prodromal markers by examining 698 individuals aged between 50 and 85 years with selected prodromal markers (SPM) with no neurodegeneration. Individuals with SPM show higher prevalence of various prodromal symptoms making SPMs as better diagnostic markers [39].

- The Parkinson's Progression Markers Initiative (PPMI) is a global cohort, having at least 50 data collection sites, started back in 2010. It has now more than 4000 participants, the major involved countries include North America, Australia, Europe, and Israel. PPMI is interested in collecting various data that comprises of motor assessments, non-motor assessments, brain imaging, cognitive impairments, blood samples, genetic and various omics data which are publicly available. The main aim of PPMI includes finding novel biomarkers, new and better treatments for PD [40].

These cohorts offer valuable pre-diagnosis information from at-risk subjects who may experience PD in the course of study period or who have recently received a diagnosis. Studies based on these cohorts pay particular attention to the emergence of prodromal symptoms and epidemiologic traits based on biofluids or biopsies. However, a basic barrier in research on neurodegenerative diseases is the inability to characterize disease at molecular level and infer disease progression from these parameters [41]. Animal models are therefore necessary since they are the only way to directly and longitudinally analyze any disease-relevant tissue. Additionally, by standardizing and closely observing living conditions, they enable the assessment of environmental and behavioral influences on etiologically complicated disorders like PD.

In addition to identification of novel biomarkers for early and accurate diagnosis, better diagnostic methods are needed to identify PD earlier in the course of disease progression. By the time a patient exhibits clinical symptoms and is diagnosed with PD, neurons and autonomic nervous system functions have been lost. An earlier diagnosis may provide a therapeutic window to slow or alleviate PD before onset of motor deficits (**Figure 1**). Even with the varying methodologies, there is a clear indication with promising results which can detect cases with strong manifestation of "pre-diagnostic" PD via clinical, imaging, and other risk markers. As many of these cohorts mature, the numbers of "high-risk" individuals "converting" to established PD provide proof of concept and will assist to establish the optimum approach to "early" detection. We must redraft our strategy and amalgamate the above-mentioned approaches to early diagnose the disease with high accuracy, sensitivity, and specificity. If PD is detected at the early stages, disease progress can be slowed or at best can be halted, consequently reducing the economic burden and improve the quality of life.

Early PD diagnosis will be beneficial in many terms such as (i) Early diagnosis will give ample time to the patient, the caregivers, the family and the clinicians to understand the disease and to decide the course of treatment and plan their future goals

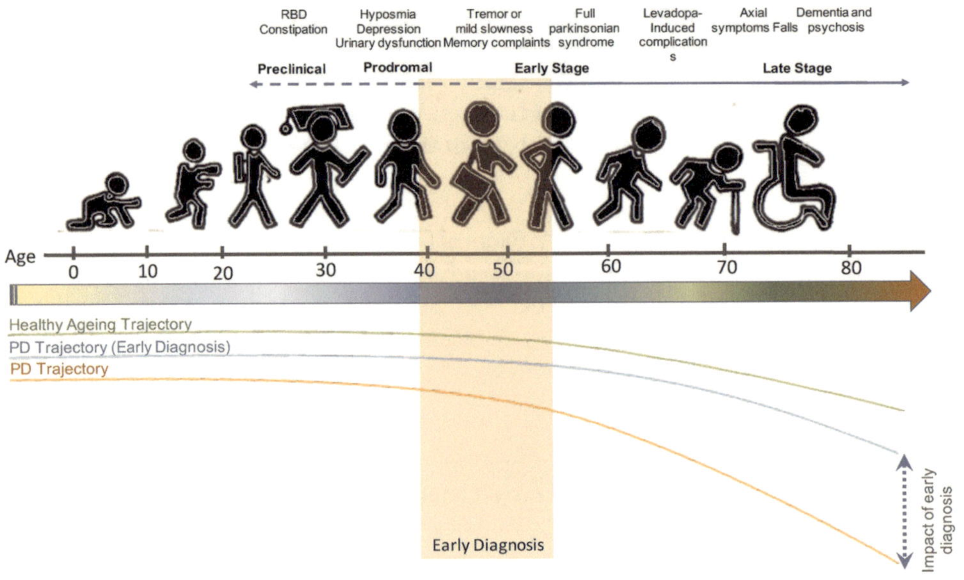

Figure 1.
Parkinson's disease symptoms during the course of a human's life, both prodromal and clinical. Diagram illustrating the progression of life from early to old age and the related brain health curves in PD cases compared to the healthy condition. The distinctive motor phenotypes that show up in late stages of the disease are the basis for the current clinical diagnosis of PD. Contrary to the prodromal phase, which might last between 10 and 15 years, the length of the preclinical phase is unclear, as shown by the dotted arrow. A prodromal diagnosis of PD might be made by following altered molecular trajectories from preclinical to clinical stages, which would increase the positive effects of neuroprotective lifestyle modifications or available therapeutic alternatives.

accordingly, (ii) It will help the patient to modify their lifestyle such that progression of the symptoms can be halted, a few non-drug treatments might be a possibility in that situation, (iii) Early diagnosis will improve the chance of cure for the disease, (iv) The classic drugs will be more effective in the patients whose symptoms have been detected at the early stages (v) Early diagnosis will reduce the economic burden on both the patient and the state.

4. Animal models in Parkinson's disease

The animal model of PD has been extensively used to study the pathophysiology of PD progression and design new therapeutic intervention. Several models have been developed by various methods in model animals (rodents, non-human primates and non-mammalians) to recapitulate clinical phenotypic features and parkinsonian manifestations (**Table 1**). Highly reproducible models have occurred in rodent such as rats and mice due to their short life of span, low maintenance, and easy handling. There are two ways to culminate the PD model in animals: one is the systemic injection of PD-inducing drugs and the local administration of the drug (intracerebral, intracerebroventricular, intrastriatal, Intra-*SNpc*. Etc.) with the use of the stereotaxic instrument.

Over the last decade, the advent of the genetic era of PD gives out phenomenal insight into the genetic model of PD. These models are solemnly based on mammalian and non-mammalian transgenic models that propagate disease-causing mutation considered to be a monogenetic form of familial PD. Neurotoxic, herbicides, and

DOI: http://dx.doi.org/10.5772/intechopen.107887

Model	Treatment	Rodents		Non-human primates	Non-mammalian species			Advantages	Disadvantages	References (PMID)
		Rat	Mice	Monkey	Zebrafish	Drosophila	Nematode			
Pharmacological model	Reserpine	✓	✓	✗	✗	✗	✗	Approx. 85% loss in DA neurons	No pathological characters	25203719, 26514557
	Haloperidol	✓	✓	✓	✓	✗	✗	Induce motor symptoms	No pathological characters	29634484, 25203719, 19940105
Neurotoxin model	6-OHDA	✓	✓	✓	✓	✗	✗	Behavioral studies	Special skill required, lack of lewy bodies	24333330, 28130746, 29809058
	MPTP	✓	✓	✓	✓	✗	✗	Mimics PD biochemical features	Reproducibility is difficult	29809058, 29515360, 28978077
Pesticide model	Rotenone	✓	✗	✗	✓	✓	✗	Replicate all biochemical hallmarks of PD	Mortality is high, other deleterious effects	26013581, 29209747, 29809058
	Paraquat	✓	✓	✗	✗	✗	✗	Selective for SNc dopaminergic neurons, leads to a 50% loss with multiple doses	High mortality rates	24483602, 20079141, 29809058
α-Synuclein model	α-Synuclein	✓	✓	✓	✗	✗	✓	Formation of lewy bodies, used for evaluation of neuroprotective stratergies	No DA neuron loss in SNpc	27658420, 25565982, 25954517
Genetic model	LRRK-2	✗	✓	✗	✗	✓	✗	Evalute role of LRRK-2 in PD, DA neurotoxicity	Nuclear abnormalities, No lewy odies	23799078, 24957201
	PINK1	✗	✓	✗	✗	✗	✗	No DA neurotoxicity	Lack of lewy bodies and neurodegeneration	25037286, 25954517
	PARKIN	✗	✓	✗	✗	✗	✓	Dose dependent DA cell death	No significant DA anormalities	20126261, 24423640
	DJ-1	✗	✓	✗	✗	✗	✗	Understand ubqiuitin protease system	Further evaluation required to support this model	23019375, 31484320

Table 1.
Advantages and disadvantages of various PD models in different animals.

transgenic models have their characteristics and limitations, which must be taken very carefully chosen to be our model. Here, in particular, we discuss the neurotoxin-based model in rodent animals. There are many chemicals are being used in the development of PD such as MPTP (1-methyl-4-phenyl-1,2,3,6-tetrahydropyridine) a prodrug that readily crosses the BBB due to its lipophilic nature. It is bound to complex 1 of electron transporter and reduces the conversion ATP from molecular oxygen, which consequently embarks the production of ROS, lipid peroxidation, irregular homeostasis in iron metabolism, and leads to cell death. MPTP has all hallmarks of PD in primates compared to non-primates. Therefore, MPTP could be the most suitable compound for PD development in Primates. Another, drug that has been used in the PD model is 6-hydroxy dopamine, it does not cross the BBB and consider non-systemic. So, it has to be injected directly into the SN region of the midbrain. Apart from the neurotoxin model herbicide and insecticide drugs are also used frequently in the development of PD such as Paraquat, and Rotenone. Transgenic models are also available in the form of monogenetic mutation. *α-synuclein* is abundantly expressed at 1% of total cytosolic brain protein. Overexpression of *α-synuclein* and its role in dopaminergic neurons has to be observed in the genetic model of PD. Mutation in α-synuclein, and LRRK2 leads to autosomal dominant disease while PINK, Parkin, and DJ1 are probably considered for Autosomal recessive disease.

4.1 Neurotoxin-based model in PD

The emergence of technology and advancement of biological research revealed the reduced levels of Dopamine in the striatum region of PD in human patients opened the window of research and treatment interventions. There are several models of PD in animals that have been characterized by the low amount of Dopamine in the SN region and striatum. Many neurotoxins and herbicide compounds ameliorate ATP production subsequently leading to cell death. Deprivation of dopamine-producing neurons is directly proportional to the less amount of dopamine in the SN region. This vital characteristic seems to be a cardinal hallmark of PD in the various animal models.

4.1.1 MPTP-based PD model

MPTP is a non-toxic, lipophilic compound that readily crosses the BBB. After entering the brain, especially in Astrocyte cells it metabolizes by monoamine oxidase B into MPP^+ (1-methyl-4-phenylpyridinium ion). MPP^+ enters in dopamine-producing neurons with the help of Dopamine transporter in *substantia nigra pars compacta* (*SNpc*) region. Active MPP+ binds to Complex1 of ETC and reduces ATP production [42]. This suggests that mitochondria are a preferential target of neurotoxicity. Administration of MPTP in primates through bilateral carotid injection causes L-DOPA responsive Parkinsonian syndrome characterized by all the clinical manifestations of PD which showed the best model of PD in Primates [43]. Intraperitoneally administration of MPTP in mice at certain doses (four MPTP every 2 hours. Over a day) gives the similar kind of lesions and phenotypic characters as in primates [44]. MPTP model has certain limitations such as, administration of MPTP in an animal model fails to mimic the progressive nature of PD [45]. Long term chronic treatments of MPTP may overcome this issue however, the smaller doses for long term resulted in the recovery of motor behavior deficit in animals when the treatment was discontinued. Another limitation of this model is that *SNpc* lesions are rarely accompanied by the formation of Lewy bodies [46].

4.1.2 6-Hydroxydopamine-based PD model

6-Hydroxydopamine (6-OHDA) is a chemical compound that is also known as oxidopamine or structurally known as 2, 4,5 trihydroxy phenethylamine is the first-ever generated PD model in animals [47]. This neurotoxin destroys the dopaminergic neurons in the *SNpc* region. 6-OHDA was a noble chemical compound that had a neurotoxic effect on catecholaminergic pathways [48]. Due to its lack of lipophilic nature 6-OHDA does not penetrate BBB hence it has to be directly administered stereotactically to a specific region of the brain such as *SNpc* or striatum. 6-OHDA effectively destroys the dopaminergic neurons in 12 hrs in the *SNpc* region while striatum-based neurons are conventionally lost within 2–3 days [49]. This kind of degeneration replicates the PD phenotypes. 6-OHDA agonistically binds to DA & NAT transporter respectively that facilitate to move inside of the cell where it auto-oxidizes in the cytoplasm, therefore, generating intracellular oxidative stress [50, 51]. 6-OHDA infused in neurons thus elevated cytotoxic molecules that are produced by an enzymatic and non-enzymatic process in which intrinsic trace element like Mg, and Fe is completely involved in cellular homeostasis [50, 52]. Moreover, 6OHDA generates H_2O_2 by the oxidation process in which it is highly toxic to cellular environments. Aside of its toxicity, it plays a vital role in free radicals' formation, ROS species, and quinone intermediate products [53]. Dopamine is a neurotransmitter and is metabolized into 6-OHDA. It acts as a neurotoxin and therefore produces lesions in the nigrostriatal pathway. In spite of that, 6-OHDA does not promote protein aggregation of alpha-synuclein protein with other fibrils, thus Lewy neurites inclusion bodies are not produced in 6-OHDA-based animal models [49].

4.2 Herbicides-based PD model

Several reports suggest that farmers who are exposed to herbicides such as Rotenone and Paraquat suffered with symptoms similar to familial PD [54]. This finding suggests the role of this chemical in the development of the PD model in animals.

4.2.1 Paraquat-based PD model in animals

Unlike MPTP, Paraquat (PQ) does not cross BBB, but it has a similar structure to MPP+ (an active metabolite of MPTP). Due to its structural resemblance, it behaves like MPP+. PQ acts through the involvement of the redox cycle and subsequently induces oxidative stress. Therefore, it produced Reactive oxygen species, particularly: superoxide radical, peroxide, and hydrogen radicals that lead to damage to lipid molecules, protein, DNA, and RNA. A recent study proposed dilemmatic evidence on paraquat exposure in rats. One report mentioned arbitrary statements chronic systemic injection of paraquat in mice reduced the motor activity and subsequently loss of the tyrosine hydroxylase-positive striatal fibers and *SNpc* neurons. On the other hand, Cory-Slechta et al. reported that prolonged treatment of PQ does not have any effect on the nigrostriatal DA region in mice model [55].

4.2.2 Rotenone-based PD model in animals

Rotenone is a naturally occurring herbicide/insecticide. Its half-life is generally 3–5 days depending on the exposure to natural light. Like MPTP neurotoxin, Rotenone has similar chemical properties and crosses the BBB readily and uniformly inhibits the complex-1 of ETC [56] In this retro-aspect, MPTP inhibits dopaminergic neurons due to the dependence of the DAT transporter in dopaminergic neurons while Rotenone inhibits complex 1 selectively in the nigrostriatal dopaminergic pathway. Thus, Rotenone seems to recapitulate all kinds of PD hallmarks such as systemic complex 1 inhibition, inflammation, ubiquitin-*α-synuclein* aggregation in nigral cells that look like Lewy bodies in PD, oxidative stress, and GI problems [57]. Behaviorally, rotenone-treated rats have hypokinetic characteristics along with flexed posture similar to stooped posture in human PD patients. Few rats have severe rigidity and few have spontaneously shaken which is similar to a resting tremor. The existing beauty of this model is that like paraquat, it also introduced *α-synuclein* aggregation and Lewy body-like formation. The limitation of this model is that it does augment the DA oxidation but the evidence is narrow about the depletion of dopaminergic neurons in the nigrostriatal system [58].

4.3 Genetic model of PD

According to Cedric Bardy (2020), 85% of the PD population are sporadic and the remaining are familial PD [59]. Familial PD is generally based on genetic defects that are counted as autosomal dominant (AD) or autosomal recessive (AR). *α-synuclein* gene (SNCA) and LRRK2 are experimentally proven to be involved in AD in Parkinson's Disease. *α-synuclein* is a small (14kD) protein, present abundantly in brain tissue, while a lesser tone of protein is present in the heart, muscle, and other tissue. Currently, its peculiar role is not clear but plays an important role in the membrane, vesicular dynamics, and intracellular trafficking within the ER/Golgi network. The identification of *α-synuclein* mutation was the first to be involved in familial PD thereafter many researchers try to overexpress in Drosophila and yeast resulting in that hampers the ER-Golgi network trafficking and toxic *α-synuclein* leads to neuropathology and amyloid aggregation in nigral cells which are the key features of familial PD [60, 61]. Mutations in *α-synuclein* create a high propensity for protein misfolding. *α-synuclein* exists in various structures including oligomers, protofibrils, fibrils, and, filaments. The amalgamation of filamentous and fibril structures seems to be a more toxic form [62]. Mashliah et al. (2000) developed the first-ever model using mutated SNCA (A53T, A30P, and E46K) and observed the inclusion kind of bodies in the hippocampus, *SNpc*, and neocortex region but they do not have any evidence of *α-synuclein* inclusion bodies like LB in human patients. Meanwhile, the same group had done another experiment to confirm the previous findings but unfortunately, the result was the same no dopaminergic neuron degeneration has been observed in mice [63]. Another group developed a double mutant (A30P, A53T) model in mice and apparent neurotrophy was reported. This key feature was retorted motor activity and promotes neuronal aggregates [63].

LRRK2 (leucine-rich repeat kinase 2) is a multidomain having 286 Kd protein. It is also known as dardarin and PARK8. One part of the dardarin protein that enriches the protein building block amino acid is known as leucine. LRRK2 is a large multimeric protein that is localized to an outer membranous structure. LRRK2 protein plays various roles in the cell but neuronal outgrowth and guidance [64]. Mutation in LRRK2 is associated with autosomal dominant PD with varying occurrence in the population [65]. The most common mutation is G2019S has a low frequency of 1% of sporadic PD patients while 4% of familial PD. The risk of PD in the person of LRRK2 G2019S is age-dependent: 28% at 59 years old, 51% at 69 years old 74% at 79 years old

[66]. The two most important mutant model G2019S and R 1441C/G have failed to recapitulate the PD hallmarks. Przedborski, S.; et al., use BCA-R 1441C mutant mice to show motor deficit and axonal pathology in the striatum, however, loss of DA neurons in *SNpc* and alpha-synuclein is not seen clearly [67]. Another team developed the LRRK2 model using a viral vector-like Herp simplex virus (HSV) and an adenoviral vector. Transfection of G2019S is more effective than WTR1441C in stimulating neuronal pathology and Lewy body aggregation [68]. In Addition, infusion of HSV-LRRK2-G2019S in mouse striatum achieved 50% DA neuronal loss in the SN region [67, 69]. So, the LRRK2 model could provide a good platform to understand the neuropathology, mechanism of neuronal loss in the mid-brain region, and their function in PD.

5. Diagnostic biomarkers for PD

Despite decades of research, PD is currently diagnosed primarily on motor symptoms. Majority of dopaminergic neurons are degenerated by the time PD is confirmed, complicating treatment. Due to intersection of symptoms between PD and other atypical parkinsonian disorder the misdiagnosis rates by the clinicians for PD are quite high. Misdiagnosis and delayed diagnosis undermine disease-modifying therapy. Therefore, identification and quantification of biomarkers are vital for evaluating individual physiological and clinical responses, supporting therapeutic decisions, defining treatment and management programs, and managing causes of individual or group changes. Although motor and non-motor symptoms are visible clinically, the brain pathology in humans can only be established by evaluating post-mortem tissue samples or body fluids. The use of humans as a PD model for the identification of early diagnostic biomarkers is complicated by the fact that we do not know the time of PD onset, which may span between 10 and 15 years [18]. This can be circumvented by utilizing animal models, as we can monitor them from the moment of neurotoxic injection until the onset of symptoms, as well as identify the molecular alterations preceding the onset of symptoms. In addition, the identification of markers from non-invasive or minimally invasive techniques necessitates the use of animal models for early diagnostics. Consequently, there is a huge demand for experimental models to enhance our comprehension. To date, however, only a handful of putative biomarkers have been tested in clinical settings.

5.1 Non-invasive biomarkers

Two main techniques fluorodopa positron emission tomography (F-DOPA PET) and dopamine transporter single-photon emission computed tomography (DAT-SPECT) are used to measure the neurochemical differences dopamine system [70, 71]. Another technique called the susceptibility-weighted imaging (SWI) also works with high sensitivity and specificity on Nigrosome-1 (N1) cluster in differentiating PD from control and other non-PD parkinsonism [72]. An important prodromal PD marker is RBD which occurs at a high risk of 45% in early prodromal stages and 76% in late prodromal stages. As per a report on RBD cohort, 39.7% of RBD patients were found to develop PD or dementia with Lewy bodies. Another study on the same cohort, demonstrated the conversion of prodromal stages into PD with high sensitivity (81.3%) and a specificity (67.9%) [73, 74].

5.2 Invasive biomarkers

Biomarkers obtained via invasive technique are blood-based biomarkers which include *α-synuclein*, Extracellular Vesicles, miRNAs and inflammation related biomarkers. *α-synuclein* is a promising biomarker that is a key protein found in the Lewy bodies. Its malformation and aggregation due to both post translational modification and genetic factors in PD is a good indicator of PD pathogenesis [75]. This pathogenic protein is mainly transported from cells to cells through extracellular vesicles which makes them a candidate to use as a biomarker. A study performed by Majbour et al. using Oligomeric α-synuclein/total *α-synuclein* in CSF was not able to classified PD from DATATOP cohort whereas Oligomeric α-synuclein/total α-synuclein, phosphorylated was able to distinguish PD from healthy controls by sensitivity and specificity of 79% and 67% respectively [76]. Another promising candidate are the miRNAs, which are a class of non-coding RNA and the combination of different biomarkers can readily differentiate PD from healthy cases. For example, a study performed by using MiR-19a, miR-19b, miR-24, miR-30c, miR-34b, miR-133b, and miR-205 from CSF classified PD from control cases with AUC of 0.98 [77]. In various studies it been stated that inflammation is a major deriver of PD and certain kinds of cytokines like TNF α, IL-1, IL-4, IL-6, and IL-10 are highly expressed in PD patients. In a recent study IFN-γ, IL-10, and TNF-α obtained from blood serum distinguished patient with cognitive impairment, postural instability and PD have high expression levels than in the control samples [78]. In recent times, gut-inflammation related biomarkers have also been discovered which are found to be linked with severe constipation and motor phenotype which includes high expression of TRL4, CD3+ T cells, and cytokines in colonic biopsies of PD patients [79].

Combination of above mentioned biomarkers can increase the sensitivity of prediction accuracy. Developing a system to aggregate the diverse types and intensities of these biomarkers into a single set of criteria is difficult. Plasma aggregated *α-synuclein* and various ESWAN imaging indicators were integrated in the prediction model of a cohort research, and it was revealed that it has a sensitivity and specificity of 0.80 and 0.80, respectively, for predicting PD [80]. Analysis of age with the combination of CSF oligomeric/total *α-synuclein* ratio and β-glucocerebrosidase activity distinguished PD cases from non-dementia cases with 82% sensitivity and 71% specificity [81]. Matsusue et al. used combination of imaging methods, including NM-MRI and DAT-SPECT, demonstrated a good diagnosis accuracy with an AUC of 0. 935 [82].

6. Utility of animal models

As discussed in the earlier sections, PD is idiopathic with multiple genetic and environmental risk factors. In humans, motor symptoms are noticeable at advanced disease stages; the pathology starts much earlier than the diagnosing time. In these situations, animal models can play a vital role where we can induce such types of disease pathology and monitor the disease from the beginning. Motor and non-motor symptoms are easily detected, but brain pathology is only possible with post-mortem brain tissue. The heterogeneous nature of PD in terms of etiology & pathology demands a range of animal models [83]. Therefore, it is crucial to deepen our understanding through various experimental models to scale up the limited available treatment options. We need a diverse range of animal models to recapitulate different aspects of PD in humans. Thus studying PD with an appropriate animal model is very important to understand the biology of disease in every aspect. Humans share most of the genetic information with different animals. There is about 96% genetic similarity between a human and a chimpanzee and 90% between humans and rats. Mouse shares about 85% of their genome with humans regarding protein-coding genes, while fruit fly shares about 61% of genetic information with humans. The handling and ease of propagation of these small animals make them valuable research tools.

Three categories of PD models are used in research so far. This includes rodents, non-human primates, and non-mammalian species [84]. By 2018 the major percentage of animal models used for PD is a rodent (85%), followed by non-human primates (10%) and non-mammalian species (5%). In another study, out of 1851 papers screened for PD, 996 used a mouse model followed by 805 rat model. Others include Drosophila-43, C. elegans-14, non-human primates-69, Chinese Hamster-6, Yeast-17, E.coli-6, Zebrafish-24, and others 27 [85]. These animal models and their advantages and disadvantages have been discussed briefly in the **Table 1**. The array of animal models available today ranges from small worms (nematodes) to flies (drosophila) to rodents (mice and rats) and primates (monkey and chimpanzee). The worms and flies model can be used to study individual pathological pathways. Still, when it comes to getting closer to the relevance of the human disease features, we need to switch to higher-order animals like rodents (mice or rats) or Primates (chimpanzees, gorillas, orangutans, etc.) [86].

Three different modeling pathologies are most common in the case of PD. These include Nigrostriatal tract degeneration, outside the nigrostriatal tract neuron dysfunction, and Lewy body pathology. Here we have summarized the different models and their respective modeling pathologies along with other features like Mitochondrial Dysfunction, Oxidative stress, Motor deficit, Cognitive deficit, Autophagy, Proteasomal Dysfunction, Neuroinflammation, Response to L-DOPA, Sensory abnormalities, Somnolescent alterations, Psychiatric Changes and Organ system dysfunction based on the latest review by Joana Lama (**Figure 2**) [87].

Small animal models and rodents partially replicate human PD's clinical and pathological features [88, 89]. In one of the studies, it has been reported that most transgenic rats show no dopaminergic neuron loss [90]. Rodent models have been widely used to model selective pathological pathways in PD like how the α-synuclein aggregate and spread, mitochondria damage and malfunction, faulty degradation of misfolded proteins, and immune system activation in PD state [91, 92]. As primates (chimpanzees, orangutans, etc.) are closer to humans than rodents, they classify as good models for identifying critical pathological events in humans than small animals. Higher-order animal models have played a key role in understanding PD so far [93]. In large animal models like the rhesus monkey, by expressing mutant α-synuclein in the fertilized embryos, the obtained progeny after 2.5 years show age-dependent non-motor symptoms like anxiety, cognitive defects, poor dexterity, and finger coordination [94]. Monkeys with stereotaxically injected Lentiviral vectors carrying A53T mutant (A53T α-synuclein) in *substantia nigra* at differing ages disclosed that aging is the major factor that promotes neuropathology in non-human primate brain [95]. Thus, large transgenic animals provide us with critical information regarding neuropathology and disease pathogenesis which is difficult to understand from rodent models. With the latest gene-editing technology like CRISPR Cas9, large animal models for PD, like non-human primates, can be easily created with a genetic mutation in one of the critical PD genes to understand the disease's pathology better [93].

All the models discussed above have contributed significantly to understanding PD. But none of the models completely replicate PD in humans exactly. Neurotoxic

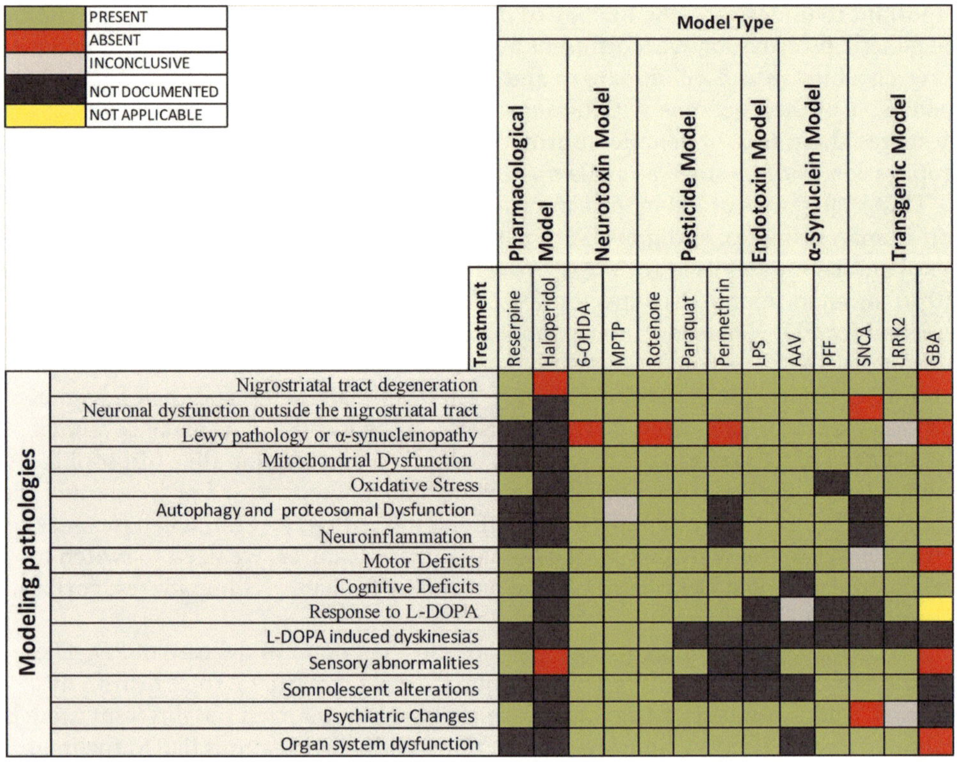

Figure 2.
Occurrence of PD pathologies in different animal models.

models are an excellent candidate because they replicate the nigrostriatal neurodegeneration and motor dysfunction but lack proper Lewy body formation. While transgenic animal models show Lewy body pathogenesis, but lacks the loss of dopaminergic neurons [96]. Many mutation studies have been performed in cell lines, but those results seem inconsistent. After the discovery that reduced dopamine levels was responsible for the motor symptoms in PD, most of the animal models focused on mimicking this dopamine loss through the use of neurotoxins. These animal studies led to the discovery of pathways related to the DA loss in *substantia nigra* and L-Dopa drug development for PD related motor symptoms treatment. But as discussed earlier, PD is a multifactorial disease that affects both CNS and PNS along with multiple organs like the gut, heart, skin, etc., and symptoms affecting these organs called the prodromal symptoms that appear much before the visible motor symptoms. These prodromal symptoms include hyposmia, constipation, hypertension, and sleep disorders which results due to the accumulation of *α-synuclein* pathology in the gut, skin, heart and lower brain regions. The prodromal phase act as a golden opportunity; if we can recapitulate and model animals in a way that mimics these symptoms, we can identify novel disease targets and treatments.

After the Braak's gut-first hypothesis [97], which states that the *α-synuclein* pathology first starts in the enteric nervous system decades before the motor symptoms start to appear and travels upto the brain stem and dopaminergic neurons through the vagus nerve, researchers started focusing on the gastrointestinal tract to model gut dysfunction in PD in animals [98, 99]. Other possible initiation sites have also been explored simultaneously for example targeting autonomic ganglia in mice mimics hyposmia, orthostatic hypotension and constipation without any motor symptoms [100] whereas targeting lower brainstem regions mimics RBD, depression, and anxiety [101]. Many transgenic rodent models that express *α-synuclein* pathology through BAC vectors show RBD-like dysfunction without atonia and hyposmia and loss of dopaminergic neurons later [102]. BAC-developed mice with A30P *α-synuclein* mutation show gut dysfunction before motor dysfunction. *α-synuclein* preformed fibrils (PFFs) injected in GI tract in mice is one of the most successful animal model since it recapitulates symptoms like gut dysfunction, anxiety, and Dopaminergic neuron loss [98]. PFFs injected in RBD-responsible region of mice also results in RBD-like behavior followed by decreased olfaction, GI dysfunction, and motor deficits [101]. VMAT-2 deficient animal models show *α-synuclein* aggregation and later DA neuron loss with increased anxiety and reduced olfaction [103]. These prodromal models have helped us gain insights into the cellular and molecular mechanism of PD initiation and progression, but it is not specific and limited. Thus, we see a plethora of symptoms overlapping in different animal models.

One of the key risk factor for PD is aging but majority of animal model used, are quite young which fail to relate to the cellular and molecular metabolism to this age. However certain studies compare treatment between young and old age animals, and have shown that the treatments are not so effective in old animals. The heterogenic nature of PD is seen in symptoms wherein some patients experience dementia much earlier than others. Pathological characters of PD include existence of *α-synuclein* Lewy bodies and loss of Lewy neurites and nigrostriatal dopaminergic pathway. But these pathologies are not restricted to only CNS but are spread outside CNS, which is extremely difficult to model in animals. Though the neurotoxin model has helped us study the dopaminergic system in PD, it is not similar to studying the complex pathology, temporal progression, and clinical expression seen in human PD. Likewise, overexpression studies of *α-synuclein* can explain its functions and other effects because of its overexpression in that part. However in PD cases with normal expression level of *α-synuclein,* the question remains unanswered through these models. Transgenic animal models are good in indicating about a particular gene or protein function, but that does not necessarily mean studying PD. Similarly, injecting *α-synuclein* PFF explains the seed pathology in that area and how it spreads, but the same pathology is seen is human PD is still not proved [104, 105]. Thus all these models failed to recapitulate the age of onset of disease, the spectrum of pathologies, and the temporal pattern of disorder similar to PD in humans. These models, as such cannot help us in understanding human PD's core pathologies to treat the sporadic form of the disease. One such example is GDNF, which is used in rodents and non-human primates to recover the loss of dopaminergic neuron system but when tried in human PD patient was unsuccessful. It was also shown that in the *α-synuclein* PD model, this toxin protein interfere with the GDNF signaling pathway indicating the clinical efficacy of these models [106, 107]. Thus we can say that animals can be used to model only specific pathologies of PD but not the disease as it is. Since animal models and humans represent two different disease states, the therapies that work on animals do not necessarily work on humans.

Despite these limitations, animal models have not failed us. From the starting, these models have helped to develop previous and current drugs and treatments. For example, reserpine-treated rats and rabbits helped develop L-DOPA therapy, the rodent neurotoxin model helped develop dopamine-receptor antagonists, and MPTP-treated monkeys have paved the path of identifying sub-thalamic nucleus for deep brain stimulation therapy. This led to the fascinating first L-DOPA trial in human PD patients in 1961–1962 only in a window of 5 years of animal experimentation [108]. The prosecution was proposed based on three simple observations (i) a single shot of L-DOPA can reverse the sedative effect of reserpine in rats and mice [109], (ii) striatum harbors the highest amount of brain dopamine [110], and (iii) reduction of dopamine levels in caudate nucleus and putamen of Parkinsonian patients [111]. This happened much before the discovery of the neurotoxin PD animal model. It also led to the discovery of a variety of dopaminergic drugs and DBS (Deep Brain Stimulation). In 1997 *α-synuclein* pathogenesis was discovered, which enlisted PD in the category of protein misfolded disease. So accordingly, the disease modeling has also changed and adapted with time. Therefore, a single model no longer can serve the purpose, and even though the neurotoxin model is beneficial, it must be accompanied by models replicating the disease pathology and its progression. Appropriately using the currently available animal models can lead to new drug interventions. Though they are expensive and time-consuming, when it comes to the ethical background, only animal models can be used for preclinical trials. PD patient-derived stem cells and organoid culture are promising concepts, but they cannot replace the need for animal trials.

It is challenging to amalgamate all the complex biochemical pathways of PD in one animal model; therefore, we can use different models for different pathological aspects of PD. Thus the utility of animal models is indispensable for PD research. But there is no single model that can be used in all conditions. We need to choose the appropriate animal models according to our needs.

7. Conclusion

The early diagnosis of PD is still a major challenge as PD symptoms are very specific to human particularly in the later stage of the disease at which the PD is typically diagnosed in the patients. Diagnosis in early/prodromal stage is difficult due to the inaccessibility of patients. The use of` animal in PD research an also be debated considering the accuracy of the results in animal and human subject. Broadly we can categories the use of animal in PD research in two categories on the basis of purpose of the study i.e. either to develop new therapeutic interventions or to discover novel biomarkers for early diagnosis. Roger A. Barker and Anders Bjorklund (2020), discussed two sides of using animal model in PD. Barker discusses why the animal models are not useful and it is waste of resources on the other hand Anders Bjorklund explains the how the animal models are significantly useful and provide good insights for PD [112]. For therapeutic purpose the use of animal can be debated but for studies intended to discover early diagnostic marker the use of animal models appear to be the best choice. Despite of several failed attempt and the diversity of PD progression between animal models and human, cannot be the reason not use the animal models for further PD research particularly to identify early diagnostic markers. To discover the early diagnostic markers it necessary to have the case and control data from human subject. The major challenge in this step is that it is difficult to have early stage data from human subject because of inaccessibility of the PD patients at prodromal stage. PD is clinically diagnosed in human patients only when motor symptoms appear and has passed the prodromal stage nearly a decade before. Even if we collect the data from patients at prodromal stage it is difficult to say that they are going to show PD in future, which would again take years to develop. Also the symptoms at prodromal stage are very common to other ailments and overlap with the normal aging symptoms. For this reason using animal model has always been a best choice to study the early changes in the group of subject which are given a specific treatment to develop PD. The group of animals subjected to the PD induction can be monitored from very early stage and compared with the control group of similar age.

Acknowledgements

We acknowledge UGC-SAP to the Department of Biotechnology & Bioinformatics, School of Life Sciences, University of Hyderabad, for providing necessary support and infrastructure. We also acknowledge IoE Phase-II, University of Hyderabad (Grant no. 97020066) and DBT, India (No. BT/PR25787/GET/119/96/2017. We also acknowledge DBT, CSIR, UGC, and ICMR for provide fellowship to the NS, MZA, BK and MA respectively.

Conflict of interest

The authors declare no conflict of interest.

Acronyms and abbreviations

6-OHDA	6-Hydroxydopamine
α-synuclein	Alpha-synuclein
AD	Autosomal Dominant
AR	Autosomal Recessive
BBB	Blood-Brain Barrier
CNS	Central Nervous System
DAT	Dopamine Transporter
DBS	Deep Brain Stimulation
GBA	Glucocerebrosidase Gene A
GDNF	Glial cell line-Derived Neurotrophic Factor
LB	Lewy Body
L-DOPA	Levodopa and l-3,4-dihydroxyphenylalanine
MPTP	1-methyl-4-phenyl-1,2,3,6-tetrahydropyridine
NAT	Noradrenaline Transporter
PD	Parkinson's disease
PFFs	Preformed Fibrils
PNS	Peripheral Nervous System
PQ	Paraquat
RBD	Rapid eye movement (REM) sleep Behavior Disorder
SNpc	*Substantia Nigra pars compacta*
VMAT2	Vesicular Monoamine Transporter 2

Author details

Neha S[†], Mohammad Ahmad[†], Baby Kumari[†], MD. Zainul Ali[†]
and Pankaj Singh Dholaniya*[†]
Department of Biotechnology and Bioinformatics, School of Life Sciences, University of Hyderabad, Hyderabad, India

*Address all correspondence to: pankaz@uohyd.ac.in

† These authors contributed equally.

References

[1] Dorsey ER, Sherer T, Okun MS, Bloemd BR. The emerging evidence of the Parkinson pandemic. Journal of Parkinson's Disease. 2018;**8**:S3-S8. DOI: 10.3233/JPD-181474

[2] Yang W, Hamilton JL, Kopil C, Beck JC, Tanner CM, Albin RL, et al. Current and projected future economic burden of Parkinson's disease in the U.S. NPJ Parkinsons Disease. 2020;**6**:6-15. DOI: 10.1038/s41531-020-0117-1

[3] Marsden CD. Parkinson's disease. Lancet. 1990;**335**:948-949. DOI: 10.1016/0140-6736(90)91006-V

[4] Jennings D, Siderowf A, Stern M, Seibyl J, Eberly S, Oakes D, et al. Conversion to Parkinson disease in the PARS Hyposmic and dopamine transporter-deficit prodromal cohort. JAMA Neurology. 2017;**74**: 933-940. DOI: 10.1001/JAMANEUROL.2017.0985

[5] Postuma RB, Gagnon JF, Bertrand JA, Génier Marchand D, Montplaisir JY. Parkinson risk in idiopathic REM sleep behavior disorder: Preparing for neuroprotective trials. Neurology. 2015; **84**:1104-1113. DOI: 10.1212/WNL.0000000000001364

[6] Postuma RB, Berg D. Advances in markers of prodromal Parkinson disease. Nature Reviews. Neurology. 2016;**12**: 622-634. DOI: 10.1038/NRNEUROL.2016.152

[7] Noyce AJ, Bestwick JP, Silveira-Moriyama L, Hawkes CH, Giovannoni G, Lees AJ, et al. Meta-analysis of early nonmotor features and risk factors for Parkinson disease. Annals of Neurology. 2012;**72**:893-901. DOI: 10.1002/ANA.23687

[8] Ugrumov M. Development of early diagnosis of Parkinson's disease: Illusion or reality? CNS Neuroscience & Therapeutics. 2020;**26**:997-1009. DOI: 10.1111/CNS.13429

[9] Haehner A, Boesveldt S, Berendse HW, Mackay-Sim A, Fleischmann J, Silburn PA, et al. Prevalence of smell loss in Parkinson's disease—A multicenter study. Parkinsonism & Related Disorders. 2009;**15**:490-494. DOI: 10.1016/J.PARKRELDIS.2008.12.005

[10] Haehner A, Masala C, Walter S, Reichmann H, Hummel T. Incidence of Parkinson's disease in a large patient cohort with idiopathic smell and taste loss. Journal of Neurology. 2019;**266**: 339-345. DOI: 10.1007/S00415-018-9135-X

[11] Murphy C, Schubert CR, Cruickshanks KJ, Klein BEK, Klein R, Nondahl DM. Prevalence of olfactory impairment in older adults. JAMA. 2002; **288**:2307-2312. DOI: 10.1001/JAMA.288.18.2307

[12] Zhang J. Mining imaging and clinical data with machine learning approaches for the diagnosis and early detection of Parkinson's disease. NPJ Parkinsons Disease. 2022;**8**:13_1-13_15. DOI: 10.1038/s41531-021-00266-8

[13] Shao Y, Le W. Recent advances and perspectives of metabolomics-based investigations in Parkinson's disease. Molecular Neurodegeneration. 2019;**14**: 3(1)-3(12). DOI: 10.1186/s13024-018-0304-2

[14] Agrawal M, Biswas A. Molecular diagnostics of neurodegenerative disorders. Frontiers in Molecular

Biosciences. 2015;**2**:54(1)-54(10). DOI: 10.3389/fmolb.2015.00054

[15] Loh HW, Hong W, Ooi CP, Chakraborty S, Barua PD, Deo RC, et al. Application of deep learning models for automated identification of Parkinson's disease: A review (2011-2021). Sensors. 2021;**21**:7034(1)-7034(25). DOI: 10.3390/s21217034

[16] Schrag A, Horsfall L, Walters K, Noyce A, Petersen I. Prediagnostic presentations of Parkinson's disease in primary care: A case-control study. The Lancet Neurology. 2015;**14**:57-64. DOI: 10.1016/S1474-4422(14)70287-X

[17] Cabreira V, Massano J. Parkinson's disease: Clinical review and update. Acta Medica Portuguesa. 2019;**32**:661-670. DOI: 10.20344/AMP.11978

[18] Kalia L, v., Lang AE. Parkinson's disease. Lancet. 2015;**386**:896-912. DOI: 10.1016/S0140-6736(14)61393-3

[19] Kilzheimer A, Hentrich T, Burkhardt S, Schulze-Hentrich JM. The challenge and opportunity to diagnose Parkinson's disease in midlife. Frontiers in Neurology. 2019;**10**:1328(1)-1328(9). DOI: 10.3389/FNEUR.2019.01328

[20] Bandres-Ciga S, Diez-Fairen M, Kim JJ, Singleton AB. Genetics of Parkinson's disease: An introspection of its journey towards precision medicine. Neurobiology of Disease. 2020;**137**: 104782(1)-104782(9). DOI: 10.1016/j.nbd.2020.104782

[21] Riboldi GM, Fonzo AB Di. GBA, Gaucher disease, and Parkinson's disease: From genetic to clinic to new therapeutic approaches. Cells. 2019;**8**:364(1)-364(16). DOI: 10.3390/cells8040364

[22] Beavan M, McNeill A, Proukakis C, Hughes DA, Mehta A, Schapira AHV. Evolution of prodromal clinical markers of Parkinson disease in a GBA mutation-positive cohort. JAMA Neurology. 2015; **72**:201-208. DOI: 10.1001/JAMANEUROL.2014.2950

[23] Mirelman A, Alcalay RN, Saunders-Pullman R, Yasinovsky K, Thaler A, Gurevich T, et al. Nonmotor symptoms in healthy Ashkenazi Jewish carriers of the G2019S mutation in the LRRK2 gene. Movement Disorders. 2015;**30**:981-986. DOI: 10.1002/MDS.26213

[24] Gatto EM, Parisi V, Converso DP, Poderoso JJ, Carreras MC, Martí-Massó JF, et al. The LRRK2 G2019S mutation in a series of Argentinean patients with Parkinson's disease: Clinical and demographic characteristics. Neuroscience Letters. 2013;**537**:1-5. DOI: 10.1016/J.NEULET.2013.01.011

[25] Gunzler SA, Riley DE, Chen SG, Tatsuoka CM, Johnson WM, Mieyal JJ, et al. Motor and non-motor features of Parkinson's disease in LRRK2 G2019S carriers versus matched controls. Journal of the Neurological Sciences. 2018;**388**: 203-207. DOI: 10.1016/J.JNS.2018.03.025

[26] Zhang J, Zeng H, Zhu L, Deng L, Fang X, Deng X, et al. The potential mutation of GAK gene in the typical sporadic Parkinson's disease from the Han population of Chinese mainland. Molecular Neurobiology. 2016;**53**: 7119-7136. DOI: 10.1007/S12035-015-9595-2

[27] Schrag A, Ben-Shlomo Y, Quinn N. How valid is the clinical diagnosis of Parkinson's disease in the community? Journal of Neurology, Neurosurgery, and Psychiatry. 2002;**73**:529-534. DOI: 10.1136/JNNP.73.5.529

[28] Rajput AH, Rajput A. Accuracy of Parkinson disease diagnosis unchanged in 2 decades. Neurology. 2014;**83**:

386-387. DOI: 10.1212/WNL.0000000000000653

[29] Hughes AJ, Daniel SE, Kilford L, Lees AJ. Accuracy of clinical diagnosis of idiopathic Parkinson's disease: A clinico-pathological study of 100 cases. Journal of Neurology, Neurosurgery, and Psychiatry. 1992;**55**:181-184. DOI: 10.1136/JNNP.55.3.181

[30] Tolosa E, Garrido A, Scholz SW, Poewe W. Challenges in the diagnosis of Parkinson's disease. Lancet Neurology. 2021;**20**:385-397. DOI: 10.1016/S1474-4422(21)00030-2

[31] Rizzo G, Copetti M, Arcuti S, Martino D, Fontana A, Logroscino G. Accuracy of clinical diagnosis of Parkinson disease: A systematic review and meta-analysis. Neurology. 2016;**86**: 566-576. DOI: 10.1212/WNL.0000000000002350

[32] Höglinger GU, Respondek G, Stamelou M, Kurz C, Josephs KA, Lang AE, et al. Clinical diagnosis of progressive supranuclear palsy: The movement disorder society criteria. Movement Disorders. 2017;**32**:853-864. DOI: 10.1002/MDS.26987

[33] Wenning GK, Litvan I, Tolosa E. Milestones in atypical and secondary Parkinsonisms. Movement Disorders. 2011;**26**:1083-1095. DOI: 10.1002/MDS.23713

[34] Koga S, Aoki N, Uitti RJ, van Gerpen JA, Cheshire WP, Josephs KA, et al. When DLB, PD, and PSP masquerade as MSA: An autopsy study of 134 patients. Neurology. 2015;**85**: 404-412. DOI: 10.1212/WNL.0000000000001807

[35] Hughes AJ, Daniel SE, Ben-Shlomo Y, Lees AJ. The accuracy of diagnosis of parkinsonian syndromes in a specialist movement disorder service. Brain. 2002; **125**:861-870. DOI: 10.1093/BRAIN/AWF080

[36] Adler CH, Beach TG, Hentz JG, Shill HA, Caviness JN, Driver-Dunckley E, et al. Low clinical diagnostic accuracy of early vs advanced Parkinson disease: Clinicopathologic study. Neurology. 2014;**83**:406-412. DOI: 10.1212/WNL.0000000000000641

[37] Jennings D, Siderowf A, Stern M, Seibyl J, Eberly S, Oakes D, et al. Imaging prodromal Parkinson disease: The Parkinson associated risk syndrome study. Neurology. 2014;**83**:1739-1746. DOI: 10.1212/WNL.0000000000000960

[38] Berg D, Godau J, Seppi K, Behnke S, Liepelt-Scarfone I, Lerche S, et al. The PRIPS study: Screening battery for subjects at risk for Parkinson's disease. European Journal of Neurology. 2013;**20**: 102-108. DOI: 10.1111/J.1468-1331.2012.03798.X

[39] Gaenslen A, Wurster I, Brockmann K, Huber H, Godau J, Faust B, et al. Prodromal features for Parkinson's disease—Baseline data from the TREND study. European Journal of Neurology. 2014;**21**:766-772. DOI: 10.1111/ENE.12382

[40] Marek K, Jennings D, Lasch S, Siderowf A, Tanner C, Simuni T, et al. The Parkinson progression marker initiative (PPMI). Progress in Neurobiology. 2011;**95**:629-635. DOI: 10.1016/J.PNEUROBIO.2011.09.005

[41] Rees RN, Acharya AP, Schrag A, Noyce AJ. An early diagnosis is not the same as a timely diagnosis of Parkinson's disease. F1000Research. 2018;7:1106(1)-1106(9). DOI: 10.12688/f1000research.14528.1

[42] Annepu J, Ravindranath V. 1-Methyl-4-phenyl-1,2,3,6-tetrahydropyridine-induced complex I inhibition is reversed by disulfide reductant, dithiothreitol in mouse brain. Neuroscience Letters. 2000; **289**:209-212. DOI: 10.1016/S0304-3940(00)01300-8

[43] Elsworth JD, Deutch AY, Redmond DE, Sladek JR, Roth RH. Effects of 1-methyl-4-phenyl-1,2,3,6-tetrahydropyridine (MPTP) on catecholamines and metabolites in primate brain and CSF. Brain Research. 1987;**415**:293-299. DOI: 10.1016/0006-8993(87)90211-3

[44] Peña-Oliver Y, Buchman VL, Stephens DN. Lack of involvement of alpha-synuclein in unconditioned anxiety in mice. Behavioural Brain Research. 2010;**209**:234-240. DOI: 10.1016/J.BBR.2010.01.049

[45] Bhathena SJ. Comparison of effects of decapitation and anesthesia on metabolic and hormonal parameters in Sprague-Dawley rats. Life Sciences. 1992;**50**:1649-1655. DOI: 10.1016/0024-3205(92)90451-T

[46] Fornai F, Lenzi P, Ferrucci M, Lazzeri G, di Poggio AB, Natale G, et al. Occurrence of neuronal inclusions combined with increased nigral expression of alpha-synuclein within dopaminergic neurons following treatment with amphetamine derivatives in mice. Brain Research Bulletin. 2005; **65**:405-413. DOI: 10.1016/J.BRAINRESBULL.2005.02.022

[47] Behavioral, Physiological, and Neurochemical Changes after 6-Hydroxydopamine-Induced Degeneration of the Nigro-Striatal Dopamine Neurons—PubMed. n.d. Available from: https://pubmed.ncbi.nlm.nih.gov/4531217/ [Accessed: July 14, 2022]

[48] Hernandez-Baltazar D, Zavala-Flores LM, Villanueva-Olivo A. The 6-hydroxydopamine model and parkinsonian pathophysiology: Novel findings in an older model. Neurologia (Barcelona, Spain). 2017;**32**:533-539. DOI: 10.1016/J.NRL.2015.06.011

[49] Blandini F, Armentero MT. Animal models of Parkinson's disease. The FEBS Journal. 2012;**279**:1156-1166. DOI: 10.1111/J.1742-4658.2012.08491.X

[50] Cadet JL, Brannock C. Free radicals and the pathobiology of brain dopamine systems. Neurochemistry International. 1998;**32**:117-131. DOI: 10.1016/S0197-0186(97)00031-4

[51] Blum K, Febo M, Badgaiyan RD, Braverman ER, Dushaj K, Li M, et al. Neuronutrient amino-acid therapy protects against reward deficiency syndrome: Dopaminergic key to homeostasis and neuroplasticity. Current Pharmaceutical Design. 2016;**22**: 5837-5854. DOI: 10.2174/1381612822666160719111346

[52] Ostrerova N, Petrucelli L, Farrer M, Mehta N, Choi P, Hardy J, et al. Alpha-Synuclein shares physical and functional homology with 14-3-3 proteins. The Journal of Neuroscience. 1999;**19**: 5782-5791. DOI: 10.1523/JNEUROSCI.19-14-05782.1999

[53] Itier JM, Ibáñez P, Mena MA, Abbas N, Cohen-Salmon C, Bohme GA, et al. Parkin gene inactivation alters behaviour and dopamine neurotransmission in the mouse. Human Molecular Genetics. 2003;**12**:2277-2291. DOI: 10.1093/HMG/DDG239

[54] Brown TP, Rumsby PC, Capleton AC, Rushton L, Levy LS. Pesticides and Parkinson's disease—Is there a link? Environmental Health

Perspectives. 2006;**114**:156-164. DOI: 10.1289/EHP.8095

[55] Thiruchelvam M, Brockel BJ, Richfield EK, Baggs RB, Cory-Slechta DA. Potentiated and preferential effects of combined paraquat and maneb on nigrostriatal dopamine systems: Environmental risk factors for Parkinson's disease? Brain Research. 2000;**873**:225-234. DOI: 10.1016/S0006-8993(00)02496-3

[56] Betarbet R, Sherer TB, MacKenzie G, Garcia-Osuna M, Panov A, v., Greenamyre JT. Chronic systemic pesticide exposure reproduces features of Parkinson's disease. Nature Neuroscience. 2000;**3**:1301-1306. DOI: 10.1038/81834

[57] Greenamyre JT, Cannon JR, Drolet R, Mastroberardino PG. Lessons from the rotenone model of Parkinson's disease. Trends in Pharmacological Sciences. 2010;**31**:141-142. DOI: 10.1016/J.TIPS.2009.12.006

[58] Wu YN, Johnson SW. Dopamine oxidation facilitates rotenone-dependent potentiation of N-methyl-D-aspartate currents in rat substantia nigra dopamine neurons. Neuroscience. 2011; **195**:138-144. DOI: 10.1016/J.NEUROSCIENCE.2011.08.041

[59] Tran J, Anastacio H, Bardy C. Genetic predispositions of Parkinson's disease revealed in patient-derived brain cells. NPJ Parkinsons Disease. 2020;**6**: 8(1)-8(18). DOI: 10.1038/s41531-020-0110-8

[60] Bell S, Rousseau J, Peng H, Aouabed Z, Priam P, Theroux JF, et al. Mutations in ACTL6B cause neurodevelopmental deficits and epilepsy and Lead to loss of dendrites in human neurons. American Journal of Human Genetics. 2019;**104**:815-834. DOI: 10.1016/J.AJHG.2019.03.022

[61] Lautenschläger J, Stephens AD, Fusco G, Ströhl F, Curry N, Zacharopoulou M, et al. C-terminal calcium binding of *α-synuclein* modulates synaptic vesicle interaction. Nature Communications. 2018;**9**:712(1)-712(13). DOI: 10.1038/s41467-018-03111-4

[62] Lee VMY, Trojanowski JQ. Mechanisms of Parkinson's disease linked to pathological alpha-synuclein: New targets for drug discovery. Neuron. 2006;**52**:33-38. DOI: 10.1016/J.NEURON.2006.09.026

[63] Masliah E, Rockenstein E, Veinbergs I, Mallory M, Hashimoto M, Takeda A, et al. Dopaminergic loss and inclusion body formation in alpha-synuclein mice: Implications for neurodegenerative disorders. Science. 2000;**287**:1265-1269. DOI: 10.1126/SCIENCE.287.5456.1265

[64] Multisociety Consensus Quality Improvement Revised Consensus Statement for Endovascular Therapy of Acute Ischemic Stroke—PubMed n.d. Available from: https://pubmed.ncbi.nlm.nih.gov/29786478/ [Accessed: July 14, 2022]

[65] Cilia R, Siri C, Rusconi D, Allegra R, Ghiglietti A, Sacilotto G, et al. LRRK2 mutations in Parkinson's disease: Confirmation of a gender effect in the Italian population. Parkinsonism & Related Disorders. 2014;**20**:911-914. DOI: 10.1016/J.PARKRELDIS.2014.04.016

[66] Healy DG, Falchi M, O'Sullivan SS, Bonifati V, Durr A, Bressman S, et al. Phenotype, genotype, and worldwide genetic penetrance of LRRK2-associated Parkinson's disease: A case-control study.

Lancet Neurology. 2008;7:583-590. DOI: 10.1016/S1474-4422(08)70117-0

[67] Li Y, Liu W, Oo TF, Wang L, Tang Y, Jackson-Lewis V, et al. Mutant LRRK2(R1441G) BAC transgenic mice recapitulate cardinal features of Parkinson's disease. Nature Neuroscience. 2009;**12**:826-828. DOI: 10.1038/NN.2349

[68] Alessi DR, Sammler E. LRRK2 kinase in Parkinson's disease. Science. 1979; **2018**(360):36-37. DOI: 10.1126/science.aar5683

[69] Lee BD, Shin JH, Vankampen J, Petrucelli L, West AB, Ko HS, et al. Inhibitors of leucine-rich repeat kinase-2 protect against models of Parkinson's disease. Nature Medicine. 2010;**16**: 998-1000. DOI: 10.1038/NM.2199

[70] Bajaj N, Hauser RA, Grachev ID. Clinical utility of dopamine transporter single photon emission CT (DaT-SPECT) with (123I) ioflupane in diagnosis of parkinsonian syndromes. Journal of Neurology, Neurosurgery, and Psychiatry. 2013;**84**:1288-1295. DOI: 10.1136/JNNP-2012-304436

[71] Suwijn SR, van Boheemen CJM, de Haan RJ, Tissingh G, Booij J, de Bie RMA. The diagnostic accuracy of dopamine transporter SPECT imaging to detect nigrostriatal cell loss in patients with Parkinson's disease or clinically uncertain parkinsonism: A systematic review. EJNMMI Research. 2015;**5**: 12(1)-12(8). DOI: 10.1186/s13550-015-0087-1

[72] Calloni SF, Conte G, Sbaraini S, Cilia R, Contarino VE, Avignone S, et al. Multiparametric MR imaging of Parkinsonisms at 3 tesla: Its role in the differentiation of idiopathic Parkinson's disease versus atypical parkinsonian disorders. European Journal of Radiology. 2018;**109**:95-100. DOI: 10.1016/J.EJRAD.2018.10.032

[73] Fereshtehnejad SM, Montplaisir JY, Pelletier A, Gagnon JF, Berg D, Postuma RB. Validation of the MDS research criteria for prodromal Parkinson's disease: Longitudinal assessment in a REM sleep behavior disorder (RBD) cohort. Movement Disorders. 2017;**32**:865-873. DOI: 10.1002/MDS.26989

[74] Iranzo A, Tolosa E, Gelpi E, Molinuevo JL, Valldeoriola F, Serradell M, et al. Neurodegenerative disease status and post-mortem pathology in idiopathic rapid-eye-movement sleep behaviour disorder: An observational cohort study. Lancet Neurology. 2013;**12**:443-453. DOI: 10.1016/S1474-4422(13)70056-5

[75] Fayyad M, Salim S, Majbour N, Erskine D, Stoops E, Mollenhauer B, et al. Parkinson's disease biomarkers based on α-synuclein. Journal of Neurochemistry. 2019;**150**:626-636. DOI: 10.1111/JNC.14809

[76] Majbour NK, Vaikath NN, van Dijk KD, Ardah MT, Varghese S, Vesterager LB, et al. Oligomeric and phosphorylated alpha-synuclein as potential CSF biomarkers for Parkinson's disease. Molecular Neurodegeneration. 2016;**11**:7(2)-7(15). DOI: 10.1186/s13024-016-0072-9

[77] Marques TM, Kuiperij HB, Bruinsma IB, van Rumund A, Aerts MB, Esselink RAJ, et al. MicroRNAs in cerebrospinal fluid as potential biomarkers for Parkinson's disease and multiple system atrophy. Molecular Neurobiology. 2017;**54**:7736-7745. DOI: 10.1007/S12035-016-0253-0

[78] Rathnayake D, Chang T, Udagama P. Selected serum cytokines and nitric oxide

as potential multi-marker biosignature panels for Parkinson disease of varying durations: A case-control study. BMC Neurology. 2019;**19**:56(1)-56(10). DOI: 10.1186/s12883-019-1286-6

[79] Perez-Pardo P, Dodiya HB, Engen PA, Forsyth CB, Huschens AM, Shaikh M, et al. Role of TLR4 in the gut-brain axis in Parkinson's disease: A translational study from men to mice. Gut. 2019;**68**:829-843. DOI: 10.1136/GUTJNL-2018-316844

[80] Chen XQ, Niu JP, Peng RQ, Song YH, Xu N, Zhang YW. The early diagnosis of Parkinson's disease through combined biomarkers. Acta Neurologica Scandinavica. 2019;**140**:268-273. DOI: 10.1111/ANE.13140

[81] Parnetti L, Chiasserini D, Persichetti E, Eusebi P, Varghese S, Qureshi MM, et al. Cerebrospinal fluid lysosomal enzymes and alpha-synuclein in Parkinson's disease. Movement Disorders. 2014;**29**:1019-1027. DOI: 10.1002/MDS.25772

[82] Matsusue E, Fujihara Y, Tanaka K, Aozasa Y, Shimoda M, Nakayasu H, et al. The utility of the combined use of 123 I-FP-CIT SPECT and neuromelanin MRI in differentiating Parkinson's disease from other parkinsonian syndromes. Acta Radiologica. 2019;**60**: 230-238. DOI: 10.1177/0284185118778871

[83] Foltynie T, Brayne C, Barker RA. The heterogeneity of idiopathic Parkinson's disease. Journal of Neurology. 2002;**249**:138-145. DOI: 10.1007/PL00007856

[84] Stoker TB, Greenland JC. Parkinson's Disease: Pathogenesis and Clinical Aspects [Internet]. Codon Publications; 2018. DOI: 10.15586/codonpublications.parkinsonsdisease.2018. Available from: https://pubmed.ncbi.nlm.nih.gov/30702835/

[85] Aerts L, Miccoli B, Delahanty A, Witters H, Verstraelen S, Strooper B De, et al. Do we still need animals? Surveying the role of animalfree models in Alzheimer's and Parkinson's disease research. The EMBO Journal. 2022;**41**: 1-8. DOI: 10.15252/embj.2021110002

[86] Breger LS, Fuzzati Armentero MT. Genetically engineered animal models of Parkinson's disease: From worm to rodent. The European Journal of Neuroscience. 2019;**49**:533-560. DOI: 10.1111/EJN.14300

[87] Lama J, Buhidma Y, Fletcher EJR, Duty S. Animal models of Parkinson's disease: A guide to selecting the optimal model for your research. Neuronal. Signals. 2021;**5**:1-24. DOI: 10.1042/NS20210026

[88] Schwarting RKW, Huston JP. The unilateral 6-hydroxydopamine lesion model in behavioral brain research. Analysis of functional deficits, recovery and treatments. Progress in Neurobiology. 1996;**50**:275-331. DOI: 10.1016/S0301-0082(96)00040-8

[89] Bugos O, Bhide M, Zilka N. Beyond the rat models of human neurodegenerative disorders. Cellular and Molecular Neurobiology. 2009;**29**: 859-869. DOI: 10.1007/S10571-009-9367-5

[90] Beal MF. Parkinson's disease: A model dilemma. Nature. 2010;**466**: S8-S10. DOI: 10.1038/466S8a

[91] Cenci MA, Björklund A. Animal models for preclinical Parkinson's research: An update and critical appraisal. Progress in Brain Research. 2020;**252**:27-59. DOI: 10.1016/BS.PBR.2020.02.003

[92] Jiang P, Dickson DW. Parkinson's disease: Experimental models and reality. Acta Neuropathologica. 2018;**135**: 13-32. DOI: 10.1007/S00401-017-1788-5

[93] Tu Z, Yang W, Yan S, Guo X, Li X-J. CRISPR/Cas9: A powerful genetic engineering tool for establishing large animal models of neurodegenerative diseases. Molecular Neurodegeneration. 2015;**10**:35(1)-35(8). DOI: 10.1186/s13024-015-0031-x

[94] Niu Y, Guo X, Chen Y, Wang CE, Gao J, Yang W, et al. Early Parkinson's disease symptoms in *α-synuclein* transgenic monkeys. Human Molecular Genetics. 2015;**24**:2308-2317. DOI: 10.1093/HMG/DDU748

[95] Yang W, Wang G, Wang CE, Guo X, Yin P, Gao J, et al. Mutant alpha-synuclein causes age-dependent neuropathology in monkey brain. The Journal of Neuroscience. 2015;**35**: 8345-8358. DOI: 10.1523/JNEUROSCI.0772-15.2015

[96] Potashkin JA, Blume SR, Runkle NK. Limitations of animal models of Parkinson's disease. Parkinson's Disease. 2010;**2011**:658083(1)-658083(8). DOI: 10.4061/2011/658083

[97] Holmqvist S, Chutna O, Bousset L, Aldrin-Kirk P, Li W, Björklund T, et al. Direct evidence of Parkinson pathology spread from the gastrointestinal tract to the brain in rats. Acta Neuropathologica. 2014;**128**:805-820. DOI: 10.1007/S00401-014-1343-6

[98] Kim S, Kwon SH, Kam TI, Panicker N, Karuppagounder SS, Lee S, et al. Transneuronal propagation of pathologic *α-synuclein* from the gut to the brain models Parkinson's disease. Neuron. 2019;**103**:627-641.e7. DOI: 10.1016/J.NEURON.2019.05.035

[99] van den Berge N, Ferreira N, Mikkelsen TW, Alstrup AKO, Tamgüney G, Karlsson P, et al. Ageing promotes pathological alpha-synuclein propagation and autonomic dysfunction in wild-type rats. Brain. 2021;**144**: 1853-1868. DOI: 10.1093/BRAIN/AWAB061

[100] Wang X-J, Ma M-M, Zhou L-B, Jiang X-Y, Hao M-M, Teng RKF, et al. Autonomic ganglionic injection of *α-synuclein* fibrils as a model of pure autonomic failure α-synucleinopathy. Nature Communications. 2020;**11**: 934(1)-934(13). DOI: 10.1038/s41467-019-14189-9

[101] Shen Y, Yu WB, Shen B, Dong H, Zhao J, Tang YL, et al. Propagated α-synucleinopathy recapitulates REM sleep behaviour disorder followed by parkinsonian phenotypes in mice. Brain. 2020;**143**:3374-3392. DOI: 10.1093/BRAIN/AWAA283

[102] Taguchi T, Ikuno M, Hondo M, Parajuli LK, Taguchi K, Ueda J, et al. *α-synuclein* BAC transgenic mice exhibit RBD-like behaviour and hyposmia: A prodromal Parkinson's disease model. Brain. 2020;**143**:249-265. DOI: 10.1093/BRAIN/AWZ380

[103] Taylor TN, Caudle WM, Shepherd KR, Noorian AR, Jackson CR, Iuvone PM, et al. Nonmotor symptoms of Parkinson's disease revealed in an animal model with reduced monoamine storage capacity. The Journal of Neuroscience. 2009;**29**:8103-8113. DOI: 10.1523/JNEUROSCI.1495-09.2009

[104] Irwin DJ, Abrams JY, Schonberger LB, Leschek EW, Mills JL, Lee VMY, et al. Evaluation of potential infectivity of Alzheimer and Parkinson disease proteins in recipients of cadaver-derived human growth hormone. JAMA

Neurology. 2013;**70**:462-468. DOI: 10.1001/JAMANEUROL.2013.1933

[105] Strohäker T, Jung BC, Liou S-H, Fernandez CO, Riedel D, Becker S, et al. Structural heterogeneity of *α-synuclein* fibrils amplified from patient brain extracts. Nature Communications. 2019; **10**:5535(1)-5535(12). DOI: 10.1038/s41467-019-13564-w

[106] Decressac M, Kadkhodaei B, Mattsson B, Laguna A, Perlmann T, Björklund A. α-Synuclein-induced down-regulation of Nurr1 disrupts GDNF signaling in nigral dopamine neurons. Science Translational Medicine. 2012;**4**:163ra156(1)-163ra156(15). DOI: 10.1126/scitranslmed.3004676

[107] Kirkeby A, Barker RA. Parkinson disease and growth factors—Is GDNF good enough? Nature Reviews. Neurology. 2019;**15**:312-314. DOI: 10.1038/S41582-019-0180-6

[108] The L-3,4-dioxyphenylalanine (DOPA)-effect in Parkinson-akinesia—PubMed n.d. Available from: https://pubmed.ncbi.nlm.nih.gov/13869404/ [Accessed: July 14, 2022]

[109] Carlsson A, Lindqvist M, Magnusson T. 3,4-Dihydroxyphenylalanine and 5-hydroxytryptophan as reserpine antagonists. Nature. 1957;**180**:1200. DOI: 10.1038/1801200A0

[110] Bertler Å, Rosengren E. Occurrence and distribution of dopamine in brain and other tissues. Experientia. 1959;**15**: 10-11. DOI: 10.1007/BF02157069

[111] Ehringer H, Hornykiewicz O. Distribution of noradrenaline and dopamine (3-hydroxytyramine) in the human brain and their behavior in diseases of the extrapyramidal system. Klinische Wochenschrift. 1960;**38**: 1236-1239. DOI: 10.1007/BF01485901

[112] Barker RA, Björklund A. Animal models of Parkinson's disease: Are they useful or not? Journal of Parkinson's Disease. 2020;**10**:1335-1342. DOI: 10.3233/JPD-202200

Chapter 5

Sexual Dysfunction in Neurological Disorders with Special Emphasis on Parkinson's Disease: Insights from Clinical Studies and Animal Models

Zevelou Koza, Padmanabhan S. Rajani, Muralidhara, Ajaikumar B. Kunnumakkara and Sarat Chandra Yenisetti

Abstract

Epidemiological studies illustrate that sexual dysfunction (SD) is common among the majority of patients suffering from neurological disorders (NLDs). However, our understanding of the SD in NLDs is in its infancy. Our effort in this review article reveals how the clinical studies illustrate different phenotypes relating to SD in both men and women suffering from NLDs, with special reference to PD, and how the development of animal models will provide a fantastic opportunity to decipher mechanistic insights into the biological and molecular processes of SD, understanding of which is critical to figure out the causes of SD and to develop therapeutic strategies either by targeting molecular players or altering and/or regulating the profiles of involved genetic targets. Specific emphasis is placed on dopamine-dependent and independent mechanism(s) of SD among PD patients, which is important because certain critical dopamine-independent phenotypes are yet to be characterized and understood in order to decipher the comprehensive pathophysiology of PD. Synergic efforts of both clinicians and bench scientists in this critical direction would significantly improve the quality of life of sufferers of NLDs who are already burdened. This knowledge relating to SD will help us to make one more step in reducing the burden of disease.

Keywords: sexual dysfunction, neurodegenerative disorders, Parkinson's disease, dopamine, animal models, drosophila, rat, mice

1. Introduction

In humans, sexual behavior is classified into two main activities: sexual desire and sexual arousal. Sexual desire is represented by libido/sexual drive [1], whereas sexual arousal is the ability to respond to an appropriate sexual stimulus with a sequence of stereotyped vascular, neural, and muscular reactions [2]. The typical sexual response cycle of men consists of libido, erection, ejaculation, orgasm, and

IntechOpen

detumescence [3]. In women, the sexual cycle follows a parallel framework as in men, such as libido, arousal, orgasm, and satisfaction [4]. A problem occurring during any phase of this sexual response cycle, which prevents the individual from experiencing satisfaction from the sexual activity, is referred to as sexual dysfunction (SD). The human sexual response cycle, therefore, sets the foundation for studying and categorizing SD in men and women. As reported by Hatzimouratidis and Hatzichristou [5], numerous measures have been taken since 1992 to define and classify SD in a precise manner. Although a number of classification systems were proposed for SD, the two most widely used classification systems are the International Classification of Diseases (ICD)-10 provided by the World Health Organization [6] and the Diagnostic and Statistical Manual of Mental Disorders (DSM)-IV provided by the American Psychiatric Association [7]. The four major categories of SD as described by both systems include disorders of sexual desire/interest, arousal, orgasm, and sexual pain.

These dysfunctions of sexual function are extremely common in patients with neurological disorders (NLD). NLDs are diverse forms of central nervous system disorders distinguished by the continuing loss of neural tissues because they alter the normal sexual functions in both men and women patients [8].

2. Prevalence of sexual dysfunction in neurological disorders

Disorders of sexual function are common among men of all ages, ethnicities, and cultural backgrounds. SD is highly prevalent in both sexes, ranging from 10 to 52% of men and 25 to 63% of women [9–11]. It is reported that more than 18 million men in the United States alone and 40 million men in the European Union are affected by erectile dysfunction (ED), and individuals suffering from this dysfunction are estimated to reach 322 million by 2025. Aberrant sexual function is reported in several diseases, namely, arterial hypertension, diabetes, metabolic syndrome, coronary diseases, neurological diseases (stroke, epilepsy, multiple sclerosis, Parkinson's disease), and psychiatric disorders [12]. Below are some of the neurological disorders and the prevalence of SD in these patients.

2.1 Multiple sclerosis

Multiple sclerosis (MS) is a continual inflammatory demyelinating disease of the central nervous system along with the presence of relapsing–remitting attacks of inflammation, demyelination, and axonal damage, causing a broad spectrum of neurological symptoms and impairment both in men and women. The symptoms of MS include weakness and imbalance, visual abnormalities, changes in cognition, bladder, and sexual dysfunction (SD) [13], which affect young adults in their sexually active phase of life [14]. MS occurs due to the integrated effects of genetic, environmental, infectious factors, and vascular problems but chiefly due to an autoimmune mechanism [15].

SD is extremely common in MS sufferers, affecting 40–80% of women and 50–90% of men [16] and has an adverse impact on the quality of life (QoL) of these patients. Although SD is a painful symptom, most often it goes underreported and underdiagnosed in MS, because of the patients and physicians' reluctance with the topic [17]. The symptoms of SD in MS men include ED, ejaculatory dysfunction, orgasmic dysfunction, and reduced libido [17]. Whereas low libido, orgasmic dysfunction, reduction in the tactile sensations originating from the thigh and genital regions, and vaginal dryness with subsequent dyspareunia (difficulty in sexual activity) are some of the sexual symptoms in MS women [18]. SD in MS is mainly due to the lesions affecting the neural pathways involved in physiologic function and also the psychological impact of the disease on the patients [14]. All these studies show that SD is highly prevalent in MS patients, and there is a need for both the patients and the neurologist to discuss more about this symptom, which otherwise is neglected.

2.2 Epilepsy

Epilepsy is the most prevalent chronic NLD, represented by an episodic seizure that demands lifelong management with medication [19]. Mameniškienė et al. [20] reported in their study the high prevalence of sexual problems in one third of epileptic patients and only a quarter of them seeking medical help. Dysfunctions such as decrease in sexual desire, potency, orgasm, and ED were reported by male epileptic patients [21]. Sexual symptoms in epileptic women include decreased sexual arousal, vaginismus, and dyspareunia [22]. The most common SD in males were ED and early ejaculation, whereas female's lack of sexual interest and failure to reach orgasm were the most common sexual problems based on several studies on epilepsy [23].

The cause of SD in epileptic patients is multifactorial in nature, such as the effects of antiepileptic drugs on neurotransmission, the epilepsy itself, and psychosocial factors associated with it, but the presence of hormonal changes in epileptic patients is believed to be one of the prominent factors for SD [24]. All these studies illustrate the common presence of SD in both male and female epileptic patients and highlight the multifactorial nature of this dysfunction.

2.3 Multiple system atrophy

Multiple system atrophy (MSA) is a progressive neurodegenerative disease of unspecified etiology, affecting both males and females [25]. Symptoms of the disease include motor symptoms (gait, coordination, and muscle tone) and non-motor features (cardiovascular, gastrointestinal, genitourinary, sleep disorders, cognitive, mood, and behavioral problems, dysphagia, SD, and visual abnormalities [26]). SD such as impairment in ED was reported to be the first symptom of the disease in men [27]. In another study, reduced genital sensitivity in female MSA patients was one of the early manifestations of the disease [28]. Sexual problems in MSA are believed to be due to abnormalities in the central and peripheral nervous systems in MSA patients [29]. All these studies elucidate the importance of SD in the early diagnosis of the disease.

2.4 Huntington's disease

Huntington's disease (HD) is a chronic disabling disease caused by a single defective gene on chromosome 4 affecting the basal ganglia region of the brain and is linked with aberrant sexual behaviors. A total of 85% of men and 75% of women complain of sexual problems, such as hypoactive and hyperactive sexual disorders and paraphilia in certain cases [30]. Huntington's female patients suffer from sexual problems, such as difficulty in arousal, lubrication, orgasm, and sexual dissatisfaction, that impair their quality of life [31]. Whereas in male patients, problems with erection, reduced sexual desire, and performance are some of the common sexual problems [32]. SD in HD is reported to be due to the progression of the disease and its associated symptoms, such as depression or dementia, the decline in patient's motor functions, and side effects of medication [31]. Although only a few studies have been conducted on sexuality in HD, all these studies show that SD is extremely common in these patients and that sexual disorders may take the form of hypoactive to increased sexual interest or paraphilias.

2.5 Amyotrophic lateral sclerosis

Amyotrophic lateral sclerosis (ALS) is a progressive disorder of motor neurons in the brain and spinal cord [33]. ALS patients were found to have problems with their sexual relationship due to impaired sexual function such as decreased libido [34], with studies indicating that ALS had the worst rates of SD when compared with other NLDs [35]. Shahbazi et al. [36] reported that although SD affected the QoL in ALS patients, 75% of their clinicians were not familiar with any strategies or interventions to help the patients. This shows the need to further explore sexuality in both ALS men and women. The change in sexual functions in ALS patients was due to the physical and psychosocial factors associated with the disease [34]. All these studies show that sexuality in patients with ALS has received little attention, and sexual function is rarely assessed in both male and female ALS patients.

2.6 Schizophrenia

Schizophrenia is a severe psychiatric disorder that attacks close to about 1% of the world's population with no concrete etiology [37]. The neurodevelopmental postulation of schizophrenia caused by genetics or environmental elements is one of the glaring reasons for the disease, which leads to the alteration of important and fine signaling pathways, resulting in the initial presentation of the disease [38]. It is identified by positive symptoms such as delusions and hallucinations, negative symptoms such as emotional withdrawal and apathy, and cognitive deficits such as impaired attention, learning, and memory [39]. The age of onset of schizophrenia in men is between the ages of 16 and 25 years, and in women from 25 to 35 years.

Schizophrenia affects individuals at their prime reproductive age, with a negative impact on sexual functions of both male and female patients [40]. The extensiveness of SD in schizophrenic patients was 31.1–82.7%. In males, the prevalence of SD was 82–84.5%; and in female patients, the prevalence was 78.6–92% [41]. Reduced sexual desire was frequently reported by the patients [42]. Dysfunction such as ED (95.2%) was the most common complaint in men followed by pleasure dysfunction (94.2%). In female patients, pleasure dysfunction (94.7%) was the most prevalent SD followed by arousal/excitement dysfunction (93.2%) [41]. The use of antipsychotic medication is believed to be one of the important causes of SD. Postsynaptic dopamine antagonism, prolactin elevation, and α1-receptor blockade are some of the factors behind the pathogenesis of antipsychotic-induced SD [40]. All these studies illustrate the high existence of SD in both male and female schizophrenic patients and its negative impact on the quality of life of these young patients.

2.7 Alzheimer's disease

Alzheimer's disease (AD) is one of the most widespread forms of dementia, consisting of 60–70% of all dementia cases [43] and affecting 35 million individuals worldwide with 5.4 million Americans alone [44]. AD has a significant effect on the sexual behavior of the patients [45], and loss of sexual interest and decreased sexual activity are the two common types of sexual disorders in AD patients [46]. Studies have shown that 53% of male AD patients suffer erectile failure or loss of erection [47]. Thus, the onset of the disease affects the relationship between the patient and their partner because of the presence of high sexual dissatisfaction [48]. The cause of this sexual impairment in AD is believed to be due to a decline in the patient's ability to consent, physical vulnerability, depression, anxiety, and medical conditions related to the disease [49]. All these studies show that SD is not uncommon in AD patients, which deteriorates the relationship between patients and their spouses.

2.8 Parkinson's disease

Parkinson's disease (PD) is the second most prevalent neurodegenerative disorder that affects about 1% of the population over the age of 50 [50]. PD was first reported by James Parkinson in 1817, and symptoms such as trembling, difficulty walking and standing, tiredness, sleep disturbances, drooling, difficulty swallowing, gastrointestinal dysfunction, and bladder dysfunction were all described by James Parkinson in his early study [51]. Today, symptoms of PD are classified into motor and non-motor symptoms (NMS). Motor problems such as resting tremors, bradykinesia, rigidity, and postural abnormalities [52] are some of the symptoms with which clinicians diagnose PD. However, over the years, the NMS of PD has gained a lot of interest because several studies have supported that non-motor issues preceded the motor manifestation of the disease [53] and may even project the future development of PD years or even decades earlier than a motor-based diagnosis [54]. The spectrum of NMS in PD includes loss of sense of smell, rapid eye movement (REM) sleep disturbances, daytime drowsiness, delusions, difficulty in concentration, drooling, difficulty swallowing, episodes of confusion, fatigue, impulse control disorders (ICDs), memory problems, depression and anxiety, pain paranoia, sensation of breathlessness, sweating, postural hypotension, urinary problems, gastrointestinal dysfunction, and SD [55].

Data from a number of studies report the prevalence of non-motor disorders affecting PD patients [56], but unless specifically investigated, it goes unreported with no adequate treatment available [57]. Epidemiological studies of non-motor symptoms of PD such as the presence of REM sleep behavior disorder, olfactory dysfunction, urinary disorder, and constipation [58] are known to clearly increase the future chance of developing PD. Symptoms such as constipation, anxiety disorders, RBD, and anemia were shown to precede the motor dysfunction by at least 20 years, whereas olfactory impairment and depression preceded the motor symptoms with a lag time of 2 to 10 years [53]. Therefore, such studies show that NMS of PD can play an important role as a predictive biomarker for the identification of a population at greater risk of developing the disease.

3. Sexual dysfunction in Parkinson's disease subjects

Sexual dysfunction in men is generally defined as the inability to achieve or maintain an erection until the completion of sexual activity. Whereas in women, SD is the disruption in sexual desire and in the psychophysiological changes that identify the sexual response cycle and cause marked distress and interpersonal difficulty [7]. SD is one of the most common non-motor disorders affecting Parkinsonian patients [59]. Although SD remains one of the prominent symptoms of PD, it is the most neglected, underreported, and under-recognized aspect of PD [59].

Singer and colleagues [60] conducted the first study on PD men to show that these men had worse sexual problems when compared with non-Parkinsonian healthy individuals. Thereafter, several studies have reported the widespread presence of sexual impairments in Parkinsonian patients [61, 62]. Some of the most common sexual malfunctions in PD men were a decrease in libido/ loss of sexual interest, decrease in frequency of sexual intercourse, decrease in orgasm/inability to experience orgasm/ orgasmic dissatisfaction, decrease in erection/ED, difficulties/delayed in ejaculation, premature ejaculation [59, 62]. In PD women, the sexual impairment ranged from decrease in libido/loss of sexual interest, decrease in frequency of sexual intercourse, inability to experience orgasm/difficulty reaching orgasm, orgasmic dissatisfaction, difficulty with arousal, and dyspareunia [61, 62]. All these studies and findings in PD subjects indicate the extent of sexual impairments in PD sufferers and the urgency of effective therapeutic intervention in the management of SD in PD. The nature of SD among male and female patients and its prevalence are elaborated in **Table 1**.

SD, such as ED, was shown to act as an early marker for detection of individuals who are at higher risk of developing PD in the near future. A study conducted by

Sexual dysfunction in PD men		
Nature of sexual problems	**Prevalence in PD patients**	**References**
Erectile dysfunction (ED)	42.6–79%	[60, 61, 63, 64]
Premature ejaculation	40.6%–51.4%	[61, 62]
Difficulties ejaculating	27.3–79%	[61, 64]
Difficulties reaching orgasm	39.5–87%	[61, 63]
Low sexual desire	23.3–84%	[61, 63–65]
Reduced sexual activity	33.4–55%	[63, 65]
Dissatisfaction with sexual life	59–65.1%	[61, 66]
Sexual dysfunctions in PD women		
Nature of Sexual Problems	Prevalence in PD patients	References
Dyspareunia (painful sex)	12.5%	[61]
Difficulties in getting aroused	87.5%	[61]
Difficulties reaching orgasm	72–75%	[61, 62]
Low sexual desire	46.9–83%	[61, 63, 65]
Orgasmic Dissatisfaction	76%	[62]
Reduced sexual activity	75–88%	[63–65]
Dissatisfaction with sexual life	36–37.5%	[61, 66]

Table 1.
Nature of sexual dysfunction in Parkinson's disease patients.

[67] reported that individuals with ED were 3.8-fold more likely to develop PD when compared to subjects without ED. Medical record review found that ED was more prevalent in individuals who later developed PD compared with non-PD individuals at 5 years and 2 years prior to diagnosis [68]. In PD patients with idiopathic RBD, ED was noticed 7 years before the disease conversion, with an extrapolated prodromal interval of 11 years [69]. Thus, the above studies show that sexual malfunction such as ED is a good marker for early detection of individuals at risk of developing PD. Therefore, people with any type of SD must take preventive measures and check for necessary assistance.

4. Factors responsible and insights into the mechanism of sexual dysfunction in Parkinson's disease

4.1 Age

In PD, advancing age of an individual is one of the major risk factors for the development and progression of the disease [70]. Even in the absence of any clinical or medical conditions, aging process was shown to play a key role in the development of SD such as a decrease in potency and ED [71]. However, a study conducted on PD patients and non-PD individuals shows that with age, sexual function was worse in PD patients than in the normal elderly population [72]. In addition, in aged PD patients, disease severity or disease duration did not have any effect on PD-related changes in sexual function [73]. Thus, all these studies suggest that SD is more prevalent in the PD population, and age has little effect on the sexual function of these patients.

Dysfunction in normal sexual functions is not only limited to aging Parkinson's patients but also young PD individuals were reported to be affected more often by this dysfunction [8, 70, 73]. In addition, SD was one of the greatest concerns of the disease in young patients [74]. Another study was conducted to see the effect of PD's age of onset on the sexual function of the patients and reported that 59% of early-onset PD (EOPD) patients suffer from sexual problems as compared to 80.3% of late-onset PD (LOPD) patients [75]. Thus, suggesting that SD is not only limited to aging Parkinson's patients but also very prevalent even in young PD patients.

4.2 Involvement of dopamine and dopaminergic pathways

Dopamine (DA), the chief neurotransmitter in the central nervous system (CNS), plays a role in facilitating sexual motivation, copulation, and genital reflexes [76] by regulating sexual behaviors through the determination of the strength of libido, arousal, and erection. Early clinical studies show that l-3, 4-dihydroxyphenylalanine (L-DOPA), the precursor of DA, induces penile erection in men with PD [77], supporting the involvement of DA in sexual behavior. However, disruptions in the hypothalamic area in PD in relation to SD have not been well studied [62]. Moreover, the use of various DA agonists in animal models for the treatment of SD provides strong evidence of the involvement of the dopaminergic system in the control of sexual function in mammals such as humans.

Below are the several studies done on animal models to show the involvement of DA in the normal sexual function:

4.2.1 Rat model

Rat models were used to understand the SD caused by death in the dopaminergic neurons of the *substantia nigra* (SN). In rats, the central dopaminergic neurons project in the medial preoptic area and paraventricular nucleus and travel from the hypothalamus to the lumbosacral spinal cord, controlling both the autonomic and somatic components of penile reflexes [78]. Experimental rats injected with 6-hydroxydopmaine, a DA antagonist, mimic PD by destroying dopaminergic SN cells. These rats showed a decrease in the number of erections and a complete absence of SN *pars compacta* in the brain when compared to normal rats. Quantification of DA and its metabolites using HPLC (high-performance liquid chromatography) also showed a significant decline in their levels in both hemispheres of the brain, with a significant reduction in the right hemisphere when compared to normal rats [79]. As also shown, the right hemisphere is involved in the sexual functions of mammals including humans [80]. This study suggests DA in the hemisphere plays a vital role in the observed SD in the rat models and could likely be the possibility among human PD patients.

Several other studies show that DA antagonist inhibits sexual behaviors such as copulation, genital reflexes, and sexual motivation in rats [81]. Whereas DA agonists restored the copulation activity of male rats by reducing the latency of ejaculation, producing spontaneous ejaculation and enhancing penile erection [18]. Male rats with 6-hydroxydopamine or radiofrequency lesions in the nucleus accumbens showed a low incidence of noncontact erection, indicating the role of DA in arousal processes in responding to remote cues from estrous females [82]. All these studies suggest that DA is the crucial neurotransmitter in the regulation of sexual functions involved in both sexual motivation and sexual performance, which is likely the case in humans.

4.2.2 Mice model

A study was done on a mice model to show the effect of DA and its agonist on the sexual behavior of the mice. DA was shown to influence the rewarding aspects of intromissions in both male and female mice, and DA receptors were essential for the actions of DA on the receptivity of male and female sexual behavior [83]. Apomorphine, a DA agonist shows pro-erectile effects (erection, erection-like responses, and genital grooming) in mice models by activating the central dopaminergic receptors (D2) [84]. All these studies illustrate that dopamine agonists can be a possible therapeutic agent to address ED-related SD in PD subjects.

4.2.3 Drosophila model

Study using *Drosophila* as model animal has shown that dopamine regulates the male courtship intensity via the dopaminergic neurons PPL2ab (protocerebral posteriolateral dopaminergic cluster neuron 2ab); and by increasing the DA levels in these neurons, the decreased courtship activity in aged male flies was reinstated [85]. Kuo and co-workers demonstrated it both quantitatively and qualitatively by observing the behavioral assay of male fly via courtship index (percentage of time spent on courtship behavior), which is a quantitative expression of courtship duration; and courtship bout length (indicates the degree to which the courtship period was fragmented between courtship and non-courtship behavior), which quantifies courtship episode duration. Whereas when DA levels were downregulated, there was a significant decrease in the courtship index and courtship bout length in males. This study therefore highlights the importance of DA in regulating sexual activity in flies. Disruption in the dopaminergic neurotransmission also shows a significant reduction in the male's courtship behavior towards a female [86]. A *Drosophila* model of SD of PD was first reported by Shaltiel-Karyo et al. [87]. They used the *Drosophila* α-syn model where there is a loss of DA neurons and showed that this male fly has impaired sexual function and performs an overall less sexual activity in the courtship parameters of orientation, wing vibration, licking, attempted copulation, nonsexual encounter, and copulation [87]. All these studies illustrate the direct involvement of dopamine in the regulation of sexual behavior, which is likely the case in humans.

4.3 Non-dopaminergic pathways and sexual dysfunction

Because degeneration of dopaminergic neurons is the critical pathological hallmark associated with PD, I have primarily focused on the involvement of dopaminergic pathways in SD. However, it has been reported that other various factors/pathways are involved in human sexual function. Meston and Frohlich [88] provided a concise review of several factors that influence male and female sexual function such as (a) the endocrine factors: androgens, estrogens, progesterone, prolactin, oxytocin, cortisol, and pheromones; and (b) neurotransmitters and neuropeptides: nitric oxide, serotonin, epinephrine, norepinephrine, opioids, acetylcholine, histamine, and g-aminobutyric acid. In spite of their involvement in sexual function, no detailed information is available whether these factors/pathways are involved in SD of PD.

Of all these non-DA pathways, it has been demonstrated that PD patients over the age of 60 were reported to have low levels of testosterone [89]). Testosterone deficiency encompasses several domains, namely, sexual, physical, psychological, and cognitive. SD such as decreased or lost sexual desire diminished nocturnal and morning erections, and ED are often among the most recognized symptoms of testosterone deficiency [90]. In a case study involving five PD patients over the age of 60 with symptoms of testosterone deficiency, patients experienced significant improvement in their sexual functions following testosterone replacement therapy [91]. A daily dose of transdermal testosterone gel given to PD patients with testosterone deficiency showed improvement in their sexual function such as libido [91]. Apart from this, not much/nothing has been studied about the involvement of other factors with reference to SD in PD.

5. Conclusion and future aspects

SD, such as a decrease in desire and ED, are extremely common in NLD. SD greatly impacts the quality of life of patients and their spouses. Although SD is common in NLDs such as PD, it remains one of the most neglected and understudied symptoms of the disease. SD affects some 80% of PD patients, and the cause of this dysfunction can be multifactorial in nature and a mechanism that is poorly understood to date. However, several studies have implicated the role of dopamine in the regulation of sexual function in a wide variety of animal models including humans. But little progress has been made in the area of exploring sexuality in these diseases, which greatly hampers the overall quality of life of the patients. The multifactorial causes of SD in NLD make it difficult for an effective therapeutic treatment. Further studies to understand the mechanisms of SD in NLD such as PD will greatly help in identifying therapeutic targets for sexual problems. Here lies the challenge and great opportunity for both clinicians and bench scientists.

Acknowledgements

This work is supported by DBT (Department of Biotechnology), India Grant nos. BT/405/NE/U-Excel/2013, 11/12/2014; and NECBH/2019-2020/153, (Eureka category), 29-4-2019).

Author details

Zevelou Koza[1], Padmanabhan S. Rajani[2], Muralidhara[2], Ajaikumar B. Kunnumakkara[3] and Sarat Chandra Yenisetti[1*]

1 Drosophila Neurobiology Laboratory, Nagaland University (Central), Nagaland State, India

2 CSIR-Central Food Technological Research Institute (CFTRI), Mysuru, India

3 Cancer Biology Laboratory and DBT-AIST International Laboratory for Advanced Biomedicine (DAILAB), Department of Biosciences and Bioengineering, Indian Institute of Technology Guwahati, Guwahati, Assam, India

*Address all correspondence to: sarat@nagalanduniversity.ac.in; yschandrays@rediffmail.com

References

[1] Montouris G, Morris GL III. Reproductive and sexual dysfunction in men with epilepsy. Epilepsy & Behavior. 2005;**7**:7-14

[2] Morrell MJ. Sexual dysfunction in epilepsy. Epilepsia. 1991;**32**:38-45

[3] Kandeel FR, Koussa VK, Swerdloff RS. Male sexual function and its disorders: Physiology, pathophysiology, clinical investigation, and treatment. Endocrine Reviews. 2001;**22**:342-388

[4] Ho CC, Singam P, Hong GE, Zainuddin ZM. Male sexual dysfunction in Asia. Asian Journal of Andrology. 2011;**13**:537-542

[5] Hatzimouratidis K, Hatzichristou D. Sexual dysfunctions: Classifications and definitions. The Journal of Sexual Medicine. 2007;**4**:241-250

[6] World Health Organization. ICD-10: International Statistical Classification of Diseases and Related Health Problems. Geneva: World Health Organization; 1992

[7] American Psychiatric Association. Diagnostic and Statistical Manual of Mental Disorders DSM-IV. 4th ed. Washington, DC: American Psychiatric Press; 1994. pp. 493-522

[8] Rees PM, Fowler CJ, Maas CP. Sexual function in men and women with neurological disorders. Lancet. 2007;**369**:512-525

[9] Spector IP, Carey MP. Incidence and prevalence of the sexual dysfunctions: A critical review of the empirical literature. Archives of Sexual Behavior. 1990;**19**:389-408

[10] Rosen RC, Taylor JF, Leiblum SR, Bachmann GA. Prevalence of sexual dysfunction in women: Results of a survey study of 329 women in an outpatient gynecological clinic. Journal of Sex & Marital Therapy. 1993;**19**:171-188

[11] Laumann EO, Paik A, Rosen RC. Sexual dysfunction in the United States: Prevalence and predictors. Journal of the American Medical Association. 1999;**6**:537-544

[12] Grant JG, Baig I, Quin J. Erectile dysfunction in general medicine. Clinical Medicine (London, England). 2013;**13**:136-140

[13] Gauthier SA, Glanz BI, Mandel M, Weiner HL. A model for the comprehensive investigation of a chronic autoimmune disease: The multiple sclerosis CLIMB study. Autoimmunity Reviews. 2006;**5**:532-536

[14] Kessler TM, Fowler CJ, Panicker JN. Sexual dysfunction in multiple sclerosis. Expert Review of Neurotherapeutics. 2009;**9**:341-350

[15] Fletcher JM, Lalor SJ, Sweeney CM, Tubridy N, Mills KH. T cells in multiple sclerosis and experimental autoimmune encephalomyelitis. Clinical and Experimental Immunology. 2010;**162**:1-11

[16] Marck CH, Jelinek PL, Weiland TJ, Hocking JS, De Livera AM, Taylor KL, et al. Sexual function in multiple sclerosis and associations with demographic, disease and lifestyle characteristics: An international cross-sectional study. BMC Neurology. 2016;**16**:210

[17] Prévinaire JG, Lecourt G, Soler JM, Denys P. Sexual disorders in men with

multiple sclerosis: Evaluation and management. Annals of Physical and Rehabilitation Medicine. 2014;**57**: 329-336

[18] Demirkiran DJ, Riolo JV, Xu Z, Hull EM. Regulation by the medial amygdala of copulation and medial preoptic dopamine release. The Journal of Neuroscience. 2001;**21**:349-355

[19] Atif M, Azeem M, Sarwar MR. Potential Problems and Recommendations Regarding Substitution of Generic Antiepileptic Drugs: A Systematic Review of Literature. Vol. 5. London: Springerplus; 2016. p. 182

[20] Mameniškienė R, Guk J, Jatužis D. Family and sexual life in people with epilepsy. Epilepsy & Behavior. 2017;**66**:39-44

[21] Nikoobakht M, Motamedi M, Orandi A, Meysamie A, Emamzadeh A. Sexual dysfunction in epileptic men. Urology Journal. 2007;**4**:111-117

[22] Demerdash A, Shaalan M, Midani A, Kamel F, Bahri M. Sexual behavior of a sample of females with epilepsy. Epilepsia. 1991;**32**:82-85

[23] Atif M, Sarwar MR, Scahill S. The relationship between epilepsy and sexual dysfunction: A review of the literature. Springer Plus. 2016;**5**:2070

[24] Yogarajah M. Epilepsy and sexual dysfunction. In: Mula M, editor. The Comorbidities of Epilepsy. Amsterdam: Academic Press; 2019. pp. 51-76

[25] Watanabe H, Riku Y, Hara K, Kawabata K, Nakamura T, Ito M, et al. Clinical and imaging features of multiple system atrophy: Challenges for an early and clinically definitive diagnosis. Journal of Movement Disorders. 2018;**11**:107

[26] Jung YJ, Kim HJ, Yoo D, Choi JH, Im JH, Yang HJ, et al. Various motor and non-motor symptoms in early multiple system atrophy. Neurodegenerative Diseases. 2019;**19**:238-243

[27] McKay JH, Cheshire WP. First symptoms in multiple system atrophy. Clinical Autonomic Research. 2018;**28**:215-221

[28] Oertel WH, Wachter T, Quinn NP, Ulm G, Brandstadter D. Reduced genital sensitivity in female patients with multiple system atrophy of parkinsonian type. Movement Disorders. 2003;**18**:430-432

[29] Papatsoris AG, Papapetropoulos S, Singer C, Deliveliotis C. Urinary and erectile dysfunction in multiple system atrophy (MSA). Neurourology and Urodynamics. 2008;**27**:22-27

[30] Reininghaus E, Lackner N. Relationship satisfaction and sexuality in Huntington's disease. Handbook of Clinical Neurology. 2015;**130**:325-334

[31] Kolenc M, Kobal J, Podnar S. Female Sexual Dysfunction in Presymptomatic Mutation Carriers and Patients with Huntington's Disease. Journal of Huntington's Disease. 2017;**6**:105-113

[32] Kolenc M, Kobal J, Podnar S. Male sexual function in presymptomatic gene carriers and patients with Huntington's disease. Journal of the Neurological Sciences. 2015;**15**:312-317

[33] Statland JM, Barohn RJ, McVey AL, Katz J, Dimachkie MM. Patterns of weakness, classification of Motor Neuron Disease & Clinical Diagnosis of sporadic ALS. Neurologic Clinics. 2015;**33**:735-748

[34] Wasner M, Bold U, Vollmer TC, Borasio GD. Sexuality in patients with amyotrophic lateral sclerosis and

their partners. Journal of Neurology. 2004;**251**:445-448

[35] Nasimbera A, Rosales J, Silva B, Alonso R, Bohorquez N, Lepera S, et al. Everything you always wanted to know about sex and Neurology: neurological disability and sexuality. Arquivos de Neuro-Psiquiatria. 2018;**76**:430-435

[36] Shahbazi M, Holzberg S, Thirunavukkarasu S, Ciani G. Perceptions of sexuality in individuals with amyotrophic lateral sclerosis (ALS) and their treating clinicians. Neurological Rehabilitation. 2017;**41**:331-342

[37] Insel TR. Rethinking schizophrenia. Nature. 2010;**468**:187-193

[38] Bychkov E, Ahmed MR, Gurevich EV. Sex differences in the activity of signalling pathways and expression of G-protein-coupled receptor kinases in the neonatal ventral hippocampal lesion model of schizophrenia. The International Journal of Neuropsychopharmacology. 2011;**14**:1-15

[39] Faludi G, Dome P, Lazary J. Origins and perspectives of schizophrenia research. Neuropsychopharmacologia Hungarica. 2011;**13**:185-192

[40] de Boer MK, Castelein S, Wiersma D, Schoevers RA, Knegtering H. The facts about sexual (Dys)function in schizophrenia: An overview of clinically relevant findings. Schizophrenia Bulletin. 2015;**41**:674-686

[41] Fanta T, Haile K, Abebaw D, Assefa D, Hibdye G. Assessment of sexual dysfunction and associated factors among patients with schizophrenia in Ethiopia. BMC Psychiatry. 2018;**18**:158

[42] Aizenberg D, Zemishlany Z, Dorfman-Etrog P, Weizman A. Sexual dysfunction in male schizophrenic patients. The Journal of Clinical Psychiatry. 1995;**56**:137-141

[43] Reitz C, Brayne C, Mayeux R. Epidemiology of Alzheimer disease. Nature Reviews. Neurology. 2011;**7**:137

[44] LaFerla FM, Green KN. Animal models of Alzheimer disease. Cold Spring Harbor Perspectives in Medicine. 2012;**2**:a006320

[45] Davies HD, Zeiss A, Tinklenberg JR. Til death do us part: Intimacy and sexuality in the marriages of Alzheimer's patients. Journal of Psychosocial Nursing and Mental Health Services. 1992;**30**:5-10

[46] Ostrowski M, Mietkiewicz MC. Approach of the sexuality of Alzheimer's disease patients according to caregivers' guides approach. Gériatrie et Psychologie Neuropsychiatrie du Vieillissement. 2015;**13**:434-440

[47] Zeiss AM, Davies HD, Wood M, Tinklenberg JR. The incidence and correlates of erectile problems in patients with Alzheimer's disease. Archives of Sexual Behavior. 1990;**19**:325-331

[48] Nogueira MM, Neto JP, Sousa MF, Santos RL, Lacerda IB, Baptista MA, et al. Perception of change in sexual activity in Alzheimer's disease: Views of people with dementia and their spouse-caregivers. International Psychogeriatrics. 2017;**29**:185-193

[49] Davies HD, Sridhar SB, Newkirk LA, Beaudreau SA, O'Hara R. Gender differences in sexual behaviors of AD patients and their relationship to spousal caregiver well-being. Aging & Mental Health. 2012;**16**:89-101

[50] Modi P, Mohamad A, Phom L, Koza Z, Das A, Chaurasia R, et al.

Understanding pathophysiology of sporadic Parkinson's disease in drosophila model: Potential opportunities and notable limitations. In: Dorszewska J, Kozubski W, editors. Challenges in Parkinson's Disease. London: IntechOpen; 2016

[51] Parkinson J. An essay on the shaking palsy 1817. The Journal of Neuropsychiatry and Clinical Neurosciences. 2002;**14**:223-236

[52] Gelb DJ, Oliver E, Gilman S. Diagnostic criteria for Parkinson disease. Archives of Neurology. 1999;**56**:33-39

[53] Savica R, Rocca WA, Ahlskog JE. When does Parkinson disease start. Archives of Neurology. 2010;**67**:798-801

[54] Palma JA, Kaufmann H. Autonomic disorders predicting Parkinson's disease. Parkinsonism & Related Disorders. 2014;**1**:94-98

[55] Palma JA. Autonomic dysfunction in Parkinson's disease and other synucleinopathies: Introduction to the series. Movement Disorders. 2018;**33**:347-348

[56] Kovács M, Makkos A, Aschermann Z, Janszky J, Komoly S, Weintraut R. Impact of sex on the nonmotor symptoms and the health-related quality of life in Parkinson's disease. Parkinson's Disease. 2016;**2016**:7951840

[57] Chaudhuri KR, Prieto-Jurcynska C, Naidu Y, Mitra T, Frades-Payo B, Tluk S, et al. The non declaration of nonmotor symptoms of Parkinson's disease to health care professionals: An international study using the nonmotor symptoms questionnaire. Movement Disorders. 2010;**25**:704-709

[58] Gao X, Chen H, Schwarzschild MA, Ascherio A. A prospective study of bowel movement frequency and risk of Parkinson's disease. American Journal of Epidemiology. 2011;**174**:546-551

[59] Bhattacharyya KB, Rosa-Grilo M. Sexual dysfunctions in Parkinson's disease: An underrated problem in a much discussed disorder. International Review of Neurobiology. 2017;**134**:859-876

[60] Singer C, Weiner WJ, Sanchez-Ramos JR, Acker- MM. Sexual dysfunction in men with Parkinson's disease. Journal of Neurologic Rehabilitation. 1989;**3**:199-204

[61] Bronner G, Royter V, Korczyn AD, Giladi N. Sexual dysfunction in Parkinson's disease. Journal of Sex & Marital Therapy. 2004;**30**:95-105

[62] Jitkritsadakul O, Jagota P, Bhidayasiri R. Postural instability, the absence of sexual intercourse in the past month, and loss of libido are predictors of sexual dysfunction in Parkinson's disease. Parkinsonism & Related Disorders. 2015;**21**:61-67

[63] Sakakibara R, Shinotoh H, Uchiyama T, Sakuma M, Kashiwado M, Yoshiyama M, et al. Questionnaire based assessment of pelvic organ dysfunction in Parkinson's disease. Autonomic Neuroscience. 2001;**92**:76-85

[64] Kummer A, Cardoso F, Teixeira AL. Loss of libido in Parkinson's disease. The Journal of Sexual Medicine. 2009;**6**:1024-1031

[65] Wermuth L, Stenager E. Sexual problems in young patients with Parkinson's disease. Acta Neurologica Scandinavica. 1995;**91**:453-455

[66] Brown RG, Jahanshahi M, Quinn N, Marsden CD. Sexual function

in patients with Parkinson's disease and their partners. Journal of Neurology, Neurosurgery, and Psychiatry. 1990;**53**:480-486

[67] Gao X, Chen H, Schwarzschild MA, Glasser DB, Logroscino G, Rimm EB. Erectile function and risk of Parkinson's disease. American Journal of Epidemiology. 2007;**166**:1446-1450

[68] Schrag A, Horsfall L, Walters K, Noyce A, Petersen I. Prediagnostic presentations of Parkinson's disease in primary care: A case-control study. Lancet Neurology. 2015;**14**:57-64

[69] Postuma RB, Gagnon JF, Pelletier A, Montplaisir J. Prodromal autonomic symptoms and signs in Parkinson's disease and dementia with Lewy bodies. Movement Disorders. 2013;**28**:597-604

[70] Reeve A, Simcox E, Turnbull D. Ageing and Parkinson's disease: Why is advancing age the biggest risk factor? Ageing Research Reviews. 2014;**14**:19-30

[71] Wylie K, Kenney G. Sexual dysfunction and the ageing male. Maturitas. 2010;**65**:23-27

[72] Kim HS, Cheon SM, Seo JW, Ryu HJ, Park KW, Kim JW. Nonmotor symptoms more closely related to Parkinson's disease: Comparison with normal elderly. Journal of the Neurological Sciences. 2013;**324**:70-73

[73] Buhmann C, Dogac S, Vettorazzi E, Hidding U, Gerloff C, Ju¨rgens T. P. The impact of Parkinson disease on patients' sexuality and relationship. Journal of Neural Transmission. 2016;**124**:983-996

[74] Hand A, Gray WK, Chandler BJ, Walker RW. Sexual and relationship dysfunction in people with Parkinson's disease. Parkinsonism & Related Disorders. 2010;**16**:172-176

[75] Özcan T, Benli E, Özer F, Demir EY, Kaya Y, Ayyıldız A. The association between symptoms of sexual dysfunction and age at onset in Parkinson's disease. Clinical Autonomic Research. 2016;**26**:205-209

[76] Andersson KE. Mechanisms of penile erection and basis for pharmacological treatment of erectile dysfunction. Pharmacological Reviews. 2011;**63**:811-859

[77] Bowers MB, Woert MV, Davis L. Sexual behavior during L-DOPA treatment for parkinsonism. The American Journal of Psychiatry. 1971;**127**:1691-1693

[78] Andersson KE. Pharmacology of penile erection. Pharmacological Reviews. 2001;**53**:417-450

[79] Zahran AR, Simmerman N, Carrier S, Vachon P. Erectile dysfunction occurs following substantia nigra lesions in the rat. International Journal of Impotence Research. 2001;**13**:255

[80] Coslett HB, Heilman KM. Male sexual function. Impairment after right hemisphere stroke. Archives of Neurology. 1986;**43**:1036-1039

[81] Hull EM, Dominguez JM. Getting his act together: Roles of glutamate, nitric oxide, and dopamine in the medial preoptic area. Brain Research. 2006;**1126**:66-75

[82] Liu YC, Sachs BD, Salomone JD. Sexual behavior in male rats after radiofrequency or dopamine depleting lesions in nucleus accumbens. Pharmacology, Biochemistry, and Behavior. 1998;**60**:585-592

[83] Kudwa AE, Dominguez-Salazar E, Cabrera DM, Sibley DR, Rissman EF. Dopamine D5 receptor modulates male

and female sexual behavior in mice. Psychopharmacology. 2005;**180**:206-214

[84] Rampin O, Jerome N, Suaudeau C. Proerectile effects of apomorphine in mice. Life Sciences. 2003;**72**:2329-2336

[85] Kuo SY, Wu CL, Hsieh NY, Lin CT, Wen RK, Chen LC, et al. PPL2ab neurons restore sexual responses in aged drosophila males through dopamine. Nature Communications. 2015;**6**:7490

[86] Alekseyenko OV, Lee C, Kravitz EA. Targeted manipulation of serotonergic neurotransmission affects the escalation of aggression in adult male Drosophila melanogaster. PLoS One. 2010;**5**:e10806

[87] Shaltiel-Karyo R, David D, Menuchin Y, Frenkel-Pinter M, Marcus-Kalish M, Ringo J, et al. A novel, sensitive assay for behavioural defects in Pakinson's disease model drosophila. Parkinson's Disease. 2012;**2012**:1-6

[88] Meston CM, Frohlich PF. The neurobiology of sexual function. Archives of General Psychiatry. 2000;**57**:1012-1030

[89] Okun MS, McDonald WM, DeLong MR. Refractory nonmotor symptoms in male patients with Parkinson disease due to testosterone deficiency: A common unrecognized comorbidity. Archives of Neurology. 2002;**59**:807-815

[90] Buvat J, Maggi M, Guay A, Torres LO. Testosterone deficiency in men: Systematic review and standard operating procedures for diagnosis and treatment. The Journal of Sexual Medicine. 2013;**10**:245-284

[91] Okun MS, Walter BL, McDonald WM, Tenover JL, Green J, Juncos JL, et al. Beneficial effects of testosterone replacement for the nonmotor symptoms of Parkinson disease. Archives of Neurology. 2002;**59**:1750-1753

Section 3

Therapeutic Strategies Clinical Trials and Health Technologies for Parkinson's Disease

Chapter 6

Current Rehabilitation Therapies in Parkinson's Disease

Qing Zhao, Lingjing Jin, Lin Ma, Tingting Sun and Mengdie Zhou

Abstract

Rehabilitation is one of the important non-pharmacological interventions for Parkinson's disease (PD). At the time of diagnosis, an appropriate exercise regimen can be prescribed based on the patient's symptoms. Rehabilitative therapies should be continued throughout the disease course. This chapter summarized the standard specifications and research progression on PD from perspectives of assessment and treatment of rehabilitation. The physical therapy, occupational therapy, speech-language therapy, and neuromodulation therapy are the focus of the introduction. Accurate and comprehensive functional assessment is the premise of rehabilitation plan. Various approaches are used individually or in combined targeted at one or more dysfunction. Although there is still no consensus about the optimal approach about intensity, the frequency of treatment sessions, and complexity, rehabilitation is proved to be able to induce short-term, but clinically important benefits, particularly for gait and balance. The rehabilitative program for PD should be targeted to practicing and learning specific activities in the core areas and be tailored to the individual patients' characteristics. In addition to improving patient's performance, environmental modification and alleviation of caregivers are also included in rehabilitation intervention. Innovative techniques have been recently proposed: virtual reality and exergaming, motor imagery and action observation, robot-assisted physiotherapy, and nonconventional therapies.

Keywords: Parkinson's disease, rehabilitation, physical therapy, occupational therapy, speech-language therapy, self-management

1. Introduction

Rehabilitative therapy is very important across Parkinson's disease (PD) stages, which is considered as an adjuvant to pharmacological and surgical treatments for PD to maintain functional ability, minimize secondary complications, and improve quality of life. In a broad sense, rehabilitation includes exercise, physiotherapy, occupational therapy, speech-language therapy, psychological and cognitive therapy, nursing and care, dietetic intervention, as well as neuromodulation. Telemedicine and artificial intelligence are also boosting the development of PD rehabilitation. The evidence of these interventions is growing rapidly, and the following contents mainly refer to

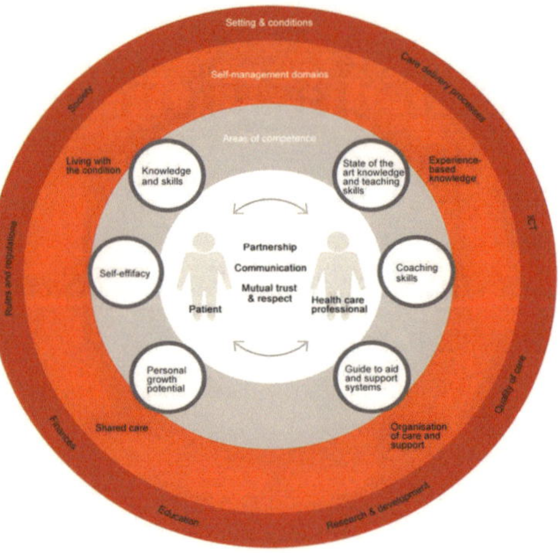

Figure 1.
Generic model of self-management [1].

authoritative guidelines as well as findings from relatively high-quality randomized clinical trial studies. No matter what kind of rehabilitation, self-management, and long-term adherence should be emphasized. Experts recommend using *5As* model (Assess, Advice, Agree, Assist, and Arrange) to foster motivation of people with PD (Pwp) (**Figure 1**).

2. Mechanisms underline benefits of physical therapy in PD

Animal experiments have shown that exercise and learning are able to induce a dynamic interplay between degenerative and regenerative mechanisms, influence dopaminergic and glutamatergic neurotransmission, increase synaptic strength and potentiate functional circuitry and induce the brain plasticity which is likely to represent neural basis of rehabilitation for PD. In addition, increasing evidence suggests that physical exercise alleviates chronic oxidative stress through increasing mitochondria biogenesis and up-regulating autophagy, stimulates the synthesis of neurotransmitters and trophic factors. All of these molecular biological changes probably contribute to neuroplasticity.

On the other hand, a combination of physical therapy and neuromodulation techniques (DBS, rTMS, tDCs) may improve retention of motor learning by modulating excitability of certain cortical areas.

So, it may be explained to some extent, exercise and physiotherapy could help not only motor and non-motor symptoms or complications but also show disease-modified potential.

3. Physical therapy (PT)

In European physiotherapy guidelines for PD, the five core areas of PT are physical capacity, transfers, manual activities, balance, and gait. Additional areas include pain and respiratory problems. Physical capacity is expressed by exercise tolerance, joint mobility plus muscle tone, power, and endurance, which is precondition for activities

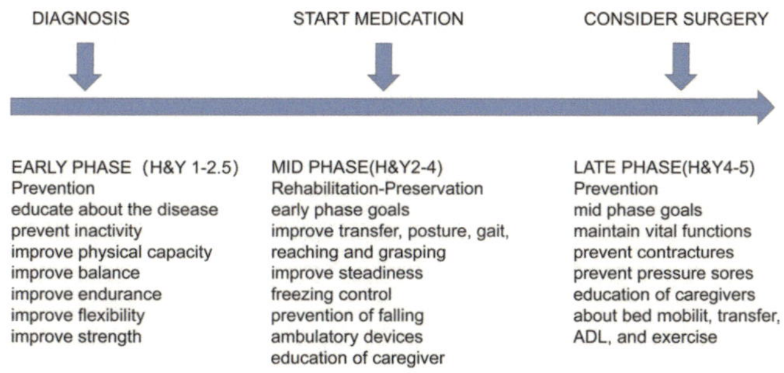

Figure 2.
Main goals in each stages of PD [2].

of daily life and participation in society. As the disease progresses, transfer and manual activities are often diminished as complex motor sequences and associated with tremor sometimes. The main hazard of balance disorders are fallen. Other associated factors of falls include freezing, reduced step height, bradykinesia, impaired postural reflexes, sedative drugs, and fear. It is recommended to establish rehabilitation goals and specific programs according to the individual differences in Pwp and stages of disease, including early, mid, and late phase corresponding to Hoehn-Yahr classification (**Figure 2**). All physiotherapists are advised to describe ***SMART*** goals:

- Specific: avoid broad goals and identify specific problems.
- Measurable: using one or more of the recommended measurement tools.
- Attainable: where both the Pwp and physiotherapist expect its feasibility as well as practicable.
- Relevant: to this individual Pwp and within the scope of physiotherapy
- Time-based: by when it is expected, these goals should be achieved.

The goal attainment scaling (GAS) provides a method to score the extent to which Pwp goal is achieved in the course of intervention.

3.1 Measurement tools

Evaluation is necessary and critical for rehabilitation of PD because it contributes to identify impairments, set goal to meet the patient's needs, develop the appropriate treatment plan, and even motivate patients in adherence to the therapy. Due to the medication intake impairments and activity limitations for Pwp can vary greatly during a day, most questionnaires and measurement tools are used at time of the day and tiredness of patients after medication intake. But for balance or applicable for specific patients who report differences in ability, it is recommended to assess in both on and off stages. Although it could be assessed for the severity of disease comprehensively by means of MDS-UPDRS from four perspectives, more detailed and targeted rehabilitative evaluations are still needed. Recommended measurement tools for physical therapy of PD are summarized in **Table 1.** And the most common ones are described below:

Physical capacity	Transfer	Manual activity	Balance	Gait	Flexibility	Fall	Quality of life
Endurance: 6MWT,GXT Borg Scale (RPE)	Bed related: M-PAS Bed	STEF	Push & Release Test, RPT FRT,SLST	10 MW 6MWT	ROM (Goniometer)	ABC	PDQ-39 EQ-5D PDQL
Aerobotic: TMST		NHPT	Stationary: BBS	Rapid Turns		FES-I	ADL
Resistance: MMT, ACT Isokinetic dynamometer	Chair related: M-PAS Chair FTSTS		Transfer related: M-PAS Chair FTSTS	M-PAS gait &TUG	SRT Bach scratch		CGI PSI-PD
FTSTS	TUG		Gait related: M-PAS gait &TUG Rapid Turns DGI FGA Mini-BESTest	FOG-Q			

6MWT: 6 Minutes' Walk Test; GXT: Graded Exercise Test; TMST: 2 Minutes Step Test; ACT: Arm Curled Test; FTSTS: 5 Times Sit To Stand; M-PAS: Modified Parkinson Activity Scale; TUG: Timed Up&Go; STEF: Simple Test for Evaluating Hand Function; NHPT: Nine-Hole Peg Test; RPT: Retropulsion Test; FRT: Functional Reach Test; SLST: Single Leg Stand Test; BBS: Berg Balance Scale; DGI: Dynamic Gait Index; FGA: Functional Gait Assessment; FOG: Freezing Of Gait; SRT: Sit and Reach Test; ABC: Activities Balance Confidence Scale; FES-I: Falls Efficacy Scale International.

Table 1.
Measurement tools for PD.

3.1.1 Modified Parkinson activity scale (M-PAS)

The M-PAS was developed as an objective evaluation tool for activity limitations within the core areas of motor rehabilitation. The M-PAS was introduced as the only rating scale recommended in the physical and occupational therapy guidelines for Pwp. It consists of 14 items divided into three domains that describe core activities related to functional mobility for Pwp: chair transfer (two items), gait akinesia (six items), and bed mobility (six items). Each item is scored on a 5-point scale (0–4), with higher scores indicating greater independence. This assessment takes into account whether to use hands when transfer, whether there is a dual task (motor or cognitive) and so on more accurately so that it can break the ceiling effects of PAS.

3.1.2 Berg balance scale (BBS)

The BBS has been the main instrument used to evaluate balance impairment in different populations and disorders. It is a 14-item scale that objectively measures static and dynamic activities of varying difficulty. Each item is scored on a 5-point ordinal scale ranging from 0 (unable to perform) to 4 (normal performance). The total score range is 0–56, and higher scores denote better balance. Scores of 0–20 refer to those patients restricted to a wheelchair; 21–40 refer to assistance during the gait; and 41–56 points correspond to independence. Scoring is based on the individual's ability to perform each task independently and/or meet certain time or distance requirements. But it is not suitable for Pwp in Hoehn-Yahr 4—5 stage, and for patients with vestibular dysfunction.

DOI: http://dx.doi.org/10.5772/intechopen.107237

3.1.3 Six minute walk test (6MWT)

The 6MWT is a sub-maximal exercise test used to assess aerobic capacity and endurance, which provides valuable information regarding all the systems during physical activity, including pulmonary and cardiovascular systems, blood circulation, neuromuscular units, body metabolism, and peripheral circulation. Turning difficulty is frequently reported in Pwp and affects ability of movement combined with hypokinesia. Locomotor assessment of straight-line walking and turning are widely clinically used when considered together rather than when assessed independently. The 6MWT is conducive to such an assessment because it generally combines numerous turns and straight-line walking within 6 minutes. It is important to standardize the track for both clinical and research purposes and it is recommended that a 30-meter or 100-foot walkway with the length of corridor be marked every 3 meters while turn-around points are to be marked by a cone [3].

3.1.4 10 meter walk (10 MW)

The 10 MWT is a performance measure used to assess walking speed in meters per second over a short distance. It can be employed to determine functional mobility, gait, and vestibular function. The individual walks without assistance for 10 meters, with the time measured for the intermediate 6 meters to allow for acceleration. It has demonstrated excellent reliability in many conditions, including PD, so it was updated by American Physical Therapy Association (APTA) in 2013. The test can be performed at preferred walking speed or fastest speed possible. The average walking speed for persons in 60–69 is 1.34–1.24 m/s, while Pwp is much slower than that.

3.1.5 Timed up and go (TUG)

The TUG test is a clinical tool widely used to determine fall risk and measure the progress of balance, sit-to-stand and walking. During the test, the patient stands up upon therapist's command, walks 3 meters, turns around, walks back to the chair, and sits down. For Pwp, some changes usually are observed such as slow tentative pace, loss of balance, short strides, little or no arm swing, and shuffling. The sensitivity and specificity have been reported to be 87%. But it demonstrates less reliability among patients suffering from cognitive impairment (**Figure 3**).

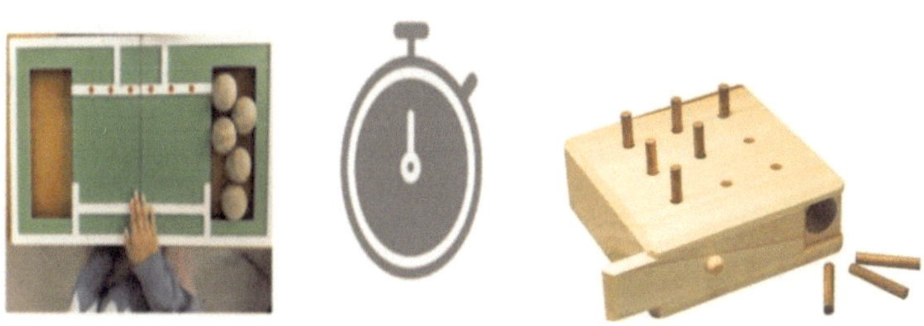

Figure 3.
Assessment tests for manual activity.

3.1.6 Mini-BESTest

The Mini-BESTest is both a clinical tool and a research outcome measure that examines postural control systems through the performance of dynamic balance tasks. Four items of it include anticipatory, reactive postural control, sensory orientation, and dynamic gait. Recent clinical study has shown that the Mini-BESTest was the strongest individual predictor of falls in individuals with PD compared with other balance scales, highlighting the importance of evaluating dynamic balance ability during fall risk assessment.

3.1.7 Five times sit to stand (FTSTS)

The FTSTS is a quick and easy test for functional lower extremity strength, ability to transition movements, balance, and fall risk. Its scoring is based on the amount of time (to the nearest decimal in seconds) a patient is able to transfer from a seated to a standing position and back to sitting five times, which was more sensitive for younger population(<60 years). The shorter the time to complete the test, the better the outcome of it. It has a moderate responsiveness to change over time and was moderately related to measures of gait and dynamic balance in vestibular and balance disorders participants.

3.1.8 New freezing of gait questionnaire (NFOG-Q)

NFOG-Q is a widely used tool to quantify freezing of gait severity. It is a self-reported questionnaire consisting of nine items that measure freezing of gait (FOG). But its reliability is influenced by the patients' difficulties with self-perceived ratings of FOG and it is currently questioned as an outcome indicator for clinical trials [4]. So, the automated video system and wearable sensor techniques are developed for Pwp to provide more objective and accurate information about FOG. For example, the Kin-FOG system uses an RGB-D sensor based on Microsoft Kinect V2 for capturing data [5]. Wearable sensor-based devices can detect freezes in progress and provide a cue to help the Pwp resume walking.

3.1.9 Borg scale 6–20

Borg rating of perceived exertion (RPE) is a tool to measure person's perception of effort and exertion, breathlessness, and fatigue during activity. It can be used in monitoring the progress and intensity of exercise for Pwp undergoing rehabilitation and endurance training. Borg's original version is a 15-point scale ranging from 6 to 20 (no exertion at all to absolutely maximum). Effort is graded using number or words. It is a significant predictor of heart rate and workload, which is not affected by age, gender, or disease severity. So, it is used in Pwp in which formal exercise testing may not be available [6].

3.2 Approaches of physiotherapy

The contents of physical therapy include three parts: exercise, practice, and movement strategy training. Functional exercise aiming to induce motor learning is called "Practice." Conventional physiotherapy is categorized as all physiotherapist-supervised active exercise interventions targeting the core areas above. To gain insight into the barriers and preferences regarding exercise of Pwp is the foundation and one of main goals of PT is encouraging Pwp strives for normal physical activity under supervision or not.

Exercise, as a subset of physical activity, is planned, structured, repetitive, and has a defined endpoint with the goal of improving physical fitness. Exercise is a universal prescription for PD. Moreover, exercise is a broad term that incorporates various activities, such as aerobic exercise, resistance training, flexibility training, and other types. Recommendations for valid exercise are shown in **Table 2** according to the APTA guideline 2022 [7].

Intervention	Quality of Evidence	Strength of Recommendation	Recommendation
Aerobic exercise	High	♦♦♦♦	Physical therapists should implement moderate- to high-intensity aerobic exercise to improve VO_2, reduce motor disease severity and improve functional outcomes in individuals with Parkinson disease
Resistance training	High	♦♦♦♦	Physical therapists should implement resistance training to reduce motor disease severity and improve strength, power, nonmotor symptoms, functional outcomes, and quality of life in individuals with Parkinson disease
Balance training	High	♦♦♦♦	Physical therapists should implement balance training intervention programs to reduce postural control impairments and improve balance and gait outcomes, mobility, balance confidence, and quality of life in individuals with Parkinson disease
Flexibility exercises	Low	♦♦◊◊	Physical therapists may implement flexibility exercises to improve ROM in individuals with Parkinson disease
External cueing	High	♦♦♦♦	Physical therapists should implement external cueing to reduce motor disease severity and freezing of gait and to improve gait outcomes in individuals with Parkinson disease
Community-based exercise	High	♦♦♦♦	Physical therapists should recommend community-based exercise to reduce motor disease severity and improve nonmotor symptoms, functional outcomes, and quality of life in individuals with Parkinson disease
Gait training	High	♦♦♦♦	Physical therapists should implement gait training to reduce motor disease severity and improve stride length, gait speed, mobility, and balance in individuals with Parkinson disease
Task-specific training	High	♦♦♦♦	Physical therapists should implement task-specific training to improve task-specific impairment levels and functional outcomes for individuals with Parkinson disease
Behavior-change approach	High	♦♦♦◊	Physical therapists should implement behavior-change approaches to improve physical activity and quality of life in individuals with Parkinson disease

Intervention	Quality of Evidence	Strength of Recommendation	Recommendation
Integrated care	High	◆◆◆◆	Physical therapist services should be delivered within an integrated care approach to reduce motor disease severity and improve quality of life in individuals with Parkinson disease
Telerehabilitation	Moderate	◆◆◇◇	Physical therapist services may be delivered via telerehabilitation to improve balance in individuals with Parkinson disease

Table 2.
Recommendations of American Physical Therapy Association (APTA) [7].

3.2.1 Aerobic exercise

Several high-quality clinical trials confirmed that moderate to high-intensity aerobic exercise can improve oxygen consumption (VO2), motor and non-motor impairments, be a benefit for improving functional activities (gait, balance) and quality of life in Pwp. As for modes of exercise walking on a treadmill or stationary cycling are frequently used but there is no evidence single form of aerobic exercise is superior to another. It should be chosen to ensure safety of Pwp, especially for those who are at high risk of falling and/or with FOG. Gradually progressing the duration and intensity of the aerobic exercise is recommended to reduce risk of injury. In Parkinson's exercise guidelines in American College of Sports Medicine (ACSM) there are elaborate introduction on the frequency, intensity and progression, time and volume, type of exercises, and even disease-related considerations for Pwp (**Table 3**), [8]. In addition, regular, long-term engagement in aerobic exercise is needed to sustain a benefit.

3.2.2 Resistance training

A progressive resistance training program was shown to be more effective than a nonprogressive exercise intervention (modified from the fitness counts booklet, Parkinson's foundation). Resistance training with instability (RTI) was favored and specific modes include free weights, weighted vests, weight machines, closed vs. open-chain activities, body weight resistance, etc.

Either alone or as a part of multimodal intervention resistance training can improve muscle power or strength, non-motor (depression, anxiety, and cognition), activities (gait speed, balance, mobility, and stability), quality of life, and reduce fall rate of Pwp.

3.2.3 Balance training

The intervention approaches used to target balance are mainly multimodal balance training that incorporated elements of strengthening, sensory integration, anticipatory postural adjustments, compensatory postural adjustments, gait, and functional task training. Its benefits are reflected in improvement of postural control, balance and confidence, mobility, gait outcomes, quality of life as well as non-motor

F.I.T.T.-V.P.	Aerobic	Strength	Balance, agility, & multi-Tasking	Flexibility
Frequency	At least 3 days per week.	2–3 days per week, challenging all major muscle groups on nonconsecutive days.	2–3 days per week focused workout, with daily integration as possible.	≥ 2–3 days/week, with dally being most effective.
Intensity & Progression	Moderate Intensity: 40% - 60% HRR (or VO_2R), RPE of 12–13/20 or 3–4/10. **Progress** to vigorous intensity: 60–85% HRR; RPE 14–17/20 or 5–7/10), when physiologically appropriate and safe. Teach client to self-assess.	40–50% of 1-RM for beginners. 60–70% 1-RM for more advanced exercisers. **Progress** number of repetitions and resistance, working muscles to fatigue.	Appropriate challenge delivered in a safe manner given the setting (individual vs. group). **Progress** motor and cognitive challenges as patient improves and can tolerate.	Full extension, flexion, or rotation stretch to the point of slight discomfort. **Progress** as patient can tolerate
Time & Volume	≥30 min of continuous or intermittent exercise per session.	10–15 repetitions starting an exercise program. ≥1 set of 8–12 repetitions (~60% 1-RM) and progress to 3 sets of 8–10 to fatigue. Build to 2–3 hours/week.	30–60 minutes per workout.	Static Stretching: 15–60 seconds per muscle; 2–4 repetitions of each stretch.
	Build to at least 150 minutes/week.		Build to 2–3 hours/week.	Dynamic Stretching: 8–10 movements in each direction.
Type	Prolonged, rhythmic activities using large muscle groups.	Major muscle groups of the upper and lower body using weight machines, resistance bands, or body weight. Focus on extensors. Could use resistance training with instability.	Multi-directional stepping, weight shifting, reaching, large amplitude movements, functional agility (steps, turning, obstacles, backwards, floor activities, sit-to-stand). Multi-task training (motor, cognitive, distractions). Static and dynamic balance with varied surfaces, limb support, perturbations.	Static Stretching: All major muscle groups after exercise, first thing in the morning or before bed. Dynamic stretching/active range of motion: Prior to intense aerobic and strengthening exercise. Include diaphragmatic breathing and meditation.
Disease-Related Considerations	Prioritize safety (ambulatory status, physical assistance, equipment). Risk of freezing of gait. Consider comorbidities (*e.g.*, musculoskeletal, cardio-respiratory). Risk of autonomic	Posture and body mechanics. Estimate 1-RM safely. Progressive with high repetitions. Timed for ON periods of optimal functioning. For safety, avoid heavy free weights.	Consider varied ability levels related to cognitive engagement and attention. Allow upper extremity support when needed. Consider comorbidities (*e.g.*, peripheral	Consider dystonia (tonic or activity-induced) and general worsening of flexed posture with disease progression. Consider comorbidities (*e.g.*,

F.I.T.T.-V.P.	Aerobic	Strength	Balance, agility, & multi-Tasking	Flexibility
	dysfunction, including orthostatic hypotension, blunted heart rate response to exercise, arrhythmias associated with PD or medications.	Consider comorbidities (*e.g.*, spinal stenosis, osteoporosis, osteopenia).	neuropathy, cognitive decline). Risk of freezing of gait. Use of gait belt for safety.	osteoporosis, pain, dystonia).
	Consider collaborating with a licensed physical therapist specializing in Parkinson's disease to assist with full functional evaluation and Individually-tailored exercise recommendations taking into account complex medical history.			2021

Table 3.
Parkinson's exercise guidelines (Parkinson's foundation) from ACSM [8].

symptoms. What should be concerned the benefits of using technology-required equipment not yet commercially available, such as wearable sensors, research-grade force plates, rotational treadmills, exergaming systems [9], and so on.

3.2.4 Gait training

The schemes of gait training are varied, including forward treadmill, downhill treadmill, curved walking rotating treadmill, robot-assisted gait training (RAGT) [10], treadmill with virtual reality (VR). Aggregate evidence demonstrates that gait training could improve severity of disease, step length and cadence, walking speed and capacity, functional mobility, and balance. But individuals who are at H&Y stages 4–5 of PD and high risk for falls should be considered more for safety and need more supervision.

3.2.5 External cueing

This is one of movement strategy training approaches that compensates for the deficits with the internal (automatic) generation of behavior. External cueing was defined as an external temporal or spatial stimulus, including rhythmic auditory cueing, visual cues, verbal cues, or attentional cues. Above cues or feedback often combined with gait and balance training, for example, rhythmic auditory stimuli (RAS) provided during balance training or treadmill are more effective and sustain longer than the general program without RAS [11]. No matter which kind of cue, combined overground or treadmill training, it has an immediate and positive impact on spatio-temporal parameters of gait and improves functional outcomes of gait and FOG. In future, optimal modes of delivery leveraging advances in technology should be further examined.

3.2.6 Task-specific training

This is an upgrade from exercise to practice. The tasks trained for PD include mental imagery, upper extremity training, turning training, fall prevention training, dual-task training, bladder training, and multimodal training. Mental imagery training with sufficient repetition uses dynamic neurocognitive imagery, with the goal of developing an individual's imagery skills, kinesthetic and proprioceptive sense, and motor self-awareness, to improve mental imagery ability. Upper extremities training may improve strength, manual dexterity, sensation, and goal attainment. Dual-task training may utilize cognitive challenge tasks during gait training to improve balance impairment and perception of FOG. In clinical practice physical therapy is usually delivered in a multimodal manner, not targeting only one specific outcome but rather designed to improve multiple deficits of Pwp.

3.2.7 Multidisciplinary team and integrated care

PD is a complex and heterogeneous disorder from prodromal to advanced stages, with a wide range of motor and non-motor symptoms, so it is necessary for teams working multidisciplinary, including movement disorder neurologists, physiotherapists, occupational therapists, speech and language therapists, psychiatrists or neuropsychologists, dietician, nurse specialist, and social workers. Besides the core care team above, there are other healthcare professionals who should be available for referral, including the gastroenterologist, geriatrician, neurosurgeon, nursing home physician, pain specialist (usually an anaesthesiologist), and urologist [12]. The multidisciplinary team (MDT) pattern improves reductions in motor severity, non-motor symptoms (anxiety, depression, and psychosocial consequences), functional outcomes (gait speed and spatio-temporal gait parameters, ADL, balance, and stability) and even health care utilization.

3.2.8 Telerehabilitation

Telerehabilitation evolved from telemedicine that means exchange of information via telecommunication systems between the provider and the patient to improve a patient's health. For instance, specifically, remotely supervised Wii-based balance training could improve activities and participation, especially for patients without cognitive impairment and low fall risk. In addition, it is available for order Pwp with other diseases and limited access to hospital. Nevertheless, telerehabilitation may increase the cost of health care and its efficacy for disease severity needs to be examined further.

3.2.9 Others

In addition to above training, there are also some effective approaches for PD, such as community-based exercise, dance/music, Tai chi, Nordic walking, Lee Silverman voice treatment physical (LSVT BIG), and acupuncture could be used alone or in combination depending on specific situation of the Pwp.

4. Occupational therapy (OT)

The aim of occupational therapy is to reduce restrictions on participation in meaningful activities and roles. OT intervention may include education and coping strategies for the individual and their families, exercise program, particularly for the upper limb, providing assistive equipment, creating supportive and functional daily routines, and suggesting and practicing compensatory strategies.

4.1 Occupational assessment scales

Similar to physical therapy, the first step of OT is evaluating Pwp's issues related to occupational performance, including living/caring, work, and leisure. The Canadian occupational performance measure (COPM) is recommended instead of using ADL questionnaires [13]. The occupational performance history interview (OPHI-II) or parts thereof is also recommended when more information and background is needed regarding occupational identity, coping, and motivation. In addition, the occupational therapist needs to assess the caregiver's burden and competencies to ensure enough caring and support for Pwp, for example by means of PD caregiver burden questionnaire (PDCB). Other aspects include analyzing the context of problems related to specific activities, assessment of the time of activities and energy distribution, observation of occupational performance, and assessment of impairments in body functions and structures as well as physical environment.

4.2 OT interventions

The strategies selected depending on the preference of the Pwp or caregiver as well as the potential for changing aspects of the person, the activity, and the environment. A combination of interventions usually applies. For Pwp, the main tasks are improving and maintaining skills during the performance of activities, applying compensatory skills or strategies during the performance of activities, increasing insight and knowledge in order to adequately deal with current and future limitations in daily activities (self-management).

4.2.1 Optimizing daily structure and activities

Setting priorities and rescheduling activities considering the medication or specific situations. To structure the day and promote the patient's motivation for occupational performance through choosing activities matches the interest and capability of Pwp. It may be effective for people who suffer from fatigue to plan a program for teaching the application of energy-saving principles.

4.2.2 Dealing with stress and time pressure

Occupational therapist will help the Pwp and caregiver to identify the factors contribute to the stress and time pressure during the assessment phase especially due to the slowed performance. Then try to give advice on reducing the time pressure in the planning and organization of activities, improving the feeling of personal effectiveness through encouraging self-management, optimizing occupational performance, and teaching the Pwp to carry out activities in a relaxed manner.

4.2.3 Practicing arm/hand motor skills

The regular practicing of fine motor skills in functional tasks is useful for maintaining and improving these skills for Pwp. Participation in the LSVT BIG program can improve perceived occupational performance and satisfaction measured by COMP, and produce gains in hand strength and dexterity for Pwp [14]. A sensory motor training intervention alongside constraint-induced movement therapy was effective in improving hand and upper extremity sensory motor function in Pwp [15].

4.2.4 Compensatory strategies in activities

Pwp can learn to perform complex tasks step-by-step with focused attention, which is called cognitive movement strategies. This is effective in facilitating the performance of transfers. But complex fine motor actions (e.g., fastening buttons and writing) cannot be adequately reduced to simple steps. In addition, external cue is also one of compensated strategies to facilitate movement.

4.2.5 Optimizing the physical environment

Aids, adaptations, and other modifications to physical environment compensate for cognitive and motor problems of Pwp reducing fall frequency and lead to more independent and safe performance. Specific methods are as follows [13]:

- Creating an unobstructed walking and turning route for Pwp who suffer from freezing, removing obstacles that increase the risk of falling;
- Setting up visual reminders, structure, and overview in the arrangement of space and objects for Pwp, especially with cognitive problems;
- Rearranging space and objects based on ergonomic principles for Pwp to promote safety, effectiveness, and efficiency of performing activities;
- Installing visual cues in places where it is important or necessary;
- Creating support points or possibilities for sitting during activities for Pwp with impaired balance;
- Using aids and adaptations according to motivation and acceptance of alternatives, safety, and skills, such as rise-and-recline armchairs, wheeled walkers, stairlifts, bed transfer aids, electric wheelchairs, and so on.

5. Speech-language therapy (ST)

With respect to PD, speech-language pathology focuses on three domains [16]:

- Problems with speech: dysarthria and the influence of cognitive impairments on language comprehension, use, and communication skills;
- Problems with chewing and swallowing: dysphagia, choking, slow chewing, and swallowing;
- Problems with controlling saliva: drooling or dribbling of saliva.

5.1 Assessment and treatment of dysarthria

The most frequently reported speech problems of Pwp are weak, hoarse, nasal or monotonous voice, imprecise articulation, slow or fast speech, difficulty starting speech, impaired stress or rhythm, stuttering, and tremor. But guideline proposes a video laryngostroboscopy by an otolaryngologist for a Pwp with hypokinetic dysarthria only when vocal fold pathology is suspected which is unrelated to PD.

The intelligibility subscale of the therapy outcomes measures (TOM) is used to quantify the severity of speech problems and treatment results. Spontaneous speech can be evaluated based on features used for all dysarthrias. The best way to evaluate the stimulability of speech is by including automatic speech tasks, maximum phonation time, pitch range, and calling.

The Robertson dysarthria profile (RDP) is a tool designed for the assessment of clients with the motor speech disorder, dysarthria which contains eight domains (respiration, phonation, facial musculature, diadochokinesis, oral reflexes, articulation, intelligibility, and prosody). VHI is a patient-rated scale that has been developed to determine the level of disability experienced by patients with different voice disorders. Recently, acoustic analysis has been developed and applied which could provide more comprehensive information of speech problem (**Table 4**) [17].

Hypophonia is one of the most common problems with speech for Pwp. Traditionally, voice therapy is based either on behavioral treatment, which involves training to strengthen muscles involved with coordination of respiration, phonation, and articulation, or using devices that provide environmental cues or biofeedback for voice amplification. Lee Silverman voice treatment, LSVT LOUD is a standardized and leading treatment of choice for hypophonia in PD. In addition, pitch limited voice treatment (PLVT) is also strongly recommended for Pwp with hypokinetic dysarthria with an intensity of four times a week for 4 weeks. Both treatments produce the same increase in loudness, but PLVT limits an increase in vocal pitch and prevents a strained or pressed voicing [18] .

5.2 Assessment and treatment of dysphagia

The swallowing disturbance questionnaire (SDQ) represents the most appropriate self-reported patient test for screening swallowing disorders in PD. The Munich dysphagia test (MDT-PD) test, swallowing clinical assessment score in PD (SCAS-PD), and Radboud oral motor inventory for PD(ROMP) may be also considered valid questionnaire-based tools for dysphagia screening in PD [19]. Fiberoptic endoscopic evaluation of swallowing (FEES) and videofluoroscopic swallowing study (VFSS) are both considered to be the gold standard to evaluate opharyngeal dysphagia. The combination of these instrumental methods allows a detailed analysis of disturbance patterns in the oral, pharyngeal, and esophageal phases of swallowing in Pwp.

Treatment of dysphagia should be started when there is clinical or instrumental evidence of impairment of swallowing safety and/or efficiency. It has a relatively high level of evidence in a clinical study on the treatment of dysphagia, including swallowing maneuvers, swallowing exercises, expiratory muscle strength training, and neuromodulation, especially DBS in STN and rTMS as well as botulinum toxin injection [20].

Deviant speech dimension [vocal task]	Acoustic feature	Definition	Pathophysiological interpretation with respect to hypokinetic dysarthria
Respiration			
Aerodynamic insufficiency [sustained phonation]	MPT	Maximum phonation time, defined as the maximum duration of sustained vowel phonation.	The rigidity of respiratory muscles leads to decrease ability to sustain vowel.
Weak inspirations [monolog]	RLR	Relative loudness of respiration, defined as the median of loudness measured relatively between respirations and speech as a difference in logarithmic scale.	Hypokinesia of respiratory muscles and decreased range of rib cage motion make respiration quieter.
Phonation			
Harsh voice [sustained phonation]	HNR	Harmonics-to-noise ratio, defined as the amount of noise in the speech signal.	Reduced rate of airflow and improper control of vocal folds causes increased turbulent noise.
Decreased voice quality [monolog]	CPP	Cepstral peak prominence, defined as the measure of cepstral peak amplitude normalized for overall amplitude.	Deteriorated control of laryngeal muscles leads to unstable periods of vocal fold opening, causing a dysphonic and breathy voice.
Articulation			
Imprecise consonants [syllable repetition]	VOT	Voice onset time, defined as the length of the entire consonant from initial burst to vowel onset.	Hypokinesia causes slowing of lip and tongue movements, leading to a longer time required to pronounce individual consonants.
Articulatory decay [monolog]	RFA	Resonant frequency attenuation, defined as the differences between the maxima of the second formant region and minima of local valley region called antiformant.	Hypokinesia leads to decrease spectral energy as a result of decayed articulatory movements.
Prosody			
Monoloudness [reading passage]	IntSD	The standard deviation of speech intensity contor extracted from voiced segments.	Hypokinesia leads to the decreased amplitude of respiratory and thyroarytenoid muscles.
Monopitch [reading passage]	FOSD	The standard deviation of fundamental frequency contor converted to semitone scale.	Hypokinesia causes the reduced amplitude of vocal cord movements, leading to glottal incompetence.
Speech timing			
Slow SMR [syllable repetition]	DDKR	Diadochokinetic rate, defined as the number of syllable vocalizations per second.	Hypokinesia of speech apparatus makes the movements of articulators slower.
Prolonged pauses [monolog]	DPI	Duration of pause intervals, defined as the median length of pause intervals.	Hypokinesia of speech apparatus makes initiating of speech difficult, leading to prolonged pause intervals.

Table 4.
Acoustic measurements [17].

5.3 Assessment and treatment of drooling

There are indications that the drooling severity and frequency scale modified for Parkinson's disease (DSFS-P) is a valid scale for quantifying the severity of drooling. The treatment of drooling by means of a self-use swallow reminder can be effective in reducing the loss of saliva and teaching the patient cognitive movement strategies can also be helpful.

6. Cognitive rehabilitation

Cognitive dysfunction is one of the common non-motor symptoms of PD, including mild cognitive impairment(PD-MCI) and Parkinson's disease dementia (PDD). The short-term and instantaneous memory decline, while the impairment of long-term memory and digital-related memory is not obvious. Visual–spatial impairment can be characterized by slower visuomotor speed, decreased visual memory and comprehensive analysis ability, motor coordination ability, as well as spatial abstraction ability. Language naming and semantic comprehension can remain intact in the early stage of PD.

6.1 Measurement tools

Neuropsychological scales for overall cognitive function assessment comprise five domains: executive function, attention and working memory, language, memory, and visuospatial skills. The following three scales with ideal clinical measurement characteristics (validity and reliability) are recommended for the assessment of global cognitive function in PD [21, 22]: Montreal cognitive assessment (MoCA), Parkinson's disease cognitive rating scale (PD-CRS), and mattis dementia Rating Scale-2 (MDRS-2). The mini-mental state examination (MMP) and scales for outcomes in Parkinson's disease cognition (SCOPA-COG) are specifically designed scales to evaluate the cognitive function of PD patients despite their assessment value in executive function and visuospatial ability is not enough.

6.2 Cognitive training (CT)

CT can be carried out for one or more cognitive domains in paper-and-pencil or computerized training forms. Multi-domain, computer-based cognitive training at a frequency of 2–3 times every week over 3–12 weeks can improve executive functions, memory, processing speed, and attention for Pwp [23]. Aerobic and resistance exercises combined with cognitive training have shown effective for mild cognitive impairment. It is recommended tailoring of CT programs to suit the cognitive domains predominantly affected in the specific sub-population of PD [24]. CT involves the repetition of standardized tasks and may be limited by motor impairment so the use of more recent integrative, adaptive, and assistive technologies, such as virtual reality, may optimize the delivery of CT in PD.

7. Rehabilitation of other non-motor symptoms

Non-motor symptoms of PD have become an important factor affecting the quality of life of Pwp (**Figure 4**). And mental, sleep, fatigue, and other general abnormal status are also the major determinants of rehabilitation outcomes.

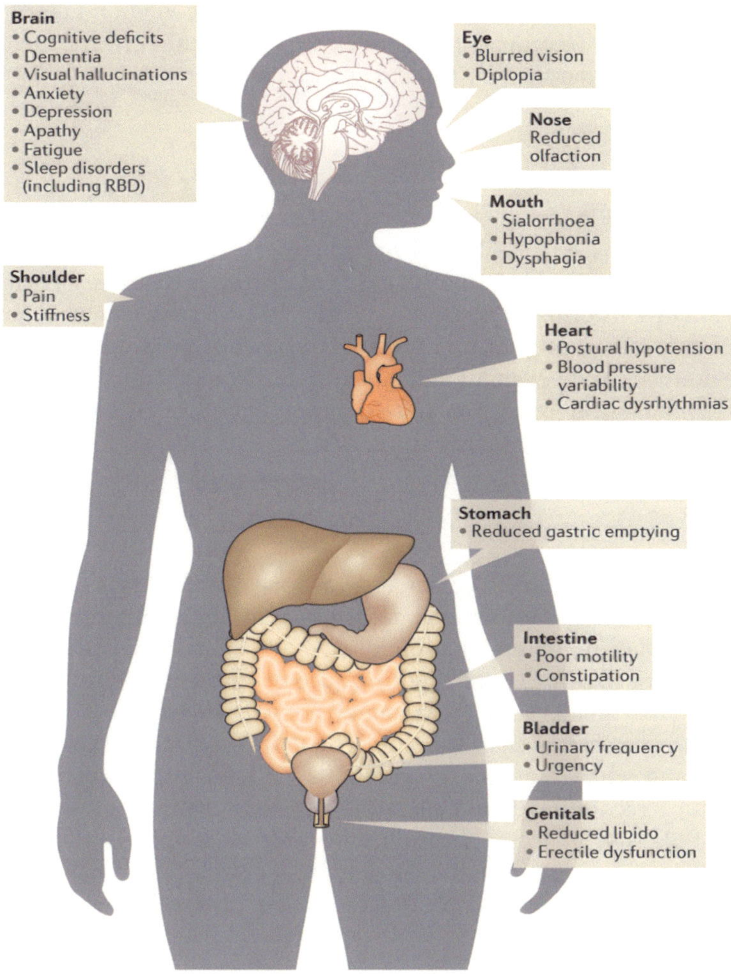

Figure 4.
Non-motor features in PD [25].

7.1 Mood disorders

Mood disorders and anxiety significantly impact the prognosis and disease course of PD, which are related to the frontal lobe caused by catecholamine and serotonin deficiency in the brain tissue. Apathy, anhedonia, and fatigue overlap with diagnostic criteria for anxiety and depression, thus making an accurate diagnosis of mood disorders in Pwp difficult. So, multidisciplinary teamwork with psychologists and psychiatrists is necessary. Beck depression inventory (BDI), Hamilton depression rating scale (HAMD-17), montgomery-asberg depression rating scale (MADRS), 15 item geriatric depression scale (GDS-15), are the most widely recognized tools. HAMD and self-report GDS are recommended for screening and measuring severity of depression in PD, while Cornell scale for depression in dementia (CSDD) can be used to screen for PD in patient with and without dementia [26]. As for anxiety, Parkinson's anxiety scale (PAS) and a PD-specific anxiety scale have higher specificity and sensitivity for their use as a screening tools than other scales [27]. Non-pharmacologic approaches in addition to classic psychotherapy, for example, cognitive-behavioral therapy (CBT) and other rehabilitative treatments are proven to have certain effects, including exercise therapy, music therapy, yoga, Tai chi, Qigong, and acupuncture.

7.2 Sleep disorders

Sleep disorders in PD include both nocturnal manifestations, such as insomnia, REM sleep behavior disorder (RBD), obstructive sleep apnea (OSA) and restless legs syndrome (RLS), and diurnal symptoms, such as excessive daytime sleepiness (EDS). Persian version of Parkinson's disease sleep scale (PPDS) has acceptable validity and reliability for measuring sleep disturbances in Pwp, while polysomnography (PSG) can provide more accurate evaluation data of sleep. Exercise and above treatments for mental and psychological problems can also improve the sleep disorder of PD to some extent.

7.3 Pain

Pain was evident in 53% of PD cases and has four different types in Pwp: musculoskeletal pain (due to rigidity, skeletal deformity), radicular–neuropathic pain (due to root lesion, focal or peripheral neuropathy), dystonic pain (related to antiparkinsonian medication), and akathisia (occurs in the off period or drug-induced). The visual analog scale (VAS) and brief pain inventory (BPI) are the commonly used assessment scales for pain. The PD-pain classification system (PD-PCS) is a valid and reliable tool for differentiating PD-related pain from PD-unrelated pain. The popular recommendation currently supports exercise as part of pain reduction treatment plans in a variety of conditions. Additionally, hydrotherapy, massage therapy, acupuncture, and neuromodulation (DBS, rTMS, tDCS) may provide appreciable results in pain management [28].

7.4 Autonomic nervous dysfunctions

Among the autonomic disorders, cardiovascular, urogenital, gastrointestinal, and thermoregulatory disorders are the most commonly occur in Pwp. The scale for outcomes in PD for autonomic symptoms (SCOPA-AUT) is a specific scale to assess autonomic dysfunction in PD patients.

7.4.1 Orthostatic hypotension (OH)

Orthostatic hypotension questionnaire (OHQ) can be used to evaluate the impact of symptoms on daily activities that require standing and/or walking.

Non-pharmacological treatment for OH includes drinking water (1.5–2.0 L/day) and increasing salt intake, compression stockings, sleeping with the head of the bed elevated (10–15 cm elevation or angle of 30–45 degrees), and physical therapy. Physical maneuvers can be used to activate the skeletal muscle pump and briefly elevate pressures, which include crossing the legs and pushing them against each other, arm flexing, and rocking up on the toes. Combination of both aerobic and resistance training, working toward a goal of performing at least 20–30 min of aerobic training or aquatic exercises three times per week [29].

7.4.2 Urinary dysfunctions

Urgency, nocturia, and incontinence are all demonstrations of overactive bladder (OAB) which is the most common lower urinary tract symptoms (LUT) in Pwp, and an objective assessment using urodynamics commonly shows detrusor overactivity (DO) in these patients. SCOPA-AUT includes six urinary items that assess both storage and voiding phases, so it is an acceptable, consistent, reliable, and valid scale. The international prostate symptom score (IPSS) has been used both in men and women for patients with neurological diseases. DBS, sacral neuromodulation (SNM), and posterior tibial nerve stimulation (PTNS) are effective therapies for improving bladder dysfunction [30]. Intradetrusor injection of botulinum toxin (BT) can be used for intractable urinary incontinence. Pelvic floor muscle exercises, behavior therapy, and acupuncture may be beneficial for urinary incontinence [31].

7.4.3 Rectal dysfunctions

Among the gastrointestinal disturbances, gastric emptying disorders and constipation are particularly noteworthy. Stool consistency in which the Bristol stool scale may be used as a practical tool, and the Knowles-Eccersley-Scott symptom (KESS) questionnaire was used to assess bowel symptoms. More accurate functional assessment requires instrumentation, such as capsule colonoscopy and EMG. Low colonic transit time (CTT) and pelvic floor dyssynergia (PFD) are major contributors to constipation in Pwp. CTT studies and defecography have been considered as "gold standard" techniques for identifying the causes of constipation as either colonic dysmotility or PFD [32].

In addition, to changing diet (30–40 grams/day of dietary fibers) and bowel habits relaxing puborectalis and pubococcygeus may alleviate this debilitating dysfunction. 30 minutes of moderate-intensity exercise per day are also advised for easing constipation [33].

8. Neuromodulation in PD

Neuromodulation is a category of treatment that involves stimulation or direct administration of medications to the nervous system for therapeutic purposes. This aims to modulate the activity of target cells as an approach to treating neurological dysfunctions, including pain, movement disorders, spasticity, and epilepsy. As for PD, it can improve motor and non-motor symptoms by regulating motor circuits and neurotransmitters in invasive or noninvasive methods.

8.1 Deep brain stimulation (DBS)

DBS is a widely acceptable revolutionized treatment for advanced levodopa-responsive PD with motor complications due to its convincing effect on motor symptoms [34]. It is summarized the different therapeutic effects for the two targets, the subthalamic nucleus (STN) and the internal part of the globus pallidus (GPi) of DBS in **Table 5**. Advancements in DBS hardware, programming, neuroimaging, and surgical techniques have led to progressive improvement in efficacy and safety profiles. By combining the precise placement of an electrode connected to a highly programmable generator of current, a therapeutic effect can be carefully tailored to the patient's specific needs.

	STN	GPi
Tremor	Improves	Improves
Bradykinesia	Improves	Improves
Rigidity	Improves	Improves
On/Off Fluctuation	Improves	Improves
Dyskinesia	Improves due to medication reduction	Greater improvement than STN
Gait/Balance	Minimal change	Minimal change, may last longer than STN
Speech	Worsens	May worsen
Cognition	May worsen. Possibly worse than GPi	May worsen
Depression	Unclear	Unclear
Anxiety	May improve	Unclear

DBS: deep brain stimulation; STN: subthalamic nucleus; GPi: globus pallidus interna.

Table 5.
Comparison of treatment effects for DBS stimulation of the STN versus the GPi [35].

8.2 Repetitive transcranial magnetic stimulation (rTMS)

rTMS is commonly used in the clinical treatment of PD. It achieves therapeutic effects mainly by varying the excitability of the central nervous system, and it is generally believed that high frequencies (HF) ≥ 5 Hz are mainly excitatory, while low frequencies (LF) < 1 Hz mainly produce inhibitory effects. Recently, a meta-analysis

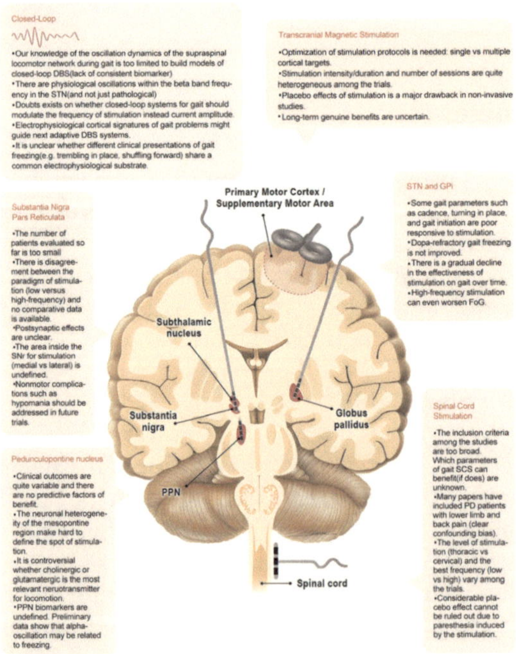

Figure 5.
Gaps of neuromodulation for gait problems in PD [27].

concluded that the pooled evidence suggested that rTMS relieves motor symptoms of Pwp and high-frequency stimulation on M1 is the most effective mode of intervention. HF rTMS has significant therapeutic effects on limb motor function, including upper limb and lower limb, akinesia, rigidity, and tremor [36]. However, for the gait impairment of PD, there are still several critical unanswered questions in the neuromodulation field that need further research [37].

In summary, the different rehabilitation approaches have in common "exercise" as a basic element and should be scheduled according to individual characteristics of the patients. Multidisciplinary collaboration maximizes the effectiveness of rehabilitation. Close monitoring and avoidance of fatigue or sports injury are paramount. Although high-intensity exercise has initially the disease-modified effects the mechanism is not clear presently. With the wide application of artificial intelligence technology and telerehabilitation technology, there will be more and more effective methods for PD, which may meet the needs of home rehabilitation in the future. At last, most of studies on rehabilitation involved mild and moderate Pwp currently so interventions to improve the patient's motor or no-motor dysfunction and quality of life in late-stage need to be explored further (**Figure 5**).

Author details

Qing Zhao*, Lingjing Jin, Lin Ma, Tingting Sun and Mengdie Zhou
Department of Neurology and Neurological Rehabilitation, Shanghai Yangzhi Rehabilitation Hospital (Shanghai Sunshine Rehabilitation Center), School of Medicine, Tongji University, Shanghai, China

*Address all correspondence to: qingzhao2010@hotmail.com

References

[1] Keus S, Munneke M, Graziano M, et al. European Physiotherapy Guideline for Parkinson's Disease. The Netherlands: KNGF/Parkinson Net; 2014. p. 38

[2] Martignon C, Pedrinolla A, Ruzzante F, et al. Guidelines on exercise testing and prescription for patients at different stages of Parkinson's disease. Aging Clinical and Experimental Research. 2021;**33**(2):221-246

[3] Crapo R, Enright P, Zeballos J. American thoracic society ATS statement: Guidelines for the six-minute walk test. American Journal of Respiratory and Critical Care Medicine. 2002;**166**(1):111-117

[4] Hulzinga F, Nieuwboer A, Dijkstra BW, et al. The new freezing of gait questionnaire: Unsuitable as an outcome in clinical trials? Movement Disorders Clinical Practice. 2020;**7**(2): 199-205

[5] Soltaninejad S, Cheng I, Basu A. Kin-FOG: Automatic simulated freezing of gait (FOG) Assessment system for parkinson's. Sensors (Basel). 2019; **19**(10):2416

[6] Penko AL, Barkley JE, Koop MM, Alberts JL. Borg scale is valid for ratings of perceived exertion for individuals with Parkinson's disease. International Journal of Exercise Science. 2017;**10**(1):76-86

[7] Osborne JA, Botkin R, Colon-Semenza C, et al. Physical therapist management of parkinson disease: A clinical practice guideline from the American physical therapy association. Physical Therapy. 2022;**102**(4):pzab302

[8] Lisa Hoffman MA. Parkinson's Exercise Guidelines for People with Parkinson's. ACSM. 2021. Available from: www.acsm.org

[9] Prosperini L, Tomassini V, Castelli L, et al. Exergames for balance dysfunction in neurological disability: A meta-analysis with meta-regression. Journal of Neurology. 2021;**268**(9):3223-3237

[10] Alashram AR, Annino G, Padua E. Robot-assisted gait training in individuals with spinal cord injury: A systematic review for the clinical effectiveness of Lokomat. Journal of Clinical Neuroscience. 2021;**91**:260-269

[11] Capato TTC, de Vries NM, Int Hout J, et al. Multimodal balance training supported by rhythmical auditory stimuli in Parkinson's disease: A randomized clinical trial. Journal of Parkinson's Disease. 2020;**10**(1):333-346

[12] Radder DLM, Nonnekes J, van Nimwegen M, et al. Recommendations for the organization of multidisciplinary clinical care teams in Parkinson's disease. Journal of Parkinson's Disease. 2020;**10**: 1087-1098

[13] Sturkenboom IHWM, Thijssen MCE, Gons-van Elsacker JJ, et al. Guidelines for Occupational Therapy in Parkinson's Disease Rehabilitation. Nijmegen, The Netherlands/Miami (FL), U.S.A.: ParkinsonNet/NPF; 2011

[14] Doucet BM, Blanchard M, Bienvenu F. Occupational performance and hand function in people with Parkinson's disease after participation in lee silverman voice treatment (LSVT) BIG®. The American Journal of Occupational Therapy. 2021; **75**(6):7506205010

[15] Taghizadeh G, Azad A, Kashefi S, et al. The effect of sensory-motor

training on hand and upper extremity sensory and motorfunction in patients with idiopathic Parkinson disease. Journal of Hand Therapy. 2018;**31**(4): 486-493

[16] Kalf JG, de Swart BJM, Bonnier M, Hofman M, Kanters J, Kocken J, et al. Guidelines for Speech-Language Therapy in Parkinson's Disease. Nijmegen, The Netherlands/Miami (FL), U.S.A.: ParkinsonNet/NPF; 2011

[17] Rusz J, Tykalová T, Novotný M, et al. Distinct patterns of speech disorder in early-onset and late-onset de-novo Parkinson's disease. NPJ Parkinsons Disease. 2021;**7**(1):98

[18] De Swart BJ, Willemse SC, Maassen BA, Horstink MW. Improvement of voicing in patients with Parkinson's disease by speech therapy. Neurology. 2003;**60**(3):498-500

[19] Cosentino G, Avenali M, Schindler A, et al. A multinational consensus on dysphagia in Parkinson's disease: Screening, diagnosis and prognostic value. Journal of Neurology. 2022;**269**(3):1335-1352

[20] Schindler A, Pizzorni N, Cereda E, et al. Consensus on the treatment of dysphagia in Parkinson's disease. Journal of the Neurological Sciences. 2021;**430**: 120008

[21] Skorvanek M, Goldman JG, Jahanshahi M, et al. Global scales for cognitive screening in Parkinson's disease: Critique and recommendations. Movement Disorders. 2018;**33**(2): 208-218

[22] Aarsland D, Batzu L, Halliday GM, et al. Parkinson disease-associated cognitive impairment. Nature Reviews. Disease Primers. 2021;**7**(1):47

[23] Nousia A, Martzoukou M, Siokas V, et al. The beneficial effects of computer-based cognitive training in Parkinson's disease: A systematic review. Archives of Clinical Neuropsychology. 2021;**28**(6): 717-726

[24] Guglietti B, Hobbs D, Collins-Praino LE. Optimizing cognitive training for the treatment of cognitive dysfunction in Parkinson's disease: Current limitations and future directions. Frontiers in Aging Neuroscience. 2021;**13**:709484

[25] Cury RG, Pavese N, Aziz TZ, Krauss JK, Moro E; Neuromodulation of Gait Study Group from Movement Disorders Society. Gaps and roadmap of novel neuromodulation targets for treatment of gait in Parkinson's disease. NPJ Parkinsons Disease. 2022;**8**(1):8. Published 2022 Jan 11

[26] Schrag A, Taddei RN. Depression and anxiety in Parkinson disease. International Review of Neurobiology. 2017;**133**:623-655

[27] Forjaz MJ, Ayala A, Martinez-Martin P, et al. Is the Parkinson anxiety scale comparable across raters? Movement Disorders. 2015;**30**(4):545-551

[28] Qureshi AR, Jamal MK, Rahman E, et al. Non-pharmacological therapies for pain management in Parkinson's disease: A systematic review. Acta Neurologica Scandinavica. 2021;**144**(2):115-131

[29] Kanjwal K, George A, Vincent M, Figueredo VM, et al. Orthostatic hypotension: Definition, diagnosis and management. Journal of Cardiovascular Medicine (Hagerstown, Md.). 2015; **16**(2):75-81

[30] Peyronnet B, Mironska E, Chapple C, et al. A comprehensive review of overactive bladder pathophysiology: On the way to tailored

treatment. European Urology. 2019; **75**(6):988-1000

[31] Moussa M, Chakra MA, Papatsoris AG, et al. Perspectives on the urological care in Parkinson's disease patients. Archivio Italiano di Urologia, Andrologia. 2022;**94**(1):107-117

[32] Wang CP, Sung WH, Wang CC, et al. Early recognition of pelvic floor dyssynergia and colorectal assessment in Parkinson's disease associated with bowel dysfunction. Colorectal Disease. 2013;**15**(3):e130-e137

[33] Van Asseldonk MJMD, Dicke HC, Van den Beemt BJW, et al. Dietetic Guideline for Parkinson's Disease. the Netherlands: Parkinson Net; 2012

[34] Lachenmayer ML, Mürset M, Antih N, et al. Subthalamic and pallidal deep brain stimulation for Parkinson's disease—meta-analysis of outcomes. NPJ Parkinsons Disease. 2021;**7**(1):77

[35] Cleary RT, Bucholz R. Neuromodulation approaches in parkinson's disease using deep brain stimulation and transcranial magnetic stimulation. Journal of Geriatric Psychiatry and Neurology. 2021;**34**(4): 301-309. DOI: 10.1177/08919887 211018269

[36] Li RY, He YJ, Qin WT, et al. Effects of repetitive transcranial magnetic stimulation on motor symptoms in parkinson's disease: A meta-analysis. Neurorehabilitation and Neural Repair. 2022;**26**:1545

[37] Cury RG, Pavese N, Aziz TZ, et al. Neuromodulation of gait study group from movement disorders society. Gaps and roadmap of novel. NPJ Parkinsons Disease. 2022;**8**(1):8

Chapter 7

Effects of Metabolic Syndrome on Parkinson's Disease and Nutraceutical Intervention Strategies

Jéssica Emy Komuro, Daniel Fabiano Barbosa dos Santos, Andreas Batista Schelp, Silvia Justina Papini and Arthur Oscar Schelp

Abstract

Hyperglycemia, insulin resistance disturbances, and other common metabolic syndrome signs are currently related to a poor outcome of Parkinson disease. There were no widely accepted nutritional intervention protocols approved for Parkinson's disease. That author exposes a brief revision of the role of insulin resistance and glycemic metabolism dysfunction in Parkinson's patients with diabetes. In an ongoing study, with a complete record of dietary habits and diet components, it was demonstrated no significant differences between diabetics (n = 19) and nondiabetics (N = 53). But body composition shows some particularities. A result that attracts attention is total fat analysis and percentage of fat of PD patients showing that diabetics are somewhat fattier. The self-reported presence of obesity does not differ from recorded data of weight and BMI, with no significant differences between the two groups. Taking into consideration that both groups have comparable degrees of disease progression, as measured by the UPDRS, it could be possible to infer that the maintenance of a relative overweight was a protective factor in this group of diabetic evaluated patients. Considerations are made about hasty intervention of nutritional approach for PD patients with diabetes, including body fat reduction, prescription of statins and therapeutic options for diabetes control.

Keywords: Parkinson's disease, metabolic syndrome, diabetes, nutraceutical intervention, cholesterol abnormalities

1. Introduction

The concurrent involvement by diabetes, a common metabolic disease, is frequent in Parkinson's disease (PD). In addition, there is strong evidence of pathological interlinking between the two entities [1, 2], and there are reports that a pre-existing diabetes could be a risk factor for more severe PD symptoms [3]. In such a relationship the mechanisms involved in the process are not fully understood [4, 5]. The same could be applied to the therapeutic and nutritional support to PD patients [6]. Just in 1992, Dirrieu et al. [7], published a study about nutritional evaluation and PD, comparing with a control group [7]. There is no unquestionably response about the influence of diabetes treatment over PD outcome. The possibility that usual therapeutic measures, per si, could be a risk factor for aggravation of that disease was discussed [8]. Only recently there have been reports of the role of diabetes medications and risk of Parkinson's disease. The effect could be so intense that the authors stated that "The incidence of Parkinson's disease in patients diagnosed with diabetes varies substantially depending on the treatment for diabetes received. The use of DPP4 inhibitors and/or GLP-1 mimetics is associated with a lower rate of Parkinson's disease compared to the use of other oral antidiabetic drugs" [9, 10]. Glucose reduction induced by hypoglycemiants could lead to less disponibility of cerebral glucose, disturbing the GLti expression in astrocyte cells. The result is a deficit in lactate and pyruvate synthesis, bearing in mind that glial astrocytes seem to play a role in the basal cell functions maintenance, especially during the events of enhanced metabolic demand or hypoglycemia [11].

Abnormalities of glucose tolerance curves associated with PD have been published over 30 years ago [12]. Many studies [1, 13, 14] had failed to demonstrate changes in glucose levels. Nevertheless, there are studies demonstrating some correlation between diabetes, metabolic syndrome and DP and their complications [1, 15–19]. Results from a survey conducted in our service showed reduced insulin resistance and low levels of plasmatic cholesterol in parkinson's patients with dementia (PPD) associated with PD, without evidence of ponderal gain compared with control patients [14]. On the other hand, hyperinsulinemia can provoke cerebral glycogen depletion, with reduction of ATP and cell death [20]. In the same way there are reports of functional dysfunctions of mitochondria related to insulin resistance and fat deposition [21].

There are few reports about the influence of severe hypoglycemia on the outcome of PD. It was found that low and high HbA1c but not diabetes was associated with faster motor symptom progression in no diabetic patients [22]. In a relatively recent study measuring glycemic levels of 11 patients, three of them with PD, only one had severe hypoglycemia (54 mg/dL; 7.5% -72 hours, closer to the critical level established by the American Society of Endocrinology (11.7% in 72 hours). The analyzed patients do not have diabetes diagnosis [23]. In a description of an isolated case, it was determined to be a severe hypoglycaemia in a diabetic patient with parkinsonian symptoms for a few months. The neuroimage evaluation shows a vasogenic lesion in basal ganglia. With antidiabetic drugs adjustment occurred glycemia normalization and clinical improvement [24]. A confounder factor could be the occurrence of hypoglycemia provoked by statins prescription to control dyslipidemia [25].

There is some evidence that the so-called Mediterranean diet is a protective factor for development of PD [26–28].

In an ongoing study, with a complete record of dietary habits and diet components, including body mass determination, it was demonstrated no significant differences between diabetics (n = 19) and non diabetics (N = 53). But body composition shows some particularities. Our goal will be a revision of literature, comments on our results and discussion about the non-individualized, standardized nutritional orientations commonly adopted to treat glycemia fluctuations in diabetic PD patients. The usual prescription of a fractionated diet with a supplement in some periods seems to be not enough and adequate to control glycemia fluctuations and other associated factors related to cholesterol metabolism. Some alimentary components and other measures will be appointed.

2. Metabolic syndrome, reverse epidemiology and Parkinson's disease

The influence of the so-called metabolic syndrome over PD was analyzed with the same conclusion in a couple of studies, that no direct correlations could be determined even with and without subgroups stratification [29, 30]. Similar results were obtained among patients with associated dementia [13, 31]. Others still question the association because it is a premorbid situation, multifactorial, and dependent on individual factors, like weight, genetic predisposition among others [32]. Even so, there are reports showing a close relationship between the modified metabolic syndrome criteria, with a poorer prognosis of motor symptoms in PD [18, 19]. A few years ago there was a publication calling attention to the so-called reverse epidemiology and the occurrence of some "abnormalities" like weight gain, among others, not as a risk factor but as a protective factor against degenerative diseases consequences [33]. On the basis of these considerations there is a place of considerations about the role of some corporal changes including weight, insulin resistance and cholesterol disturbances, either as a result of degenerative diseases like PD, or as factors related to poorer outcome of these groups of diseases [34]. The applicability of concepts of reverse epidemiology in PD was not fully discussed in current literature. In this connection, it is important to put some considerations on the role of the isolated component of metabolic syndrome on PD outcome.

2.1 Cholesterol abnormalities in PD

Some studies do not demonstrate a low if any significant association between dyslipidemia with PD [13, 33, 35]. Even so, it was possible to demonstrate that plasmatic cholesterol was lower in older patients with amnestic dementia, compared with those without cognitive dysfunctions [14]. Relevant to remember that the analyzed sample in that study was older, compared with PD patients without cognitive impairment. Others, still, point to an apparent protective effect of hypercholesterolemia in PD [36, 37]. One aspect that drew attention was that findings, cholesterol level related, was restricted to younger females and the follow-up time was twice as long as that of manns and younger. Corroborating the studies showing the apparent protector effect of cholesterol, there is a report demonstrating that increased seric cholesterol levels are associated with low levels of iron in substantia nigra and pallidus in PD patients [38]. The use of total cholesterol as a biomarker for malnourishment is also well demonstrated [39]. The question about maintenance of body mass in PD patients is still an open issue. The role of adequate nutritional advice is not questionable. Although some studies limit the importance of eggs and meat as nutritional source of cholesterol, pointing out saturated fatty acids as the highest source of cholesterol [40], it is possible to assume that that the aim is not only increase body mass, but also maintain a minimum supply of diet cholesterol, preserving striatal tissue in PD patients. A question that needs to be answered is if the "cholesterol paradox", as part of reverse epidemiology in the geriatric population, is a cause or consequence of changes observed among PD or PDD.

Abnormalities in both synthesis and absorption of cholesterol has an influence on the plasmatic cholesterol levels [41, 42]. It is also important to note that weight reduction is related with reduction in plasma cholesterol levels [43] and as it can also be artificially enhanced by increased insulin resistance observed in diabetes mellitus treated with insulin [44]. The concurrent action of cholesterol metabolic disturbances, glycemic fluctuations [45], especially hypoglycemia and concomitant insulin resistance activity must be considered as risk factors to poor outcome of PD. Is not well understood all possible interlinking between the distinct components of isolated metabolic disturbances. It seems plausible to suppose that the PD brain is sensitive to abrupt hypoglycemic variations, added to disturbances in cholesterol metabolism and the concurrent action or lack of response of insulin resistance. The presence of malnourishment or visceral fat deposition, could be considered as adjuvant risk factors in the same way as type II diabetes. The recent demonstration that cholesterol metabolic disruptions are associated with an inherited form of PD [46] open new avenues to the understanding of the apparent unsolved question of the relationship of cholesterol metabolism dysfunctions and PD.

2.2 Glycemia, insulin resistance and Parkinson's disease

The potential implications and correlation between glucose metabolism and insulin resistance, were demonstrated both in evaluation of dopamine response [47] with evidence that insulin resistance is even lower in older demented patients [14, 48]. On this topic there was demonstrated insulin immunoreactivity disturbances in PD patients compared to controls [49]. The evidence that insulin low levels lead to a reduction in lipogenesis more than food digestion and absorption [50], reinforce the relationship of loss of fat mass, insulin resistance and DP [14, 51, 52].

There is some evidence showing that higher glycaemic load and index [53] as well as total fat intake [27, 31] are not associated with PD. Increased food intake, including glycaemic load and índex, was found to be strongly correlated with aging and decreased tendency to lose weight [54]. Prospective studies were not able to confirm the association of high caloric intake and increased risk of PD [55], as well as between high caloric values or lower caloric intake and increased risk of PD [56, 57]. But a newly released study demonstrated that both low HbA1c (HR 2.7; 95% CI 1.3–6; $P = 0.01$) as well as high HbA1c (HR 3.6; 95% CI 1.5–8.9; $P = 0.005$) were independent predictors of unfavorable motor outcome in PD. In this regard euglycemia seems to be associated with a better prognosis in PD [22]. The relationship between energy and caloric consumption could explain some of the body composition changes observed in PD outcome. The fact that carbohydrates are easily chewed and digested may represent a facilitator aspect for the preference. Some epidemiological data reinforces the association between enhanced ingestion of carbohydrates and increased risk of PD, which is correlated to consumption level [15, 58].

A confounding factor could be the possible intercurrence of hypoglycemia triggered by the prescription of statins to control dyslipidemia, so common in diabetes mellitus. Despite the beneficial reduction in low-density cholesterol as well as apolipoprotein B, atorvastatin treatment results in a significant increase in baseline, fasting insulin and glycated hemoglobin levels [59]. This is consistent with insulin resistance and elevated blood glucose in hypercholesterolaemic patients.

However, the use of statins in patients with low serum albumin is associated with risk for hyperglycaemic events, independent of diabetes [60]. On the other hand the prescription of atorvastatin may inhibit glucose utilization by muscle [61], with inhibition of translocation of the transporter, GLUT4, cholesterol-dependent glucose, which may lead to the inference that such effect may also occur in the striatum. Even considering that the use and availability of glucose in the brain, mediated by GLUT 1, 2 and 3 [62] and is not directly insulin-dependent, but may be affected by elevation of insulin in the periphery, it is possible to assume that the impairment of peripheral glucose metabolism also produces effects in a striatum already compromised by PD.

Regarding this aspect, as early as 1996, when attempts to implant striatal tissue fetal cells in Parkinson's disease patients were still being made, there was a demonstration of the presence of GLUT 1 in the striatum [63]. It was demonstrated that paraquat, a recognised toxic agent for brain tissue, promotes an increase in glucose transport to the cell, displacing GLUT 4 and Na+-dependent glucose transporters (SGLT), to the cell membrane, in patients with Parkinson's disease [64], thus contributing to the death of dopaminergic cells. In any case the effect of hypoglycemia on striatal glucose transporters in the presence of hypoglycaemia has not yet been demonstrated.

It is possible to assume that both hyperglycemia, induced by toxic agents (paraquat) or even antidyslipidemic drugs (atorvastatin), and hypoglycaemia, caused by hypoglycemic drugs (insulin, oral hypoglycemic agents), have a deleterious effect on brain tissue. Evidence from studies point to a less relevant role of hyperglycaemia. Yet, even accepting the premise that we should control glycemic levels more carefully in Parkinson's patients, we have no definition or even indications of the spectrum to be achieved. As an example, the levels proposed for stroke 80–130 mg/dL may not be the most recommendable for diabetics with Parkinson's disease.

On the other hand, glucose reduction, also induced by hypoglycemic drugs, may reduce cerebral glucose availability, downregulating GLTi expression in astrocytes. The result is a deficit in lactate and pyruvate synthesis. Glial astrocytes lactate appear to play a crucial role in maintaining cellular function, especially during periods of elevated metabolic demand or hypoglycaemia [11]. In this regard, there are studies, correlating functional impairment of mitochondria with insulin resistance and abdominal fat accumulation in obese subjects [21].

The demonstration that convencional hypoglycemiant drugs are associated with increase in the incidence of PD [9, 10] is also a point of interest. An apparent inverse association of insulin use and Parkinson's incidence was found in one study. But the small sample of insulin users limits the analysis [4, 9]. The demonstration that exenatide may improve motor symptoms in PD [65], confirm the importance of adequate blood glucose control in patients with PD and prone to developing the disease, offering promising data to control the deleterious effects of commonly used oral hypoglycemic drugs. Again, the interest of cholesterol and insulin resistance gain importance in dietary intervention.

3. Nutritional habits and Parkinson's disease incidence and severity

The studies on the impact of dietary habit, Dietary Components and Supplementation effects on PD incidence and outcome are fairly recent and point to the same conclusions. Among the quoted articles, all, without exception, show a correlation between malnourishment and poor PD prognosis [66], both in relation to cognitive dysfunction [67] as to motor impairment, fatigue, anxiety and depression [68]. However, others do not find any association between motor symptoms and dietary habits [69]. Likewise, the weight gain and increased central obesity observed in newly Parkinson's diagnosed patients were not associated with cognitive impairment [70].

Still in reference to dietary components and supplementation, there are some authors showing the influence of housing and untreated waters with PD features [71]. Several mechanisms may contribute to a possible association between nutritional habits and PD, with or without metabolic impairment. The so-called brain-intestinal axis can be pointed out as one of the related factors [72]. Some medications, like pramipexole, used in the treatment of PD as a dopamine agonist, can cause hyperphagia, but they are not considered as a major factor for weight gain. [73].

The supremacy of some bacteria in the bowel, with consequent gut dysbiosis, was found to be more prevalent in patients with PD. This condition promotes a pro-inflammatory bowel offering a competitive advantage for some bacterial strains over others [74]. There is evidence that enteric α-synuclein and phosphorylated α-synuclein (αSyn) abnormalities are more common among patients with PD, and could affect both the extra-nigral structures and vagus dorsal motor region [75].

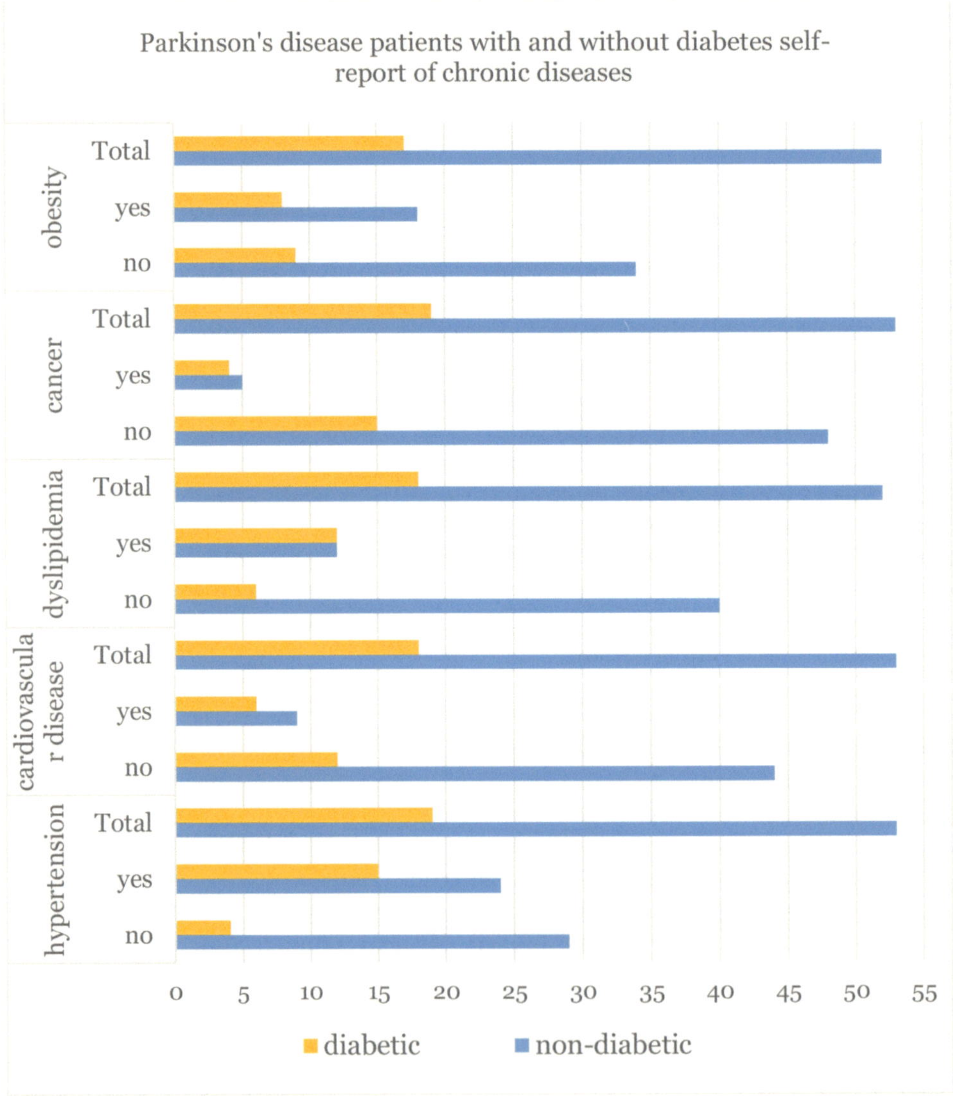

Figure 1.
Parkinson's disease patients with diabetes reported more dyslipidemia and obesity than patients without diabetes.

The bowel permeability dysfunction facilitates the entry of lipopolysaccharides into the body circulation, increasing systemic and brain inflammation [74, 76]. The findings, observed in older patients, could be associated with a greater preference for processed foods, in line with the energetic demands. The data correlate also with poor ingestion of fat, fiber-rich food, antioxidants contents and others.

Maintenance and delay of muscle mass loss may also be associated with low calorie diets, preventing sarcopenia. On the other hand, we observed in the dietary survey of our patients (unpublished results), a preference for diets rich in carbohydrates, which may lead to worsening of the sarcopenic pattern. Thus, the increase in body mass, associated with physical exercise, fatty or hypocaloric diet and even increased amino-acid supplementation, could be recommended for patients with Parkinson's disease.

In a complete record of dietary habits and diet components, including body mass determination, it was demonstrated no significant differences between diabetics (n = 19) and non diabetics (N = 53). Some data call attention, that is, a self-reporting for the presence of dyslipidemia points to dyslipidemia among diabetic patients (**Figure 1**), but the data from the medical records does not confirm it (**Figure 2**). It is still under analysis, but one hypothesis is the use of statins. Another result that draws attention is total fat analysis and percentage of fat of diabetic PD patients showing that diabetes are something fattest (**Figure 3**). The self-reported presence of obesity does not differ from recorded data of weight and BMI, with no significant differences between the two groups. Noting that both groups have comparable degrees of disease progression, as measured by the UPDRS. It could be possible to infer that the maintenance of a relative overweight was a protective factor in this group of evaluated patients.

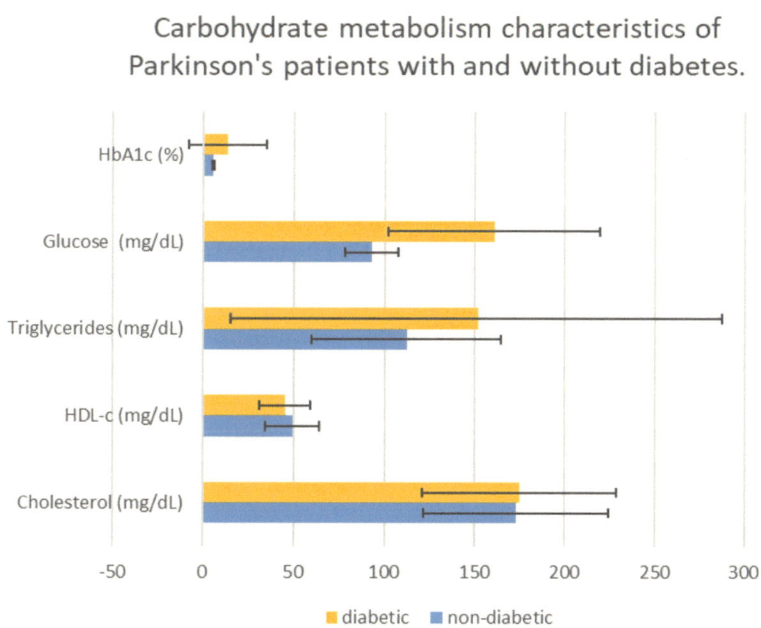

Figure 2.
Similar cholesterol laboratory tests in Parkinson's disease patients with and without diabetes but slightly lower HDL-c in patients with diabetes.

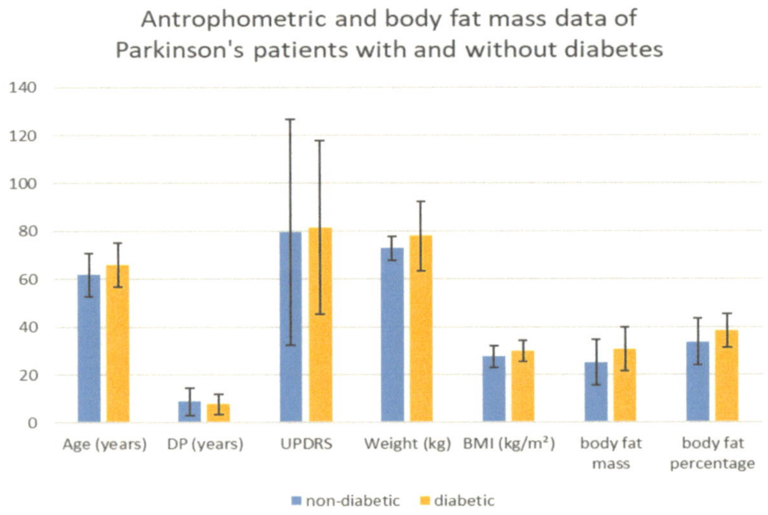

Figure 3.
Higher percentage of body fat in Parkinson's patients with diabetes did not provide an increase in disease severity.

4. Considerations about nutraceutical intervention in Parkinson's disease

The much evidence in the literature of the associations of malnutrition and low weight with poor prognosis of PD, together with the evidence that high cholesterol levels are unrelated to PD, and that low cholesterol and lack of resistance to insulin in older patients are correlated with dementia and poor outcome, enable the assistants to propose some nutritional intervention, especially in those affected by diabetes. A negative correlation between fat android mass composition and severity of parkinsonism has been evidenced [77], but the demonstration of this association is not yet well established in diabetics with Parkinson's disease, especially regarding lipid metabolism and its interactions with glucose. Again, we must keep in mind that the malnutrition observed in many PD patients may be the consequence not only of dysphagia, loss of appetite, bradykinesia and hyperkinesia, but also of abnormalities in lipid and glucose metabolism. This situation in the presence of diabetes can be an aggravating factor. As many as 90% of individuals with type 2 diabetes are overweight or obese [78], which was demonstrated, with some accumulation of fatty tissue, in our population of diabetics with PD. Although there are indications of potential therapeutic effect of ketogenic diets with different degrees of carbohydrate restriction to PD patients [79], this alternative is not viable for application in patients with PD, since it would interfere directly in the control of glycaemic levels in patients with PD and diabetes. The initial purpose should be to avoid malnourishment and, if necessary, to achieve a moderate and stable overweight status. The prescription of statins should be judicious. There is insufficient data to assume that high cholesterol levels would be worse for Parkinson's patients. In this case a mild obesity could be accepted on PD, mainly at the cost of fat accumulation. The possibility of lack of adequate insulin response in PD can also be discussed. Amid so many open questions it is feasible to affirm that obesity can be seen not as a disease but as a physiological adaptive factor to face PD, especially when associated with diabetes. The role of obesity as a functional adaptation and not as an aggravating factor in certain circumstances has been well discussed by Robert Eckel in his book [80], and should be considered. That author draws attention and exposes a revision of the role of secreted fatty tissue proteins in insulin resistance and inflammation regulation in humans. A final consideration is that the nutritional approach for PD patients with diabetes should include concern of more aggressive intervention on body fat reduction, parsimony in statin indication and therapeutic options for diabetes control. Alternative measures to control dyslipidemia in the face of cardiovascular disease should include regular physical activity.

Abbreviation

PD	Parkinson's disease
PPD	Parkinson's disease patients with dementia

Author details

Jéssica Emy Komuro[1*], Daniel Fabiano Barbosa dos Santos[2], Andreas Batista Schelp[3], Silvia Justina Papini[1] and Arthur Oscar Schelp[2]

1 Department of Nurse, São Paulo State University — UNESP Botucatu, Botucatu, SP, Brazil

2 Department of Neurology, Neurology, Psychology and Psychiatry, São Paulo State University — UNESP Botucatu, Botucatu, SP, Brazil

3 São Paulo State Public Servant Hospital - IAMSPE, São Paulo, SP, Brazil

*Address all correspondence to: jessica.komuro@gmail.com

References

[1] Palacios N, Gao X, McCullough ML, Jacobs EJ, Patel AV, Mayo T, et al. Obesity, diabetes and risk of Parkinson Disease. Movement Disorders. 2011;**26**:2253-2259

[2] Jeong SM, Han K, Kim D, Rhee SY, Jang W, Shin DW. Body mass index, diabetes, and the risk of Parkinson's disease. Movement Disorders. 2019;**35**:236-244

[3] Cereda E, Barichella M, Cassani E, Caccialanza R, Pezzoli G. Clinical features of Parkinson Disease when onset of diabetes came first. Neurology. 2012;**78**:1507-1511

[4] Guo Y, Xu W, Liu F-T, Li J-Q, Cao X-P, Tan L, et al. Modifiable risk factors for cognitive impairment in Parkinson's Disease. A systematic Review and Meta-analysis of Prospective Cohort Studies. Movement Disorders. 2019;**34**(6):876-883

[5] Cheonga JLY, de Pablo-Fernandezb E. The Association between type 2 diabetes mellitus and Parkinson's Disease. Journal of Parkinson's Disease. 2020;**10**:775-778

[6] Ma K, Xiong N, Shen Y, Han C, Liu L, Zhang G, et al. Weight loss and malnutrition in patients with Parkinson's disease: Current knowledge and future prospects. Frontiers in Aging Neuroscience. 2018;**19**(10):1

[7] Durrieu G, Lau ME, Rascol O, Senard JM, Rascol A, Montastruc JL. Parkinson's disease and weight loss: A study with anthropometric and nutritional assessment. Clinical Autonomic Research. 1992;**2**(3):153-157

[8] Schelp AO, Komuro JE, Berto SJP, Corrente JE. Interlinking dementia in Parkinson's disease: And nutritional correlates of body composition. In: Colin R. Martin Victor Preedy. (Org.), editor. The Neuroscience of Parkinson's Disease. Volucella: Academic Press; 2020. pp. 555-568

[9] Brauer R, Wei L, Ma T, Athauda D, et al. Diabetes medications and risk of Parkinson's disease: A cohort study of patients with diabetes. Brain. 2020;**143**(10):3067-3076

[10] Bayram E, Litvan I. Lowering the risk of Parkinson's disease with GLP-1 agonists and DPP4 inhibitors in type 2 di*abete*s. Brain. 2020;**143**(10):2868-2871

[11] Matsui T, Omuro H, Liu Y-F, et al. Astrocytic glycogen-derived lactate fuels the brain during exhaustive exercise to maintain endurance capacity. Proceedings of the National Academy of Sciences. 2017;**114**(24):635

[12] Lipman J et al. Glucose intolerance in Parkinson's disease. Journal of Chronic Disease. 1974;**27**(11-12):573-579

[13] Schelp AO, Mendes-Chiloff CL, Bazan B, Paduan VC, Pioltini ABM. Metabolic syndrome and dementia associated with Parkinson's disease: Impact of age and hypertension. Arquivos de Neuro-Psiquiatria. 2012;**70**(2):114-118

[14] Schelp AO, Mendes-Chiloff CL, Paduan VC, Corrente JE, Vieira A, Marchette JCN, et al. Amnestic dementia impairment in Parkinson's disease: The role of body composition, aging and insulin resistance. Clinical Nutrition ESPEN. 2017;**20**:47-51

[15] Sandyk R, Gavin I, Awerbuch GI. The association of diabetes mellitus with

dementia in Parkinson's disease. The International Journal of Neuroscience. 1992;**64**:209-212

[16] De Pablo-Fernandez E, Goldacre R, Pakpoor AJ, Warner TT. Association between diabetes and subsequent Parkinson disease: A record-linkage cohort study. Neurology. 2018;**91**(2):e139-e142

[17] Tan AH, Hewb YC, Lima S-Y, Ramlib NM, Kamaruzzamanc SB, Tanc MP, et al. Altered body composition, sarcopenia, frailty, and their clinico-biological correlates, in Parkinson's disease. Parkinsonism & Related Disorders. 2018;**56**:58-64

[18] Leehey M, Luo S, Sharma S, Wills AA, Bainbridge JL, Wong PS, et al. Association of metabolic syndrome and change in Unified Parkinson's Disease Rating Scale scores. Neurology. 2017;**89**(17):1789-1794

[19] Nam GE, Kim SM, Han K, Kim NH, Chung HS, Kim JW, et al. Metabolic syndrome and risk of Parkinson disease: A nationwide cohort study. PLoS Medicine. 2018;**15**(8):e1002640

[20] Riske L, Thoma RK, Baker GB, Dursun SM. Lactate in the Brain: An update on its relevance to brain energy, neurons, glia and panic disorder. Therapeutic Advanced in Psychopharmacology. 2017;7(2):85-89

[21] Ngo DTM, Sverdlov AL, Karki S, Mccartney-Coxson D, Stubbs RS, Farb MG, et al. Oxidative modifications of mitochondrial complex II are associated with insulin resistance of visceral fat and obesity. American Journal of Physiology. Endocrinology and Metabolism. 2019;**316**:E168-E177

[22] Markaki I, Theodora Ntetsika T, Sorjonen K, Svenningsson P. Euglycemia indicates favorable motor outcome in Parkinson's disease. Movement Disorders. 2021;**36**:1430-1434

[23] Hiroyuki T. Continuous glucose monitoring can disclose glucose fluctuation in advanced Parkinsonian syndromes. Neurology International. 2018;**10**:107-110

[24] Gil YF, Yoon JH. Hypoglycemia – induced parkinsonism with vasogenic basal ganglia lesion. Parkinsonism & Related Disorders. 2018;**49**:112-113

[25] Khanimov I, Segal G, Wainstein J, Boaz M, Shimonov M, Leibovitz E. High-Intensity Statins Are Associated With Increased Incidence of Hypoglycemia During Hospitalization of Individuals Not Critically Ill; Published online: June 21, 2019p1305-1310. 2019a

[26] Gao X, Chen H, Fung TT, Logroscino G, Schwarzschild MA, Hu FB, et al. Prospective study of dietary pattern and risk of Parkinson disease. American Journal of Clinical Nutrition. 2007;**86**:1486-1494

[27] Miyake Y, Sasaki S, Tanaka K, Fukushima W, Kiyohara C, Tsuboi Y, et al. Dietary fat intake and risk of Parkinson's Disease: A case control study in Japan. Journal of the Neurological Sciences. 2010a;**288**:117e22

[28] Barichella M, Cereda E, Cassani E, Pinelli G, Iorio L, Ferri V, et al. Dietary habits and neurological features of Parkinson's disease patients: Implications for practice. Clinical Nutrition. 2017;**36**:1054-1061

[29] Reaven GM. Banting lecture 1988. Role of insulin resistance in human disease. Nutrition. 1997;**13**:66-66

[30] Reaven GM. Syndrome X: Is one enough. American Heart Journal. 1994;**127**:1439 1442

[31] Miyake Y, Tanaka K, Fukushima W, Sasaki S, Kiyohara C, Tsuboi Y, et al. Case–control study of risk of Parkinson's disease in relation to hypertension, hypercholesterolemia, and diabetes in Japan. Journal of the Neurological Sciences. 2010b;**293**:82-86

[32] Simmons RK, Alberti KG, Gale EA, Colagiuri S, Tuomilehto J, Qiao Q, et al. The metabolic syndrome: Useful concept or clinical tool? Report of a WHO Expert Consultation. Diabetologia. 2010;**53**:600

[33] Ahmadi S-F, Streja E, Zahmatkesh G, Streja D, Kashyap M, Moradi H, et al. Reverse epidemiology of traditional cardiovascular risk factors in the geriatric population. Journal of the American Medical Directors Association. 2015;**16**(11):933-939

[34] Ahmed RM, Irish M, Piguet O, Halliday GM, Ittner LM, Farooqi S, et al. Amyotrophic lateral sclerosis and frontotemporal dementia: Distinct and overlapping changes in eating behavior and metabolism. Lancet Neurology. 2016;**15**:332-342

[35] Vikdahl M, Bäckman L, Johansson I, et al. Cardiovascular risk factors and the risk of Parkinson's disease. European Journal of Clinical Nutrition. 2015;**69**:729-733

[36] Simon KC, Chen H, Schwartzchil M, Ascherio A. Hypertension, hypercholesterolemia, diabetes and risk of Parkinson's disease. Neurology. 2007;**69**:1688-1695

[37] De Lau LML, Koudstaal PJ, Hoffmann A, Breteler MMB. Serum cholesterol levels and the risk of Parkinson's disease. American Journal of Epidemiology. 2006;**164**:998-1002

[38] Du G, Lewis MM, Shaffer ML, Chen H, Yang QX, Mailman RB, et al. Serum cholesterol and nigrostriatal R2* values in Parkinson's Disease. PLoS ONE. 2012;7:35397

[39] Zhang Z, Pereira SL, Luo MID, Matheson EM. Evaluation of blood biomarkers associated with risk of malnutrition in older adults: A systematic review and meta-analysis. Nutrients. 2017;**9**:829. DOI: 10.3390/nu9080829

[40] Cha D, Park Y. Association between dietary cholesterol and their food sources and risk for hypercholesterolemia: The 2012-2016 Korea National Hea and Nutrition: Examination Survey. Nutrients. 2009;**11**:84. DOI: 10.3390/nu11040846

[41] Santosa S, Varady KA, AbuMweis S, Jones PJH. Physiological and therapeutic factors affecting cholesterol metabolism: Does a reciprocal relationship between cholesterol absorption and synthesis really exist? Life Sciences. 2007;**80**:505-514

[42] Alphonse PAS, Jones PJH. Revisiting human cholesterol synthesis and absorption: The reciprocity paradigm and its key regulators. Lipids. 2016;**51**:519-536

[43] Di Buono M, Hannah JS, Katzel LI, Jones PJ. Weight loss due to energy restriction suppresses cholesterol biosynthesis in overweight, mildly hypercholesterolemic men. Journal of Nutrition. 1999;**129**(8):1545-1548

[44] Pihlajamaki J, Gylling H, Miettine TA, Laakso M. Insulin resistance is associated with increased cholesterol synthesis and decreased cholesterol absorption in normoglycemic men. Journal of Lipid Research. 2004;**45**(3):507-512

[45] Gorst C, Kwok CS, Aslam S, Buchan I, Kontopantelis E, Myint PK,

et al. Long-term glycemic variability and risk of adverse outcomes: A systematic review and meta-analysis. Diabetes Care. 2015;**38**:2354-2369

[46] García-Sanz P, Aerts JMFG, Moratalla R. The role of cholesterol in α-Synuclein and Lewy Body Pathology in GBA1 Parkinson's Disease. Movement Disorders. 2020;**36**:5

[47] Boyd AE, Lebovitz HE, Feldman JM. Endocrine Function and Glucose Metabolism in Patients with Parkinson's Disease and their Alteration by L-Dopa. The Journal of Clinical Endocrinology & Metabolism. 1971;**33**(5):829-837

[48] Bosco D, Plastino M, Cristiano D, Colica C, Ermio C, Bartolo MD, et al. Dementia is associated with insulin resistance in patients with Parkinson's Disease. Journal of the Neurological Sciences. 2012;**315**:39e43

[49] Wilhelm KR, Yanamandra K, Gruden MA, Zamotin V, Malisauskas M, Casaite V, et al. Immune reactivity towards insulin, its amyloid and protein S100B in blood serum of Parkinson's disease. European Journal of Neurology. 2007;**14**:327-334

[50] Kuranuki S, Arai C, Terada S, Aoyama T, Nakamura T. Possible regulatory factors for intra-abdominal fat mass in a rat model of Parkinson's disease. Nutrition. 2011;**27**:239-243

[51] Beyers PL, Palarino MY, Michalek D, Busenbark K, Koller WC. Weight changes and body composition in patients with Parkinson's disease. Journal of the American Dietetic Association. 1995;**95**:979-983

[52] Cereda E, Cassani E, Barichella M, Spadafranca A, Caccialanza R, Bertoli S, et al. Low Cardiomettabolic risk in Parkinson's disease is independent of Nutritional status, body composition and fat distribution. Clinical Nutrition. 2012b;**31**:699-704

[53] Murakami K, Miyake Y, Sasaki S, Tanaka K, Fukushima W, Kiyohara C, et al. Dietary glycemic index is inversely associated with the risk of Parkinson's disease: A case–control study in Japan. Nutrition. 2010;**26**:515-521

[54] Cheshire WP Jr, Wszolek K. Body mass index is reduced early in Parkinson Disease. Parkinsonism & Related Disorders. 2005;**11**:35-38

[55] Lorefält B, Toss G, Granérus AK. Weight loss, body fat mass, and leptin in Parkinson's disease. Movement Disorders. 2009;**24**:885-890

[56] Petroni ML, Albani G, Bicchiega V, Baudo S, Vinci C, Montesano A, et al. Body composition in advanced-stage Parkinson's disease. Acta Diabetologica. 2003;**40**:S187-S190

[57] Barichella M, Pinelli G, Iorio L, Cassani E, Valentino A, Pusani C, et al. Sarcopenia and dynapenia in patients with parkinsonism. Journal of the American Medical Directors Association. 2016;**17**:640-646

[58] Karakelides H, Irving BA, Short KR, O, Brien P, Nair KS. Age, obesity, and sex effects on insulin sensitivity and skeletal muscle miyhochondrial function. Diabetes. 2010;**59**:89-97

[59] Koh KK, Quon MJ, Han SH, Lee Y, Kim SJ, Shin EK. Atorvastatin Causes Insulin Resistance and Increases Ambient Glycemia in Hypercholesterolemic Patients. Journal of the American College of Cardiology. 2010;**55**(12):1209-1216

[60] Khanimov I, Segal G, Wainstein J, Boaz M, Shimonov LE. High-intensity statins are associated with increased

incidence of hypoglycemia during hospitalization of individuals not critically ill. The American Journal of Medicine. 2019b;**132**(11):13051310

[61] Sun B, Zhong Z, Wang F, Xu J, et al. Atorvastatin impaired glucose metabolism in C2C12 cells partly via inhibiting cholesterol-dependent glucose transporter 4 translocation. Biochemical Pharmacology. 2018;**150**:108-119

[62] Szablewski L. Glucose transporters in the brain. Journal of Alzheimer's Disease. 2017;**55**(4):1307-1320

[63] Kordower JH, Rosenstein JM, Collier TJ, Levey AE, Mufson EJ, Freeman TB, et al. Functional fetal Nigral grafts in a patient with Parkinson's Disease: Chemoanatomic, ultrastructural, and metabolic studies. The Journal of Comparative Neurology. 1996;**370**:203-230

[64] Anandhan A, Lei S, Levytskyy R, Pappa A, Panayiotidis MI, Cerny RL, et al. Glucose metabolism and AMPK signaling regulate dopaminergic cell death induced by gene (α-synuclein)-environment (paraquat) interactions. Molecular Neurobiology. 2017;**54**(5):3825-3842. DOI: 10.1007/s12035-016-9906-2

[65] Athauda D, Maclagan K, Skene SS, Bajwa-Joseph M, Letchford D, Chowdhury K, et al. Exenatide once weekly versus placebo in Parkinson's disease: A randomized, double-blind, placebo-controlled trial. Lancet. 2017;**390**:1664-1675

[66] Cumming K, Macleod AD, Myint PK, Counsell CE. Early weight loss in parkinsonism predicts poor outcomes. Evidence from an incident cohort study. Neurology. 2017;**89**:1-8

[67] Kim HH, Oh ES, Jung HL, Moon JS, Oh JE, Shin JW, et al. Relationship between changes of Body Mass Index (BMI) and cognitive decline in Parkinson's Disease (PD). Archives of Gerontology and Geriatrics. 2012;**55**:70-72

[68] Fereshtehnejad S-M, Ghazi L, Shafieesabet M, Shahidi GA, Delbari A, Lo J. Motor, psychiatric and fatigue features associated with nutritional status and its effects on quality of life in Parkinson's Disease Patients. PLOS ONE. 2014;**9**:e91153

[69] Lindskov S, Sjöberg K, Hagell P, Westergren A. Weight stability in Parkinson's Disease. Nutritional Neuroscience. 2016;**19**:11-20

[70] Vikdahl M, Carlsson M, Linder J, Forsgren L, Haglin L. Weight gain and increased central obesity in the early phase of Parkinson's disease. Clinical Nutrition. 2014;**33**:1132-1139

[71] Koller WC, Vetere-Overfield B, Gray C, et al. Environmental risk factors in Parkinson's disease. Neurology. 1990;**40**:1218-1221

[72] Felice VD, Quigley EM, Sullivan AM, O'Mahony SM. Microbiota-gut-brain signaling in Parkinson's disease: Implications for non-motor symptoms. Parkinsonism & Related Disorders. 2016;**27**:1-8

[73] Ahlskog JE. Pathological behaviors provoked by dopamine agonist therapy of Parkinson's disease. Physiology & Behavior. 2011;**104**:168-172

[74] Tan AH, Mahadeva S, et al. Small intestinal bacterial overgrowth in Parkinson's disease. Parkinsonism & Related Disorders. 2014;**20**:535-540

[75] Houser MC, Tansey MG. The gut-brain axis: Is intestinal inflammation a silent driver of Parkinson's disease pathogenesis? Nature Partner Journals Parkinson's Disease. 2017;**3**:1-9

[76] Buijs RM. The metabolic syndrome: A brain disease? Journal of Neuroendocrinology. 2006;**18**:715-716

[77] Pisciotta MS et al. Untangling the relationship between fat distribution, nutritional status and Parkinson's disease severity. Aging Clinical and Experimental Research. 2020;**32**:77-84

[78] Pi-Suyner FX, Maggio CA. The prevention and treatment of Obesity: Application to type II diabetes. Diabetes Care. 1997;**20**:744-766

[79] Choi A et al. Nutritional ketosis in Parkinson's Disease — A review of remaining questions and insights. Neurotherapeutics. 2021;**18**:1637-1649

[80] Eckel RH. Obesity: A disease or a physiologic adaptation for survival? In: Eckel RH, editor. Obesity Mechanisms and Clinical Management. Philadelphia: Lippincott Williams & Wilkins; 2003

Chapter 8

Ethical and Safety Considerations in Stem Cell-Based Therapy for Parkinson's Disease

Fangzhou Li, Jiahao Ji, Jun Xue, Jeffrey Schweitzer and Bin Song

Abstract

Stem cell-based therapy for Parkinson's Disease (PD) is entering an exciting era with many groups competing to reach the goal of safe and practical clinical application. However, the road to this goal is long and beset by challenging obstacles, among which are Good Manufacturing Practice (GMP) standards, scalability, and regulatory requirements for the final cell product. Of paramount importance is the patient safety of the stem cell-derived dopaminergic neurons, such that each stage of the cell therapy implementation process must be scrutinized for potential safety concerns before introduction to the clinic can be contemplated. In this chapter, we will critically consider the safety regulations and safety strategies of stem cell-based therapy for PD, emphasizing the principal requirements necessary for this new therapeutic approach to benefit PD patients. We will introduce the current safety challenges and the connections between these safety issues and the special characteristics of neural stem cells. In addition, we will summarize the safety standards for stem cell-based therapy currently adopted by leading cell therapy groups and international regulations. Both *in vitro* and *in vivo* safety assessment methods will be discussed as they relate to the implementation of these standards. Finally, we will speculate on strategies for further enhancing the safety of stem cell-based therapy for PD.

Keywords: Parkinson's disease, clinical trials, stem cell-based therapy, safety consideration, tumorgenicity

1. Introduction

Parkinson's disease (PD) is the second most common neurodegenerative disorder after Alzheimer's disease. Characterized by the loss of midbrain dopaminergic neurons (mDANs) in the substantia nigra pars compacta (SNpc), the condition impairs motor function with bradykinesia, tremor, and rigidity being pathognomonic symptoms [1]. Currently, treatment strategies for Parkinson's Disease, including dopamine replacement therapy and deep brain stimulation, are symptomatic and not curative interventions. They do not stop or even slow the progress of the disease. With the development of technology to create and manipulate different types of stem cells, stem cell-based therapies have become one of the most promising potential remedies for degenerative diseases, among which PD has gained particular attention due to its characteristic predominant loss of a single cell type.

Over the decades since this concept emerged, many efforts have been made to test the feasibility of using cell-based therapy to treat PD. In 1987, for the first time, researchers succeeded in transplanting human fetal midbrain tissue into the brains of PD patients in an open-label trial [2]. The apparent positive results encouraged further development of this approach. In the 2000s, double-blind multi-center clinical trials for fetal transplantation were performed in the US [3, 4]. Though these trials overall did not have positive outcomes, there were subsets of patients with clinical improvement that thus encouraged further research. This process was accelerated with the appearance of stem cell sources including both human embryonic stem cells (hESCs) and human-induced pluripotent stem cells (hiPSCs) as a source to replace fetal tissue. For example, an autologous iPSC-derived DA neuron transplantation surgery was performed by investigators at Harvard University in 2019 [5] and that same year, a clinical trial using HLA-matched hiPSC-derived DA neurons to treat PD patients was initiated at Kyoto University Hospital by researchers from the Center for iPS Cell Research and Application (CiRA) [6].

However, not all news about stem cell treatment is encouraging. The relative ease of access or production of stem cells of various types, the popularization of the stem cell idea in the public mind, and the opportunity to profit from the hopes of desperate patients can be a toxic combination. This has resulted in ill-advised and unscrupulous activity that has brought real harm to patients. A famous incident concerns a stroke patient who traveled across several countries to receive stem cell therapy in the hope that this would restore function to his left arm and leg. But in fact, the unlicensed stem cell treatments allowed the stem cells injected into his body to grow into a tumor that left him nearly paralyzed [7]. Also, in 2022, an Italian surgeon was convicted of one count of "causing bodily harm" in a Swedish court for his stem cell-embedded artificial trachea implantation surgery performed on three patients at Karolinska Institute in 2011 and 2012, all of whom died of severe complication [8]. These incidents are reminders that there are some biosafety issues unique to stem cell therapy that are not well publicized and that should receive special attention if the promise of this field is not to be cut short by such incidents.

Also, in 2022, the U.S. Supreme Court overturned Roe v. Wade, reflecting the great controversy over the right to life of embryos. It is difficult to predict where ethical and legal concerns over the capabilities of modern medicine and science will lead. Though initially an appealing alternative to the destruction of human embryos, as they have at least the theoretical ability to develop into full human bodies, stem cells, especially the hESCs, may ultimately also encounter serious ethical issues and cause conflict between people holding different beliefs.

Here we will touch upon some of the prominent ethical and safety issues of stem cell-based therapy for Parkinson's disease, and introduce some of the measures currently used or proposed to surpass the safety threshold for clinical application.

2. Ethical history of stem cells and cell therapy

With respect to PD specifically, various sources have been applied to acquire dopaminergic cells—adrenal medulla [9], carotid body [10], fetal tissue [11], fetal pig neuronal cells [12], hESCs, hiPSCs, parthenogenetic human ova [13], etc. Different types of stem cell therapy raise different levels of ethical controversy. Here, we introduce the ethical considerations for 3 major active resources for treating PD: fetal tissue, hESCs, and hiPSCs.

2.1 Fetal tissue

Fetal tissue transplantation, the first ever successful proof of the concept in cell therapy, is in a paradoxical sense the least controversial one in an ethical sense. This is because the materials used in fetal transplantation are derived from fetuses that at the point of abortion become nonviable and thus more analogous to a cadaver organ donor.

However, abortion itself is hugely controversial in many societies as already discussed, and the application of fetal transplantation may provide an incentive to increase the rate of intentional induced abortions. The economical or medical benefits behind fetal transplantation technology may thus give rise to a black market for fetal tissue, which may affect pregnant women's decisions on the fate of their babies in the womb.

Moreover, despite the nonviable status of an aborted fetus, fetal tissue transplantation is under a variety of restrictions that change over different periods. In 2019, US President Trump forbade NIH funding for research projects involving the usage of fetal tissue [14], a restriction that was then overturned 2 years later by the Biden administration [15].

2.2 Human embryonic stem cells

hESCs are derived from the pluripotent inner cell mass of 5- to 7-day-old embryos. The use of these cells for either research or medical applications, which involves the destruction of human embryos, renders this the most ethically controversial approach to stem cell therapy. Therefore, a major debate continues, as it has for decades, about whether to consider human embryos as human life.

The opponents of the application of hESCs, many of whom represent religious viewpoints, believe that human life begins at conception. For example, there is a passage in the Bible saying: "Before I formed you in the womb I knew you, before you were born, I dedicated you, a prophet to the nations I appointed you" (NAB) (Jeremiah 1:5 (calling of Jeremiah narrative)), that illustrates the basis of this thought. If we endow the embryo with all the rights of a human being, then damaging or destroying an embryo to do scientific research is assault or murder.

The proponents, on the other hand, posit that a person is defined by properties such as viable independence from the mother and that this occurs at a much later stage of development than fertilization. Ethical, moral, and religious viewpoints vary on the importance of such factors as self-awareness, further complicating the issue. Even among these proponents, few people believe that the embryo or blastocyst is just a clump of cells that can be used for research without restriction [16], and further issues arise when considering embryos that are otherwise discarded by-products of *in vitro* fertilization efforts, those produced expressly for the purpose of research or medical use, and those that derive from long term propagated cell lines; in many such scenarios no option for further development exists even if the embryo is not used for medical research.

Such contradictory views make the use of embryonic stem cells much like abortion itself, which is constantly being debated in various settings. Countries around the world have also set different restrictions on the use of embryonic stem cells according to their own religions and customs, and these restrictions are also constantly changing over time, like those for fetal tissue transplantation, due to innumerable cultural and political factors.

For instance, in the US, on August 9, 2001, U.S. President George W. Bush introduced a ban on federal funding for research on newly created hESC lines. Scientists using funding from NIH could only use cell lines created prior to that date. This policy greatly hindered research on hESCs and on stem cell therapy using such lines, since only 21 hESC lines were generally available. Hence, on March 9, 2009, President Barack Obama reversed this policy, giving researchers access to hundreds of new cell lines. However, so long as the Dickey-Wicker Amendment remains in effect, scientists are still unable to create new lines using tax dollars [17]. Moreover, actual enforcement of such laws varies between different states in ways that may also be unpredictable, and the threat of further policy reversals is underscored by the Supreme Court decision mentioned above.

The situation in the European Union is similar to that in the US. Stem cell research using human embryos is permitted in Sweden, Spain, Finland, Belgium, Greece, Britain, Denmark, and the Netherlands; however, it is illegal in Germany, Austria, Ireland, Italy, and Portugal [18].

2.3 Human induced pluripotent stem cells

hiPSCs are derived from somatic cells in mature individuals using Nobel prize-winning technology developed by Yamanaka [19]. Since no embryos are involved, it is possible to avoid many ethical problems haunting hESCs and fetal tissue transplantation.

The major "ethical" issue for hiPSC therapy is its cost. hiPSCs transplantation is more expensive and resource intensive than other forms of cell therapy as well as traditional medical or surgical therapies. How to ensure equitable access in the field of hiPSC treatment and establish a sound insurance system remains a challenge for cell therapy in PD just as it does for CAR-T and other emerging therapeutic innovations.

Even with hiPSCs there is the possibility of opinions holding that hiPSCs, with the ability to differentiate similar to ESCs, should be subject to the same regulations despite their very different origin. Furthermore, with the use of hiPSCs, the human cloning controversy would also enter the mix. Such concerns cannot be discounted as a source of ethical conflicts in the future that must be considered in clinical implementation of PD cell therapy.

3. Safety standards for stem cell-based therapy

As noted above, the core enabling feature of stem cell-based cell therapy, either ESCs or iPSCs, is that the pluripotency of the stem cell enables it to differentiate into virtually any desired cell type, thus potentially providing a stable and sustainable cell resource. With the establishment of hESCs in 1998 [20] and the advent of iPSCs from somatic cells in 2006 [19], hESCs and hiPSCs, with the ability to produce any cell type from all three germ layers, gradually became the major resource for PD cell therapy research by virtue of their pluripotency, availability in theoretically unlimited quantities, and superior logistical and ethical position compared to fetal tissue.

However, this pluripotency is also a source of significant safety concerns compared to fetal tissues. Early phase clinical trials are expressly intended to establish the safety

	Undifferentiated cell	**Neural stem cell**
Cell types generated	Pluripotent/3 germ layers	Multipotent/only neuroectodermal cells
Tumor risk	Teratoma	Neuroblastoma, medulloblastoma, primitive neuroectodermal tumor
Biological marker	OCT4, SSEA4, POU5F1	Ki67, SOX1, PAX6
Invasiveness	High	Relatively lower
H-E staining [22]	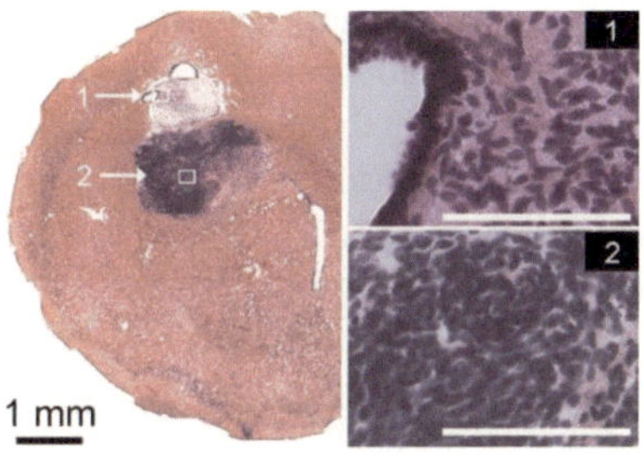	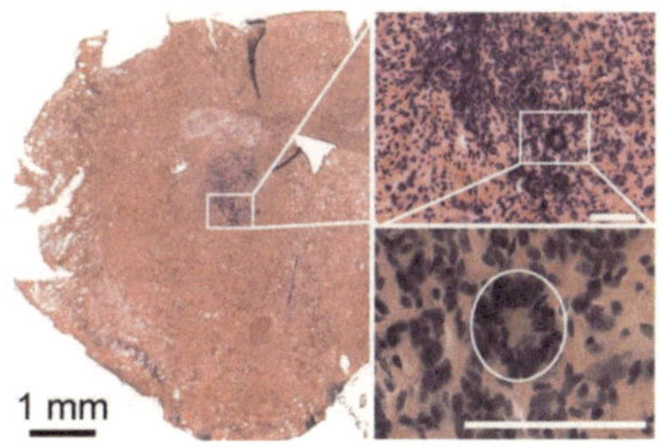

Table 1.
Differences between undifferentiated cell and neural stem cell.

of a novel therapy. But even in clinical trials, the safety of trial subjects must be prioritized, and early phase human studies must be preceded by a rigorous demonstration of safety in preclinical studies, here aimed largely at reducing the risk of generating tumors or uncontrolled proliferation. Ideally, under specific protocols, stem cells will lose their pluripotency and differentiate into specific normal mature cell type, which for PD is the SNpc mature dopaminergic A9 neuron [21]. However, stem cells exist in the tissues of mature animals—they are capable of following pathways other than differentiation and maturation, as well as of following various branches on the tree of terminal differentiation. In practice, cells may remain at various stages, from undifferentiated, to partially, to fully differentiated during the process of differentiation, and this may be affected when the cues and signals of normal embryonic differentiation are not present. This gives rise to safety concerns of potential tumorgenicity. **Table 1** illustrates two successive stages along the differentiation pathway from ESCs or iPSCs to dopaminergic neurons, either of which has unwanted proliferative potential: undifferentiated stem cells and a representative partially differentiated cell type—neural stem cells, and summarizes the distinctions between them. The identification and elimination of such cells *in vitro* is a key component of preclinical safety testing, and can guide the optimization of differentiation protocols.

4. Safety assessment methods for stem cell-based therapy for PD

To create cell therapy products that meet clinical safety criteria, various methods have been used or proposed to regulate cell quality. There has historically been no consensus on methods or thresholds to meet these criteria. To promote the development of stem cell-based cell therapy as a widely available clinical option, the establishment of uniform quality standards and acceptable methods to achieve them will be an important step. ISSCR, The International Society for Stem Cell Research, established in 2002, is a leading organization of professional stem cell scientists all around the world, and its guideline for safety studies is one proposed scheme for doing this [23]. Government regulatory bodies such as the US Food and Drug Administration (FDA) also have established standards that must be met for cell therapy products [24].

In general, cell products must be produced under Good Manufacturing Practice (GMP) conditions, with meticulous recording and complete characterization of standard operating procedures in place. Products must be fully tested for authentic target cell characteristics, microbial contamination, tumorgenicity, biodistribution, toxicology, genetic alterations, safety of ancillary therapeutic components, and in long-term animal model safety studies. In most situations, *in vitro* and *in vivo* testing should be combined for both safety and efficacy testing, but animal welfare regulations dictate that animal data should be supplied only where appropriate and informative, and that nonhuman primates should be used only if they are specifically required models [25]. Both male and female animals should be assessed in preclinical safety tests unless there is a scientifically valid reason not to do so.

4.1 Cell characterization

Transplanted cells to be used in clinical trials must first be rigorously characterized to confirm their authenticity, purity, and potential risks. Furthermore, when products fail to meet these specifications, the reasons must be understood and the production process should be refined and improved. Such reasons may include persistent epigenetic memory in iPSC lines leading to anomalous gene expression or off-target gene expression during the differentiation process. Among the characteristics used to confirm the authenticity of cell products are morphology, molecular biology, and cytogenetics.

Morphological characterization generally involves light microscopic examination and comparison to the target cell types. Molecular biological studies are used to define characteristic markers expected to be present on cells and may include analysis of expression or RNA sequencing of single or multiple cell types. Cytogenetics looks specifically at any alterations in the genetic material from karyotype to single-point mutations. Such characterization protocols should be conducted repeatedly at each stage from ESCs or parent cell type for iPSCs, through reprogramming for iPSCs, and at each step of the induced differentiation process, to monitor progress toward the desired final product.

4.2 Toxicity and microbial contamination tests

These tests are conducted on the cells, laboratory processing equipment, and reagents at every stage in accordance with GMP requirements to determine whether the product is contaminated by microorganisms or endotoxins produced by such organisms and to trace their origin if found.

4.3 Tumorgenicity studies

Because of the intrinsic nature of stem cells and the genetic manipulation required for reprogramming, (such risks for tumorigenicity would not apply so strongly to fetal tissue), these risks must be rigorously assessed for any stem cell-based products, as tumorgenicity is the most significant safety concern that needs to be addressed.

Moreover, the final product of iPSC-derived differentiated cells themselves may be tumorigenic, as there is a risk due to somatic mutations in the parent cells or later expression of any mutations acquired during reprogramming.

In vitro studies include examining rates of proliferation, with special attention to whether rapidly dividing subclones tend to take over the cultures, and looking for expression of oncogenes or loss of tumor suppressor gene activity. Although these tests may supplement *in vivo* studies, they cannot substitute for them. *In vivo* animal experiments often include histological examination of the morphology and composition of cell grafts at various stages (percentage of undifferentiated cells versus the percentage of desired cell product). Positive tumor-generating controls and negative controls are needed. It is necessary to pay attention to differences in timing and developmental patterns between animal and human species and to the special tumor risk factors in immunodeficient animal model systems. The combination of interspecies differences in tumor development between rodents and humans and the immunodeficient status of mice used for xenograft models compromises the translatability of some tumorigenic risks from animals to man. Spiking experiments using the largest feasible animal dose of the therapeutic product mixed with undifferentiated iPSCs in different quantities are usually required.

4.4 Biodistribution studies

Biodistribution studies determine the distribution, persistence, and clearance of a cell therapy product *in vivo* from the site of injection to target and nontarget tissues and biofluids. For all stem cell-based products, whether injected locally or systemically, researchers should perform detailed and sensitive biodistribution studies of cells to prevent potential risks related to abnormal migration of grafts [26]. Biodistribution studies both within the CNS and between CNS and periphery are important. In this context, the differences between autologous, allogeneic, and immunosuppressed host environments may be important and should be considered.

4.5 Ancillary therapeutic components

Cell-based interventions frequently involve materials other than cells per se, such as biomaterials, engineered scaffolds, and injection devices, as well as the carrier vehicle in which cells are prepared and suspended for transplantation. These materials or surgical instruments must also be tested for safety and effectiveness. Safety and efficacy studies should include an assessment of possible interactions between the cell products and these materials, *in vitro* and *in vivo*.

4.6 Long-term safety studies

Long-term safety studies are done after the transplantation surgery is conducted in animals. Given the intended persistence of cells and the irreversibility of some cell-based interventions, testing of the long-term fate and effect of transplanted cells in animal models is vital. As non-human animal models may not replicate the full range of human toxicities associated with stem cell-based interventions, particular care must be applied in preclinical analysis. Health conditions and mortality rates of treated animals should be carefully recorded in an unbiased fashion so that sensitive detection of unexpected adverse effects can be achieved. Beyond this, toxicities and other emerging side effects that are likely to be unique to stem cells or their progeny can also be observed.

4.7 Application of genetic alteration and genome editing technologies to stem cell products

Genetic alteration or genome editing technologies can be coupled to stem cell therapies or applied directly *in vivo* to resident tissue cells for a variety of therapeutic purposes. If gene editing technology and stem cell-based therapy are combined, researchers should comprehensively investigate the type and genomic distribution of introduced genetic alterations as well as their potential adverse effects on the genome and the biological properties of the treated cells at short and long-term time points. Special attention must be given to the effects of off-target changes in the genome and to the distribution of genetic alterations to unintended cell types in grafts.

5. Methods and technologies in stem cell-based therapy for PD

In stem cell-based therapy for Parkinson's disease, a variety of approaches have been applied to test the safety of cell products. Here, we provide examples of such approaches and some of the release criteria used by three representative teams that have obtained regulatory approval for PD cell therapy trials, including the laboratories of Kim [5], Studer [27], and Takahashi [28] (**Table 2**).

5.1 Cell characterization and counting

The composition and purity of a cell product is perhaps the most important characteristic to be measured. Differentiation protocols applied to either ESC or iPSC do not generally result in monotypic cell cultures, but rather in a mix of cell types related to the embryology of the target region [29]. Immunostaining, flow cytometry, and quantitative reverse transcriptase polymerase chain reaction (qRT-PCR) are three commonly used methods to count cells by identifying their specific genes or downstream proteins. Each method has its advantages:

- Immunostaining includes immunohistochemistry (IHC), immunocytochemistry (ICC), and immunofluorescence (IF). *In vivo* immunostaining in particular enables researchers to observe cells without damaging brain structure, thus providing more information about the relationship between graft and host.

- Flow cytometry, compared to immunostaining, is faster and more quantitative and is more often used for *in vitro* cell counting.

- PCR is a method widely used to rapidly make millions to billions of copies of a specific DNA or RNA samples, and qRT-PCR is a PCR technique used to count the amount of sample, which enables researchers to detect contrasts between samples and note specific cell type signatures.

In developing strategies for stem cell-based therapy for Parkinson's disease, biological markers for undifferentiated cells and for the end therapeutic product

Cell type	Biological marker	Release criteria (Lab)		
		Kim KS	Studer L	Takahashi J
hiPSCs/hESCs	OCT4	>90%	≥90%	N/A
	SSEA4	>90%	≥90%	N/A
	Nanog	N/A	≥90%	N/A
	TRA-1-60 & TRA-1-81	N/A	≥90%	N/A
DAPs	TRA-1-60	N/A	N/A	<1% (presort)
	CORIN	N/A	N/A	>10% (presort) >90% (postsort)
	FOXA2	>55%; >500-fold than D0	>85%	>80%
	LMX1A	>55%; >500-fold than D0	N/A	N/A
	FOXA2 & LMX1A	>50%	N/A	N/A
	TUJ1	N/A	N/A	>80%
	TH	>10%; >500-fold than D0	N/A	N/A
	OCT3	N/A	<0.1%	<0.1%
	OCT4	None detected	<0.1%	<0.1%
	SSEA4	None detected	N/A	N/A
	TRA-2-49/6E	N/A	N/A	<0.1%
	SOX1	N/A	N/A	<0.1%
	PAX6	N/A	<5%	<0.1%
	Nanog	N/A	<0.2%	N/A
	POU5F1	N/A	N/A	<1% compared to undifferentiated cells
	LIN28	N/A	N/A	<1% compared to undifferentiated cells
	TPH2	<1%	N/A	N/A
	5-HT	<1%	N/A	N/A
	DBH2	<1%	N/A	N/A

Method: red: immunostaining; green: flow cytometry; blue: qRT-PCR.
N/A: not available.

Table 2.
An overview of cell characterization release criteria.

dopaminergic cells (dopaminergic progenitors or dopaminergic neurons) are always measured. Among such markers, OCT4 and SSEA4 are representative markers for undifferentiated cells, FOXA2, and LMX1A are representative markers for dopaminergic progenitors, and TH, TUJ1 are representative markers for dopaminergic neuronal maturity.

A list of marker-based safety criteria from three major laboratories active in the field of PD cell therapy is shown in **Table 2**. A combined evaluation of biological markers with immunostaining, flow cytometry, and q-RT PCR can provide more detailed information about the composition of the culture.

5.2 Viability

Viability is a significant issue in the production process and during the transplantation of the final products. Many cells are lost during culture for reasons ranging from mechanical disruption during media changes to normal developmental apoptosis. In particular, the viability of the final cell suspension used for transplantation is a critical issue for determining how many cells are actually placed, i.e., the dose, Trypan Blue staining (criteria>70% by Kim Lab), flow cytometry (criteria>90% by Takahashi Lab), and AO/PI staining (criteria≥70% by Studer Lab) have been used for such viability testing.

5.3 Tumorgenicity, biodistribution, and toxicity studies

5.3.1 Tumorgenicity

Although cell characterization can predict the tumorgenicity of cell products through biological markers to some degree, an independent teratoma formation study is indispensable for a thorough tumorgenicity assessment. Such studies require both positive and negative controls. In positive control teratoma formation studies, the parent stem cells (ESCs or iPSCs) are usually injected into the peritoneal cavity or testes of mice to confirm their capability of forming teratomas, and similar analysis may be done with injection at the intended therapeutic target site in the brain. Here, vehicle-only injection serves as the negative control. The final proposed therapeutic product should not result in any tumor formation at the target site. For mice, a sufficient period of time (generally 6–9 months) is allowed to look for more indolent tumor formation. The number of animals used is determined by statistical consideration of the desired threshold for tumor risk which in general should be lower than the background incidence of spontaneous tumor development (**Table 3**).

5.3.2 Biodistribution

Biodistribution studies track the anatomical fate of therapeutic cell products after they are transplanted at the desired dose into the intended location in animal models. As the products are of human origin, they can be distinguished from the host using qPCR or other sensitive techniques. Tissues from different organs or, for PD cell therapy, from multiple brain regions, are collected and assessed for the presence of human genetic material. In PD cell therapy, cell products should be confined to the injection site in the brain or in a particular circuit from the substantia nigra to the striatum, but should not appear inappropriately in other organs or other regions in the brain (**Table 3**).

5.3.3 Toxicity studies

Phase I clinical trials usually include a dose escalation component designed to look for dose limitations related to toleration of side effects. This is obviously not a practical approach in cell therapy trials where the product is irretrievably implanted into the brain, and thus animal toxicity studies are critical. It is important to bear in mind that

Group	Host, administration route	Duration	Number of animals
Tumorigenicity			
Takahashi J	NOG, unlesioned, Striatum; NOG, unlesioned, Subcutaneous with Matrigel	12 months; 6 months	N = 80 (DAPs) N = 50 (Saline); N = 20 (DAPs) N = 10 (100% iPSCs) N = 50 spiked with 10% ~ 0.001% iPSCs
Studer L	NSG, unlesioned, Striatum	9 months	N = 44 (DAPs) N = 44 (with 0.01% & 0.1% hESC) N = 24 (hESCs); N = 24 (vehicle) Male and female
Kim KS	NSG, unlesioned, Striatum	9 months	N = 23 (DAPs)
Biodistribution			
Takahashi J	NOG, unlesioned, Striatum	12 months	N = 80 (DAPs) N = 50 (Saline)
Kim KS	NSG, unlesioned, Striatum	9 months	Not mentioned
Studer L	NSG, unlesioned, Striatum	1 month/ 6 months	N = 10 (High/low dose); N = 10 (Vehicle) Male and female
Toxicology			
Takahashi J	NOG, unlesioned, Striatum	12 months	N = 80 (DAPs) N = 50 (Saline)
Studer L	NSG, unlesioned, Striatum	1 month/ 6 months	N = 20 (High/low dose) N = 20 (Vehicle) Male and female

Table 3.
Summary of preclinical in vivo *safety studies.*

extrapolation to humans of certain forms of toxicity such as subtle effects on cognitive function may not be readily assessed in animal models so that conservative interpretations are used. Toxicity studies in animals, therefore, involve transplantation of doses of cell products into the target location, with comprehensive long-term analysis of the health of the animals, recording local and systemic physical and behavioral side effects and cause of death. Wide latitude is applied in drawing conclusions as to whether pathology and cause of death may be related to the cell products or transplantation procedure, with attention again paid to the autologous, allogeneic, or immunosuppressed state of the host (**Table 3**).

5.4 Contamination

Contamination tests include sensitive detection of viral, bacterial, and mycoplasma presence in the final product or in any of the reagents used to produce it, and may utilize PCR, microbial detection systems for sterility, gram staining for bacteria, endotoxin tests, and adventitious virus testing (**Table 4**).

5.5 Karyotype analysis and genetic analysis

Karyotype analysis methods include G-band analysis and standard metaphase chromosome analysis, and genetic analysis methods include DNA fingerprinting, whole-genome sequencing, whole-exome sequencing, array comparative genomic hybridization (aCGH), and single-nucleotide polymorphism array (SNP array). Such

Target	Method	Release criteria (Lab)		
		Kim KS	Takahashi J	Studer L
Mycoplasma	PCR	Negative	Negative	Negative
Sterility test	BacT/Alert® system	No organism Detected	No organism Detected	No organism Detected
Bacteria	Gram staining	Negative	Negative	Negative
Endotoxin	LAL®	<0.2EU/kg body weight/hr	≤10 EU/mL	≤1 EU/mL

Table 4.
Criteria for contamination test.

careful analyses are required to test genomic integrity and to uncover genetic changes, chromosomal aberrations, and karyotype changes in cell products that may relate both to tumorigenicity and to residual epigenetic memory in the final product or aberrant off-target effects of the reprogramming and differentiation process.

6. Strategies to enhance the safety of stem cell-based therapy for PD

6.1 Removal of unwanted cell types

To minimize the potential risks of stem cell therapy for PD, the transplanted products should differentiate to sufficiently pure ventral midbrain dopaminergic (vmDA) neurons, or at a minimum into tissue closely resembling the normal cellular composition of SNpc. To reach this goal, the first step is to remove unwanted cells from the samples.

A major potential risk of stem cell therapy is the possibility that the clinical product may still contain stem cells that are not fully differentiated. These cells have a strong capacity to divide and expand and have a high probability of developing into potentially aggressive tumors. Therefore, before further sorting of the induced mDAPs, candidate products must be treated with inhibitors of cell stemness genes such as c-Myc for the purpose of reducing the number of undifferentiated stem cells.

At the same time, however, care must be taken that the inhibitor system used is not toxic to mDAPs to ensure the survival and growth of mDAPs after transplantation. A good example is the use of the flavonoid quercetin (3,3′,4′,5,7-pentahydroxyflavone), an inhibitor of the gene BIRC5, which shows 99.99% efficiency in removing the undifferentiated hiPSCs but leaves the mDAPs intact [22].

6.2 Target cells purification

Simply removing undifferentiated cells is not sufficient to create an efficacious therapeutic product. mDAPs with specific molecular profiles indicating their commitment to vmDA neuronal fate should be further identified and purified as a second step.

The major techniques currently used to purify target cells from samples can be divided into two main categories:

Criteria methods	Price	Time cost	Versatility	Accuracy
MCS	Lower	Lower	Lower	Lower
FACS	Higher	Higher	Higher	Higher

Table 5.
The comparison between MCS and FACS.

- Bulk cell sorting methods like filtration, centrifugation, selective cultivation, and magnetic cell sorting (MCS);
- Single-cell sorting methods like fluorescence-activated cytometry sorting (FACS).

In proposed protocols for stem cell therapy, researchers use specific sequences of transcription factors and other manipulations to selectively cultivate a population enriched in the desired target cells. Then either MCS or SACS methods may be applied to further purify the products:

- FACS: This is essentially an extended version of flow cytometry, in which a nozzle creates droplets containing single cells, electrodes apply a charge to those droplets containing cells with target markers, and charged plates create electric fields in order to change the falling trajectory of the droplets so that they sort into different collecting tubes. In FACS, antibodies carrying fluorescent markers bind to specific cell surface markers to label the cells.
- MCS: This method uses magnetic beads encapsulated with antibodies that bind specifically to the target cell surface markers. The target cells with specifically bound magnetic beads are then placed in a magnetic field to separate them out of the suspension. The remaining solutions would be removed, and targeted cells are resuspended for collection.

Table 5 presents a comparison of the two methods:

Because FACS involves less manipulation of the cells and is somewhat more versatile in most respects, most published protocols using surface marker-based sorting have employed FACS to purify the cells.

The basis of sorting for both these methods is the diversity of cell surface markers and the presumed presence of specific markers or specific combinations of such markers at critical stages of differentiation to uniquely identify the desired cell types. Therefore, they depend on the ability to find such unique markers and design the corresponding antibodies for FACS. For the cell type ideally suited to our clinical requirements, e.g., dopaminergic neuronal progenitors, the goal is to search for molecular characteristics distinguishing these from other cells, with attention to unique surface markers. This may be accomplished by using single-cell RNA sequencing to look for genes specifically expressed in target cells and then to look for potential surface markers among these genes.

7. Conclusions

Despite decades of recognition of the potential benefits of cell replacement therapy for Parkinson's disease, progress in this area has been slow. This is related to both ethical and logistical issues in using human fetuses as a tissue source, and to underestimation of the complexities of the disease itself and of the ability to use embryonic tissue to restore function in the adult allogeneic brain. Nonetheless, enough evidence of the potential power of this approach emerged from these efforts that the advent of human ESC and in particular iPSC technology encouraged a renewed enthusiasm and reappraisal of the field that is currently underway. In this chapter, we have discussed some of the differences between the use of fetal tissue that was the proof of principle for these efforts and the use of human ESC or iPSC; the differences between ESC and iPSC; the shared and different risks and goals in using each; and a variety of approaches in use as of this writing to attempt to realize their potential benefits safely and efficaciously. We are optimistic that future editions of this chapter will be able to report significant continued progress toward this important goal.

Acknowledgements

This work was supported by the National Natural Science Foundation of China (32170807), and the Natural Science Foundation of Shanghai (21ZR1406300). We also thank members of the Parkinson's Disease and Cell therapy Laboratory for their discussion and suggestions.

Conflict of interest

The authors declare no conflict of interest.

Author details

Fangzhou Li[1,2], Jiahao Ji[2,3], Jun Xue[1,2], Jeffrey Schweitzer[4*] and Bin Song[1,2*]

1 Department of Neurosurgery, Huashan Hospital, China

2 Institute for Translational Brain Research, State Key Laboratory of Medical Neurobiology, MOE Frontiers Center for Brain Science, China

3 School of Basic Medical Sciences, Fudan University, Shanghai, China

4 Department of Neurosurgery, Massachusetts General Hospital, Harvard Medical School, Boston, MA, USA

*Address all correspondence to: jschweitzer1@mgh.harvard.edu; binsong@fudan.edu.cn

References

[1] Emre M. Dementia associated with Parkinson's disease. Lancet Neurology. 2003;**2**(4):229-237

[2] Lindvall O et al. Grafts of fetal dopamine neurons survive and improve motor function in Parkinson's disease. Science. 1990;**247**(4942):574-577

[3] Freed CR et al. Transplantation of embryonic dopamine neurons for severe Parkinson's disease. The New England Journal of Medicine. 2001;**344**(10): 710-719

[4] Olanow CW et al. A double-blind controlled trial of bilateral fetal nigral transplantation in Parkinson's disease. Annals of Neurology. 2003;**54**(3): 403-414

[5] Schweitzer JS et al. Personalized iPSC-derived dopamine progenitor cells for Parkinson's disease. The New England Journal of Medicine. 2020; **382**(20):1926-1932

[6] Announcement of Physician-Initiated Clinical Trials for Parkinson's Disease. 2018; Available from: https://www.cira.kyoto-u.ac.jp/e/pressrelease/news/180730-170000.html

[7] Kolata G. A Cautionary Tale of 'Stem Cell Tourism'. 2016. Available from: https://www.nytimes.com/2016/06/23/health/a-cautionary-tale-of-stem-cell-tourism.html

[8] Gretchen V. Disgraced Italian Surgeon Convicted of Criminal Harm to Stem Cell Patient. 2022. Available from: https://www.science.org/content/article/disgraced-italian-surgeon-convicted-of-criminal-harm-to-stem-cell-patient

[9] Backlund EO et al. Transplantation of adrenal medullary tissue to striatum in parkinsonism. First Clinical Trials. Journal of Neurosurgery. 1985;**62**(2): 169-173

[10] Mínguez-Castellanos A et al. Carotid body autotransplantation in Parkinson disease: A clinical and positron emission tomography study. Journal of Neurology, Neurosurgery, and Psychiatry. 2007;**78**(8):825-831

[11] Lindvall O et al. Fetal dopamine-rich mesencephalic grafts in Parkinsons-disease. Lancet. 1988;**2**(8626-7): 1483-1484

[12] Deacon T et al. Histological evidence of fetal pig neural cell survival after transplantation into a patient with Parkinson's disease. Nature Medicine. 1997;**3**(3):350-353

[13] Gonzalez R et al. Neural stem cells derived from human parthenogenetic stem cells engraft and promote recovery in a nonhuman primate model of Parkinson's disease. Cell Transplantation. 2016;**25**(11):1945-1966

[14] Kaiser J, Wadman M. Trump administration releases details on fetal tissue restrictions. 2019. Available from: https://www.science.org/content/article/trump-administration-releases-details-fetal-tissue-restrictions

[15] Amy G. Biden Administration Removes Trump-era Restrictions on Fetal Tissue Research. 2021. Available from: https://www.washingtonpost.com/health/biden-administration-removes-trump-era-restrictions-on-fetal-tissue-research/2021/04/16/71719006-9ed2-11eb-8005-bffc3a39f6d3_story.html

[16] Lo B, Parham L. Ethical issues in stem cell research. Endocrine Reviews. 2009;**30**(3):204-213

[17] Murugan V. Embryonic stem cell research: A decade of debate from Bush to Obama. The Yale Journal of Biology and Medicine. 2009;**82**(3):101-103

[18] Russo E. Follow the money-The politics of embryonic stem cell research. PLoS Biology. 2005;**3**(7):e234

[19] Takahashi K, Yamanaka S. Induction of pluripotent stem cells from mouse embryonic and adult fibroblast cultures by defined factors. Cell. 2006;**126**(4): 663-676

[20] Thomson JA et al. Embryonic stem cell lines derived from human blastocysts. Science. 1998;**282**(5391):1145-1147

[21] Arenas E, Denham M, Villaescusa JC. How to make a midbrain dopaminergic neuron. Development. 2015;**142**(11): 1918-1936

[22] Song B et al. Human autologous iPSC-derived dopaminergic progenitors restore motor function in Parkinson's disease models. The Journal of Clinical Investigation. 2020;**130**(2):904-920

[23] Lovell-Badge R et al. ISSCR guidelines for stem cell research and clinical translation: The 2021 update. Stem Cell Reports. 2021;**16**(6): 1398-1408

[24] Cellular and Gene Therapy Guidances. 2021. Available from: https://www.fda.gov/vaccines-blood-biologics/biologics-guidances/cellular-gene-therapy-guidances

[25] Goldring CEP et al. Assessing the safety of stem cell therapeutics. Cell Stem Cell. 2011;**8**(6):618-628

[26] Halme DG, Kessler DA. FDA regulation of stem cell-based therapies. The New England Journal of Medicine. 2006;**355**(16):1730-1735

[27] Piao J et al. Preclinical efficacy and safety of a human embryonic stem cell-derived midbrain dopamine progenitor product, MSK-DA01. Cell Stem Cell. 2021;**28**(2):217-229.e7

[28] Doi D et al. Pre-clinical study of induced pluripotent stem cell-derived dopaminergic progenitor cells for Parkinson's disease. Nature Communications. 2020;**11**(1):3369

[29] Kee N et al. Single-cell analysis reveals a close relationship between differentiating dopamine and subthalamic nucleus neuronal lineages. Cell Stem Cell. 2017;**20**(1):29-40

Chapter 9

Effect of Motor Learning Feedback on Cognitive Functions in Parkinsonism

Lama Saad El-Din Mahmoud

Abstract

Parkinson's disease is characterized by cognitive impairments that impair motor control. The major goal was to see how motor learning feedback with enhanced motor learning cues affected cognitive skills in Parkinson's patients. This study engaged the participation of 30 patients of both genders. The patients were split into two equal groups at random: The participants in the study were given motor learning feedback along with augmented motor learning cues and the selected cognitive therapy program, while the control group received only the selected cognitive therapy program. The patients were assessed by the computer-based cognitive assessment device (RehaCom) and the Mini-Mental State Examination (MMSE) scale. The study's findings revealed a significant difference between the study and control groups ($p = 0.0001$), The study group exhibited a larger improvement in cognitive functioning than the control group. In Parkinson's patients, motor learning feedback with enhanced cues has a significant beneficial effect on cognitive skills.

Keywords: parkinsonism, cognition, motor learning, feedback, augmented cues

1. Introduction

Parkinson's disease (PD) is characterized by deficits in cognitive functions and motor control, such as difficulties in movement initiation, scaling movement amplitudes, or modulating muscle activity. The basal ganglia, particularly those involved for "automatic execution of learnt motor plans," play an important role in the generation and monitoring of motor programmes. The basal ganglia signal the end of a preparatory activation or a previous sub-movement in the supplementary motor area (SMA) to allow a new component of a movement sequence to be initiated. However, a compensatory cortical reorganization can be achieved by modulating cortical plasticity through peripheral feedback and sensorimotor integration [1].

Motor learning is a set of processes associated with practice or experience, leading to relatively permanent changes in the capability for movement. Motor learning involves three main stages, during the first or cognitive stage of learning, the performer engages in receiving instructions and feedback from the instructor, figuring out what to do and how to do it. The second, or associative, stage of learning is indicated by linking certain environmental cues with the actions necessary to attain the goal or skill, since this is a refining stage in which the person makes fewer errors and displays more task consistency. The third stage is called the autonomous stage as the automaticity is reached, where the performers no longer think about the specific movement characteristics and can often do another task at the same time [2].

"The mental action or process of obtaining information and understanding via thinking, experience, and the senses" is what cognition is defined as. Knowledge, attention, memory, and working memory, judgment and assessment, reasoning and "computation," problem-solving, and decision-making are all included [3].

The executive functions are the most damaged by PD, resulting in a phenomenology similar to that of frontal lobe patients, with attention, planning, idea generation, and working memory deficits. Memory loss affects both spatial and non-spatial working memory domains, implicit memory, episodic memory, and procedural learning in particular, whereas the ability to construct new episodic memories is intact [4].

Visual perception and object identification problems are typically described as one of the first symptoms in people with Parkinson's disease, and they appear to be unrelated to the degree of motor dysfunctions, neuropsychiatric comorbidities, and general cognitive decline. Cognitive symptoms may be connected to the subsequent involvement of other brain areas, such as the prefrontal cortex, hippocampus, and amygdala, in addition to the loss of dopaminergic neurons in the substantia nigra [5].

Executive dysfunction is the most frequent cognitive deficit in Parkinson's disease, and it can affect planning, cognitive flexibility, abstract thinking, rule acquisition, working memory, and sensory input selection [6].

Feedback is a significant factor in motor skill acquisition. There are two forms of feedback in general. One type is sensory-perceptual information known as "task-intrinsic" (or inherent) feedback. The second type of feedback is known as "augmented" feedback, and it consists of (information, extrinsic, visual display of movement kinematics or kinetics or artificial feedback) [7].

The cueing methods such as (auditory and visual) cues are commonly applied to evoke a more goal-directed type of motor learning and reduce cognitive dysfunction severity in PD. When motor learning is coupled with external stimuli, which may become entrenched in or part of the central motor representation, at least in the near term, motor learning may be stronger (or performance increases may be greater) in people with Parkinson's disease. As a result, cue-augmented learning may only be demonstrated in situations where cues are available and allowed to the learned motor abilities. This learning's specificity has clear clinical consequences [8].

Some individuals with mental and perceptual deficits are unable to direct their performance via internal feedback. Additionally, they may be more dependent on augmented input since neurological sensory abnormalities may decrease their capacity to provide intrinsic feedback [8]. Improving task-intrinsic feedback with external cues to replace necessary internal inputs from the basal ganglia to enhance cognition and postural control during movement onset, completion, and boost task execution is known as using augmented cues [1]. It facilitates the accomplishment of the objective more rapidly, enhances one's belief in one's own expertise (motivation), and increases the likelihood that the activities will be repeated (reinforcement) [9].

So, this study was done to investigate the effect of motor learning stages combined with augmented cued of motor learning on cognitive functions in Parkinson's patients.

2. Materials and methods

2.1 Assessment methods

All the patients were evaluated pre and post-treatment program, as the assessment methods were:

2.2 Assessment of cognitive function by Reha-com device

The computerized Reha-Com device including the (reaction behavior) program was used as the patient was instructed to deal and reacted with the different items shown on the computer screen in front of him. The Reaction Behavior program included a task in which the patient was asked to press the corresponding reaction button as fast as possible whenever a relevant stimulus - a traffic sign - was shown on the screen, in addition, there were also irrelevant signs which the patient must not react to. The task contains different (16) levels of difficulty.

2.3 Mini: mental state examination (MMSE) scale

It is a series of questions and tests, each of which scores points if answered correctly. If every answer is correct, a maximum score of (30) points is possible. The MMSE a number of different mental abilities, including a person's memory, attention and language.

It is the most commonly used instrument for screening cognitive function, and can be used to indicate the presence of cognitive impairment, such as in a patient with Parkinsonism.

It includes questions that measured cognitive function including orientation, registration, attention and calculation, recall, and language. The maximum score is (30) points [10].

2.4 Intervention methods

The study group of the present study received both the functional task training using augmented cues of motor learning and a selected cognitive therapy program.

The Parkinson's patients performed a functional task training program inform of Sit to stand task, which was divided into the following subtasks: sit-to-stand initiation (leaning forward); push up off the chair, and stand up fully. This program was performed according to the three- stages motor learning strategy as the first cognitive stage at the beginning of the session where the therapist provides the patients with illustrated details on subtasks performance via verbal instructions and visual feedback cues through observing the therapist's performance, then the second associative stage which started as the patient performed the subtasks while receiving both tactile and verbal feedback cues from the therapist to detect error and correct it, finally, the third autonomous stage started as the therapist allowed the patient to perform the subtasks without the external feedback cues to be able to detect error and correct it by himself.

The control group received only the selected cognitive therapy program including the Compensatory complex task training through the step Square-Stepping Exercise (SSE): which is a simple foot placement pattern that involves forward, backward, lateral, and diagonal steps using a gridded floor squares, SSE is a physical exercise which also requires cognitive function by including intellectual activities such as attention, concentration, memory and imitation [11].

As the therapist demonstrated and performed a stepping pattern for the patient by stepping the feet on certain squares from a standing position, then the patient was asked to step on the floor squares in the same pattern that the therapist performed. Every patient in both groups received (three sessions) per week, for six weeks every other day for 60 minutes/session.

3. Results

3.1 Comparison between the results of both groups of cognitive reaction behavior level (RB) of the Reha com pre and post-intervention

- **Pre-treatment:** The mean ± SD level RB of the study group was 7 ± 1.73 and that of the control group was 7.33 ± 1.54. The mean difference between both groups was −0.33. There was no significant difference in the level of RB between the study and control groups ($p = 0.58$).
- **Post-treatment:** The mean ± SD level RB of the study group was 13 ± 2.2 and that of the control group was 9 ± 1.92. The mean difference between both groups was 4. There was a significant increase in the level RB of in the study group compared with that of the control groups ($p = 0.0001$) (**Table 1**).

3.2 Comparison between mean values of both groups pre & post-treatment of mini-mental state examination (MMSE) scale of cognitive functions

- **Pre-treatment:** The mean ± SD MMSE of the study group was 11.8 ± 1.69 points and that of the control group was 11.93 ± 2.54 points. The mean difference between both groups was −0.13 points. There was no significant difference in the MMSE between both groups pre-treatment ($p = 0.86$).
- **Post-treatment:** The mean ± SD MMSE post-treatment of the study group was 23.06 ± 0.96 points and that of the control group was 17.26 ± 2.15 points. The mean difference between both groups was 5.8 points. There was a significant increase in the MMSE of the study group compared with that of the control groups post-treatment ($p = 0.0001$) (**Table 2**).

RB Level	Pre-treatment		Post-treatment	
	Study group	Control group	Study group	Control group
$\bar{X}$	7	7.33	13	9
SD	1.73	1.54	2.2	1.92
MD	−0.33		4	
t-value	−0.55		5.29	
p-value	0.58		0.0001***	
Level of significance	NS		S	

*$\bar{X}$: Mean; MD: Mean difference; p-value: Probability value; S: Significant; SD: Standard deviation; t value: Unpaired t value; NS: Non-significant; ***: High Significance.*

Table 1.
Pre and post-treatment mean values of RB level between both groups.

MMSE (points)	Pre-treatment		Post-treatment	
	Study group	**Control group**	**Study group**	**Control group**
$\bar{X}$	11.8	11.93	23.06	17.26
SD	1.69	2.54	0.96	2.15
MD	−0.13		5.8	
t-value	−0.16		9.52	
p-value	0.86		0.0001***	
Level of significance	**NS**		**S**	

$\bar{X}$: Mean; MD: Mean difference; p-value: Probability value; SD: Standard deviation; t value: Unpaired t value; NS: Non-significant; S: Significant.

Table 2.
Pre and post-treatment mean values of MMSE between both groups.

4. Discussion

This study showed that the augmented cues of motor learning were more effective for improving cognitive dysfunction in Parkinson's patients in the study group than only the selected cognitive therapy program. The findings of the present study were supported by Heremans et al., [12] who found that Visual-motor learning cues dramatically improved the cognitive and bradykinesia symptoms of Parkinson's patients while reducing their bradykinesia. Heremans et al. [12] also showed that The participants' mental state was greatly enhanced by the visual signals, and the PD patients, who consistently performed more slowly than controls, had a greater temporal isochrony with physical execution. The precision and timing of imagined motor activities were shown to be greatly improved by the addition of enhanced external stimuli.

Cued motor development Cueing has historically been thought of as a compensatory rehabilitation technique to increase motor output by evading the PD internal motor generating system's deficiencies. Studies supporting the presence of an unique medial and lateral system with varied anatomical connections and functional relevance provide the basis of this bypassing idea. The basal ganglia and the supplementary motor area (SMA) in the medial system, along with intention and an individual's internal reference frame, would assist the creation of actions [9].

The findings of the present study were also in agreement with Price and Shin [13] who reported that Parkinson's patients with moderate cognitive impairment and those who demonstrate learning in the cognitive training program benefitted greatly from the use of enhanced feedback cues in these programs. Four weeks later, the experimental group's MMSE scores greatly outperformed those of the control group ($p < 0.05$). Especially, the improvement was significant in the moderate cognitive impairment group (MMSE = 11 ~ 21) ($p < 0.05$). In learned patients of the experimental group, the score of the MMSE was significantly more improved than the control group ($p < 0.05$).

Internal cueing processes are compromised in PD, resulting in symptoms like hypokinesia. However, by utilizing cerebral resources, external signals can enhance movement execution. Feedback signals sent by cerebro-cerebellar-cerebral neural networks can bypass damaged BG, improving the ability to move in response to the stimuli and raising cortical activity [12].

Several treatments for Parkinson's physiotherapy therapies try to instruct patients on compensating attentional/cognitive techniques that may rely on the activation of alternate motor pathways. Indeed, it has been shown that both attentional strategies, such as instructions that rely on cognitive mechanisms of motor control and are internally generated, and augmented feedback cueing strategies (based on the use of external stimuli associated with the initiation and facilitation of a motor activity), can improve performance by using alternative pathways unaffected by Parkinson disease (PD) [14].

Bypassing the ineffective medial motor system, which includes the BG, cuing activates the lateral cortical system. In order to fix their internal image of the training action, patients can learn to use signals to "Consciously focus to faulty features of the imagined movement." External cuing enhances the quality of motor imagery in PD. If this is the case, then cueing patients while they are using mental images can help them learn the task more quickly, enhancing function of that object [12].

Cueing training involves compensatory mechanisms since it is believed that externally induced movements bypass the compromised basal ganglia circuitry and instead stimulate the premotor cortex, cerebellum, and parietal cortex; and cueing training's learning-related increases in motor performance are expected to be accompanied by neural changes. Cueing training in (PD) may have rapid impacts on compensatory neural pathways that are not directly used during routine activity. The conditions for goal-based exercise training are made easier by external cueing [15].

Doyon et al. [8] stated that Improvement in motor learning may be more pronounced in Parkinson's disease (PD) (or performance gains may be stronger) when it gets coupled with external cues, which may also contribute to improvement in cognitive functioning, which, at least temporarily, may be incorporated into or made a part of the core motor image. As a result, cue-augmented learning may only be demonstrated in situations where cues are available and allow for online access to the learned motor abilities. In Parkinson's patients who also have cognitive impairment, this specificity of learning has clear clinical consequences. The explanation provided by the author backs up the findings of the current investigation.

5. Conclusion

Based on the scope and findings of this study, which concluded that the rehabilitation program that depends on the motor learning stages and included the augmented cues of motor learning showed a significant improvement in Parkinson's cognitive dysfunction, compared to the control group who received only the selected cognitive therapy program. Therefore, motor learning with augmented cues should be considered a potential rehabilitation program and must be indicated as an effective, reliable, noninvasive modality at physical therapy clinics for Parkinson's patients with cognitive dysfunctions.

Conflict of interest

The authors declare no conflict of interest.

Author details

Lama Saad El-Din Mahmoud
Faculty of Physical Therapy, Department of Neurology and Neurosurgery, October 6 University, Giza, Egypt

*Address all correspondence to: lamaelsedawyy@hotmail.com; lama.elsedawy.pt@o6u.edu.eg

References

[1] Peterson DS, Pickett KA, Earhart GM. Effects of levodopa on vividness of motor imagery in Parkinson disease. Journal of Parkinson's Disease. 2012;**2**: 127-133

[2] Flavia M, Stampatori C, Zanotti D, Parrinello G, Capra R. Efficacy and specificity of intensive cognitive rehabilitation of attention and executive functions in multiple sclerosis. Journal of the Neurological Sciences. 2010;**288**: 101-105

[3] van Wegen EEH, Hirsch MA, Huiskamp M, Kwakkel G. Harnessing cueing training for neuroplasticity in Parkinson disease. Top Geriatr Rehabil. 2014;**30**:46-57

[4] Robbins TW, Cools R. Cognitive deficits in Parkinson's disease: A cognitive neuroscience perspective. Movement Disorders. 2014;**29**:597-607

[5] Ray NJ, Strafella AP. The neurobiology and neural circuitry of cognitive changes in Parkinson's disease revealed by functional neuroimaging. Movement Disorders. 2012;**27**: 1484-1492

[6] Cools R, Miyakawa A, Sheridan M, D'Esposito M. Enhanced frontal function in Parkinson's disease. Brain. 2010;**133**: 225-233

[7] Lim I, van Wegen E, Jones D, Rochester L, Nieuwboer A, Willems A-M, et al. Does cueing training improve physical activity in patients with Parkinson's disease? Neurorehabilitation and Neural Repair. 2010;**24**:469-477

[8] Doyon J, Bellec P, Amsel R, Penhune V, Monchi O, Carrier J, et al. Contributions of the basal ganglia and functionally related brain structures to motor learning. Behavioural Brain Research. 2009;**199**:61-75

[9] Avanzino L, Gueugneau N, Bisio A, Ruggeri P, Papaxanthis C, Bove M. Motor cortical plasticity induced by motor learning through mental practice. Frontiers in Behavioral Neuroscience. 2015;**9**:105

[10] Arevalo-Rodriguez I, Smailagic NI, Figuls MR, Ciapponi A, Sanchez-Perez E, Giannakou A, et al. Mini-mental state examination (MMSE) for the detection of Alzheimer's disease and other dementias in people with mild cognitive impairment (MCI). Cochrane Database of Systematic Reviews. 2015;**2015**: CD010783

[11] Shigematsu R, Okura T, Sakai T, Rantanen T. Square-stepping exercise versus strength and balance training for fall risk factors. Aging Clinical and Experimental Research. 2008;**20**: 19-24

[12] Heremans E, Nieuwboer A, Feys P, Vercruysse S, Vandenberghe W, Sharma N, et al. External cueing improves motor imagery quality in patients with Parkinson disease. Neurorehabilitation and Neural Repair. 2012;**26**:27-35

[13] Price A, Shin JC. The impact of Parkinson's disease on sequence learning: Perceptual pattern learning and executive function. Brain and Cognition. 2009;**69**:252-261

[14] Zhang X, de Beukelaar TT, Possel J, Olaerts M, Swinnen SP, Woolley DG, et al. Movement observation improves early consolidation of motor memory. The Journal of Neuroscience. 2011;**31**: 11515-11520

[15] Spaulding SJ, Barber B, Colby M, Cormack B, Mick T, Jenkins ME. Cueing and gait improvement among people with Parkinson's disease: A meta-analysis. Archives of Physical Medicine and Rehabilitation. 2013;**94**:562-570

Chapter 10

Perspective Chapter: The Role of Dopamine Receptors in Neuropsychiatric Diseases

Burak Yaman

Abstract

Dopamine is a key regulator neurotransmitter in the important cognitive and intellectual functions of the brain. This neurotransmitter in a structure of catecholamine is responsible for motivation, movement, reward-punishment, mood, memory, attention and more functions in central nervous system. This large effect area gives dopamine high importance in the pathophysiology of neuropsychiatric diseases. Dopamine shows its effects through dopamine receptors that are G protein-coupled receptors ranging from D1 to D5. Changes in the activity of these receptors are associated with diseases like schizophrenia, Parkinson's disease and addiction. This relationship between dopamine receptors and neuropsychiatric diseases has made these receptors main target in the strategy of clinic researches. Cognitive physiological functions of dopamine and the role of dopamine receptors in the common neuropsychiatric diseases are focused in this chapter.

Keywords: addiction, dopamine, dopamine receptors, G protein, Parkinson's disease, schizophrenia

1. Introduction

1.1 General cognitive functions of dopamine

Dopamine is a monoamine neurotransmitter synthesized from tyrosine and is precursor for epinephrine and norepinephrine. Dopamine is responsible for plenty of different body functions from visual physiology in retina to motor activity controlled by basal ganglia and a lot of emotional and cognitive functions controlled by limbic system and prefrontal cortex. Among functions of dopamine in the Central Nervous System (CNS), there are voluntary movement, reward, formation of conditioned reflexes, sleep regulation, feeding, affect, attention, olfaction, vision, hormonal regulation, sympathetic regulation, penile erection and more [1]. Even in other body regions except for brain, dopamine has important effects on immune, cardiovascular, gastrointestinal and urinary system, as well [2].

Dopamine decreases signal transduction of gap junctions between retina neurons after increase in light intensity. This change provides cone receptors to be more active than rod receptors during daylight. The release of dopamine from interplexiform cells increases and stimulates the D2-like receptors on cone and rods. Intracellular Cyclic Adenosine Monophosphate (cAMP) and Protein Kinase A (PKA) activity reduces, resulting in the reduction in the conductance of gap junctions between cones and rods. This regulatory mechanism provides cones to be more active than rods during high amount of light during the daytime [3].

Dopaminergic system follows the stages of ingestion from seconds to minutes and this provides learning about the consequences of ingestion, as well [4]. According to the taste of food or drink, neurons in Ventral Tegmental Area (VTA) secrete dopamine, providing cues for next preferences of food [5]. Dopaminergic release activity in VTA is pivotal for post-ingestion-related food seeking [6].

Dopaminergic substantia nigra neurons secrete dopamine in CNS. These neurons project into the striatal region of the basal ganglia and other brain regions like prefrontal cortex. Dopamine has both inhibitory and excitatory effects on different neurons in the brain. These different effects emerge through different dopamine receptors and their different intracellular secondary messenger systems.

1.2 Dopaminergic pathways in the brain

There are four major dopaminergic pathways in the CNS. Dopaminergic neurons from A9 region supply dopamine into the nigrostriatal pathway, neurons from A10 supply dopamine into the mesolimbic and mesocortical pathways and neurons from A8 supply dopamine into the tuberoinfundibular pathway [7].

Dopaminergic pathways come from substantia nigra, VTA and arcuate nucleus of medial hypothalamus. Nigrostriatal system comes from substantia nigra to dorsal striatum. Sensorial-motor coordination, cognitive integration and habituation are related to dopaminergic neurotransmission in the nigrostriatal system. The mesolimbic pathway between the VTA and the ventral striatum and between the hippocampus and the amygdala is associated with feelings of pleasure, reward and desire. Sense originated from this pathway provides existence of the emotion. Mesocortical pathway is projected from VTA and into the prefrontal dorsolateral, temporal, parietal and anterior cingulate cortex regions. This pathway is related to addiction and memory. Tuberoinfundibular pathway is composed of dopaminergic neurons projected from arcuate nucleus of hypothalamus and into the eminentia media. Dopamine synthesized from the tuberoinfundibular pathway regulates the secretion of the prolactin from the adenohypophysis.

1.3 G protein-coupled receptors

G Protein-Coupled Receptors (GPCR) are found only in eukaryotic cells. They are also called "7 transmembrane receptors" because their protein structure folds the cell membrane seven times. This is a feature unique to G protein-coupled receptors. While ligand binds to the outer surface of the cell in the transmembrane protein, there is a G protein on the inner surface of the cell, and this protein consists of three subunits, alpha, beta and gamma. G protein alpha and gamma subunits are attached to the cell membrane by the lipid anchor (lipid raft). Dopamine receptors are among the G protein-coupled receptors. These receptors exist in the vertebrate CNS. Abnormal changes in the dopaminergic neurotransmission in the brain are related to some neuropsychiatric diseases like schizophrenia, PD and addiction.

1.3.1 Dopamine receptors

There have been detected five dopamine receptor subtypes, ranging from D1 to D5. Effects of dopamine emerge through these five GPCR [8]. D1-like receptors and D2-like receptors are two main groups in the classification of the dopamine receptors. They are grouped according to their similar intracellular mechanisms. D1 and D5 belong to D1-like receptor family. D2, D3 and D4 belong to D2-like receptor family (**Table 1**).

Effects of the same type of dopamine receptors may vary between different brain regions. This phenomenon occurs thanks to the different intracellular signal transduction pathways [9]. Gs related increase in cAMP and Gi related decrease in cAMP in the cytoplasm of the neuron, phospholipase C pathway, regulation of the arachidonic acid secretion, regulation of Na-H exchanger and Na-K ATPase activity are among these different pathways.

Neurotransmission of dopamine is regulated by autoreceptors on the dopaminergic neurons, enzymatic degradation in the neurosynaptic space, presynaptic Dopamine Transporters (DAT) and other neurotransmitters like γ-Aminobutyric Acid (GABA), glutamate and serotonin. Besides, activity of dopamine receptors is regulated by Dopamine Receptor Interacting Proteins (DRIPs).

1.3.1.1 D1 receptors

It was firstly that dopamine was shown in brain as a neurotransmitter in 1957 [10]. Besides it was found that dopamine was concentrated in basal ganglion region in the CNS thanks to spectrofluorometry technique and D1 receptor activity increased the cAMP and PKA level in the cytoplasm of target cells [9].

There are D1 receptors in different regions of the brain like limbic system, hypothalamus, thalamus, olfactory tubercle, nucleus accumbens and striatum. D1 receptors are responsible for neurotransmission in the striato-thalamo-cortical circuit. D1 receptors provide the activation of adenylate cyclase and thus increase the cAMP in the cytoplasm of the target neuron. Increase in the cAMP level stimulates

Receptor	Gene	Structure	Intracellular signal transduction	Mechanism of action	Synaptic location
D1	DRD1	D1-like	Gs/activation of adenylate cyclase	Increase in cAMP	Postsynaptic
D2	DRD2	D2-like	Gi/inhibition of adenylate cyclase	Decrease in cAMP	Presynaptic and postsynaptic
D3	DRD3	D2-like	Gi/inhibition of adenylate cyclase	Decrease in cAMP	Presynaptic and postsynaptic
D4	DRD4	D2-like	Gi/inhibition of adenylate cyclase	Decrease in cAMP	Presynaptic and postsynaptic
D5	DRD5	D1-like	Gs/activation of adenylate cyclase	Increase in cAMP	Postsynaptic

Table 1.
General properties of dopamine receptors.

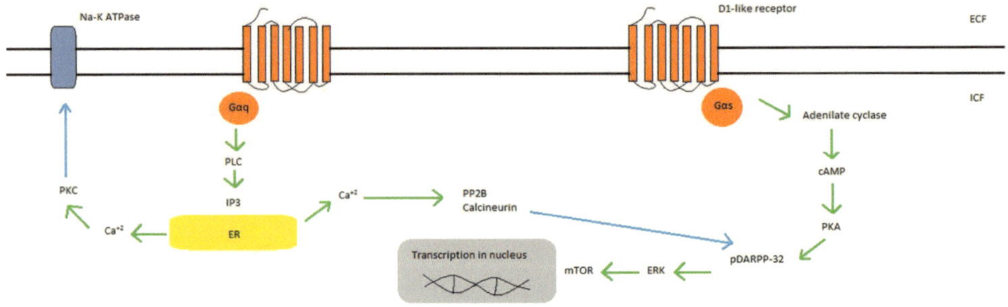

Figure 1.
Schematic representation of the intracellular signal transduction mechanism of the D1-like receptors. ECF, Extracellular Fluid; ICF, Intracellular Fluid; ER, Endoplasmic Reticulum; PLC, Phospholipase C; PKA, Protein Kinase A; DARPP-32, Dopamine and cAMP Regulated Phosphoprotein; IP3, Inositol Triphosphate; mTOR, Mammalian Target of Rapamycin; ERK, Extracellular Signal-Regulated Kinase; green arrow, activator pathway; blue arrow, inhibitor pathway.

the phosphorylation of the cAMP-related protein kinase and cAMP-regulated phosphoprotein (DARPP-32), (**Figure 1**). DARPP-32 amplifies the intracellular effects of PKA and regulates the synaptic plasticity in prefrontal cortex projected by dopaminergic neurons [11]. Some D1 and D2 receptor subtypes regulate the activity of the Ca^{+2}, K^+ and Na^+ ion currents in cell membrane through the different G protein subunits [12].

Effort-based decision-making is mostly related to dopaminergic system through D1 receptors. Neuropsychiatric disorders like schizophrenia and Major Depression (MD) continue with low desire to exert effort and psychomotor retardation [13]. Changes in the effort-based decision-making is seen in schizophrenia, MD, bipolar disorder, eating disorders and autism [14]. Unwillingness to effort for rewards is a specific characteristic of some neuropsychiatric diseases related to dopaminergic system like schizophrenia [15] and PD [16]. However, willingness to effort for food rewards is increased in some eating disorders and obesity [17].

1.3.1.2 D2 receptors

D2-like receptors, couple with Gi protein, inhibit adenylate cyclase and activate K^+ channels. D2 receptors have roles on survival of dopaminergic neurons [1] and neuronal growth [18, 19]. D2 receptors are found in the dorsal striatum, nucleus accumbens, ventral tegmental region and substantia nigra, which are areas of intense dopaminergic innervation.

D2 receptor activity provides the inhibition of the adenylate cyclase, the regulation of the activity of the ion channels like Ca^{+2} and K^+ and production of the phosphoinositide. Type of activity of the D2 receptor in the neuron depends on the type of neuron that synthesizes the receptor thanks to the different intracellular signal transducing mechanisms.

Contrary to D1 receptors, D2 receptors show both presynaptic autoreceptor and postsynaptic activity. D2 receptors are in the dopaminergic axonal terminals, soma and dendrites. D2 receptor modulator drugs are useful against schizophrenia and PD. An important amount of the highest global sales of medicines in 2017 were antipsychotic drugs like aripiprazole, olanzapine and quetiapine that target GPCR like dopamine receptors [20]. D2 receptors in the adenohypophysis regulate the inhibition of the secretion of the prolactin and alpha-MSH.

Catalepsy in patients with schizophrenia because of the antipsychotics like haloperidol may result from its effects on long form of D2 receptors [21].

There is an increase in the amount of postsynaptic D2 receptors in patients with schizophrenia. This condition leads to dopamine supersensitivity and psychotic reactions in these patients [22, 23]. While D2 receptor density is increased, D1 is not changed in the basal ganglia of patients with schizophrenia compared with control subjects [7].

Anhedonia, basic symptom of MD, is associated with the decrease in the sensitivity of the D2 and D3 receptors in the limbic system related to reward [7]. While D1 receptor density is decreased, D2 is not changed or increase in basal ganglia of patients with MD compared with control subjects [7]. In drug abusers, D2 receptor level is decreased in striatum [24]. D2 dopamine receptor density is altered, while D1 is not changed in PD. In earlier stages of PD, D2 receptor level is increased, however in the later stages level of D2 receptor is decreased [7, 25].

In some genetic studies, it has been reported that variations in D2, D3 and D4 dopamine receptor genes are related to schizophrenia and response to antipsychotic drugs [26–28]. Abnormalities in the D2 dopamine receptor gene are related to substance abuse [29].

In the clinical psychopharmacology experiments, it has been reported that D2 receptor is the main target of both typical and atypical antipsychotic drugs and drugs to treat PD [30]. However, many drugs targeting D2 are non-specific and affect unrelated receptors in therapy strategy. This condition results in some serious life threatening adverse effects in patients [31].

Aripiprazole is a partial agonist of the D2 dopamine receptors and affects the inhibition exerted by Gi on cAMP accumulation. Aripiprazole antagonizes the D2 receptor activity on the postsynaptic D2 receptors, while it activates D2 autoreceptors on the presynaptic D2 receptors and hence, antipsychotic effect occurs in a biased pharmacodynamics mechanism [7].

PKC regulates the D2 [32] and D3 [33] dopamine receptors through functional desensitization, receptor internalization and intracellular trafficking. Because of the different location of their phosphorylation and pseudosubstrate sites, D2S and D2L isoforms have different levels of sensitivity for desensitization by PKC [34]. Ethanol potentiates the D1 dopamine receptors through the phosphorylation by PKC [35].

A synonym mutation of human D2 receptor gene (C957T) is reported that results in the reduction in the dopamine induced up-regulation of the D2 receptors by changing mRNA stability [36]. C957T in a European American population is associated with schizophrenia and alcoholism [37].

In a recent animal study where male adult mice were used, it was reported that alterations in D2 receptor levels in purkinje cells in the cerebellum change sociability and preference for social novelty without affecting motor functions. In this study, it has been implied that although the regulation of reward, emotion and social interaction is largely related to monoaminergic system in limbic regions, the contribution of dopaminergic neurotransmission targeting D2 receptors on the purkinje cells in cerebellum cannot be ignored [38].

1.3.1.3 D3 and D4 receptors

D3 and D4 receptors belong to the group of D2-like receptors. Dopamine has 10–30 times more affinity to D3 and D4 receptors than D2. D3 receptors are found in the limbic system and nucleus accumbens.

D3 receptors are related to locomotor activity. Because it has important role on apathy in PD, D3 receptor may be targeted to treat motivational deficits [39]. Levodopa induced dyskinesia and psychosis in patients with PD may be prevented by antagonizing D3 receptors through new therapy strategies [40]. Activation of nicotinic acetylcholine receptors on dopaminergic neurons shows neurotrophic effects on these neurons together with D3 receptors. This functional complex composed of nicotinic acetylcholine receptors and D3 receptors is a heterodimeric modulator on dopaminergic neuronal growth [41]. This heterodimeric mechanism of action may be new target for anti-Parkinson drug design studies.

D4 receptors are found in frontal cortex, mesencephalon, amygdala, hippocampus and medulla oblongata. D4 receptors are found in the external of the CNS like heart and kidney, as well. D4 has important roles in the formation of novelty seeking behavior. Similar to D2, the amount of the D4 receptors are in a high level in the postmortem brain of the schizophrenia patients. Clozapine, an atypical antipsychotic, has high affinity to D4 receptors.

1.3.1.4 D5 receptors

D5 receptors are D1-like receptors and exist in the hippocampus, hypothalamus, prefrontal cortex and striatum in CNS. D5 receptors are responsible for the inhibition of locomotor activity [42].

1.4 Intracellular signal pathways of dopamine receptors

While Gsα increases the activity of adenylate cyclase, Gi decreases. D1-like receptors increase cAMP activity and D2-like receptors decrease it [43]. One of the most important consequences of the stimulation or suppression of cAMP formation is the activation or suppression of protein kinase A. Hence, some differences related to receptor type emerge in the cellular metabolic reactions like phosphorylation or dephosphorylation, synthesis of different cytoplasmic and nuclear proteins, activation of the different membrane channels and different G protein-coupled receptor sensitization.

Signal transduction of the dopamine receptors may result in phospholipase C activity or regulation of the arachidonic acid secretion, as well. Besides, dopamine receptors regulate Na-K ATPase and Na/H exchanger activity.

Activation of D2S isoform of D2 receptors coupling with Rho family of the G proteins results in stimulation of phospholipase D. Phospholipase D catalyzes the hydrolysis of the phosphatidylcholine to phosphatidic acid. Phosphatidic acid is an active signal molecule that plays pivotal role in cell growth, cell differentiation and regulation of cell metabolism.

Gβγ subunits of both D2S and D2L receptor isoforms are effective in the activity of protein kinase C, Mitogen-Activated Protein Kinase (MAPK), extracellular signal regulated kinase pathway (ERK) related cell growth, differentiation and apoptosis. Activation of MAPK and ERK pathways by dopamine agonists through D2 receptors provides apoptosis and cell death in tumor cells in the hypophysis.

Dopamine receptors are regulated by DRIPs [44]. Dopamine receptor interacting proteins provide movement of the receptors, emerging of the dopaminergic signals in the neurons and regulation of the receptor signals. Neurons having D1 and D2 receptors are controlled by different DRIPs.

1.5 Regulation of dopaminergic secretion

There are two basic transmission types called as intrasynaptic and extrasynaptic for dopamine in the CNS. In striatum, intrasynaptic dopamine secretion stimulates the postsynaptic dopamine receptors and extrasynaptic dopamine stimulates presynaptic D2-like autoreceptors. In extrastriatal regions, such as the prefrontal cortex, dopamine shows its extrasynaptic effect by diffusion through the gap junctions and by activating D1 receptors [45].

Dopamine regulates its self-dynamic activity through D2/D3 receptors through a (-) feedback mechanism of action. In addition, diffusion, intrasynaptic enzyme degradation through Monoamine Oxidase (MAO) and Catechol O-Methyltransferase (COMT) and transportation through presynaptic DAT all play a role in regulating dopamine levels in neurosynaptic junctions. DAT is a protein in the dopaminergic neurons and a specific marker showing dopaminergic neurons in immunohistochemically experiments [45]. There is the highest amount of DAT in the putamen, nucleus caudate and ventral striatum, meaning highest density of the dopaminergic neurons [46].

There are two types of secretion of dopamine from dopaminergic neurons. After an action potential from a presynaptic neuron, a dopamine secretion called as burst or phasic dopamine response with fast and high amplitude occurs in the first type of secretion. Mostly this type of response is associated with the dopaminergic behavior. Low-level extrasynaptic dopamine concentration called as tonic dopamine response occurs in the second type of secretion. In this response, dopamine level is too low to activate intrasynaptic dopamine receptors, but at a level to activate extrasynaptic autoreceptors. This response provides the (-) feedback suppression of high amount of phasic dopamine secretion.

Synthesize of dopamine is also regulated by other neurotransmitters. Afferent neurons synthesizing GABA from striatonigral and local circuits regulate secretion of dopaminergic neurons. N-methyl-D-aspartate (NMDA) receptor activity induced by glutamate administration results in slow Excitatory Postsynaptic Potentials (EPSP) in dopaminergic neurons in substantia nigra and VTA [45, 47].

Abnormalities in the dopaminergic system in the brain are related to diseases such as schizophrenia, Parkinson's disease (PD), addiction, depression and attention deficit hyperactivity disorder.

1.6 Cognitive effects of changes in dopaminergic neurotransmission on dopamine receptors

1.6.1 Importance of the nigrostriatal dopaminergic system on motor functions

Bilateral lesions primarily affecting the substantia nigra can result in slowness of movement and are correlated with bradykinesia in PD. The movement time in monkeys after 6-OHDA-induced lesion of the dopaminergic neurons and reaction time in a conditioned motor task in the rat administered to 6-OHDA were reported to increase. Such deficit has led to assume the importance of dopaminergic nerve terminals of dorsolateral part of the striatum on motor functions. Administration of D2 dopaminergic receptor antagonists were reported to cause similar results. However, DA and DA agonists were reported to decrease the reaction time. In Parkinsonian patients and Parkinsonian rodents constituted by lesion of the nigrostriatal dopaminergic system, increased reaction time has been reported. Besides, similar results also shown in conditioned motor task experiments in primates where 6-OHDA administration in substantia nigra or the neurotoxin MPTP were used. These results show the pivotal role of the nigrostriatal projections on the early stages of the motor control [48].

Forward locomotion is mostly controlled by the D1–3 receptors in ventral striatum. Activation of presynaptic D2 autoreceptors leads to a decrease in dopamine release, resulting in decreased locomotor activity. However, activation of postsynaptic D2 receptor activity slightly increases the locomotor activity. D3 receptors in nucleus accumbens have inhibitory role on locomotor activity. D3 agonists increase this effect while D3 antagonists decrease it [49].

1.6.2 Importance of mesocorticolimbic system on adaptation and memory

The administration of 6OHDA and lesioning of the different brain structures innervated by the mesocorticolimbic dopaminergic neurons are reported to show specific behavioral deficits. Lesions in VTA resulted in the inability to switch from one behavior to another, affecting the motivation and adaptation to behavior. Lesions of the dopaminergic terminals at septal level, the level of amygdala, hippocampus and habenula of the limbic system resulted in impaired performances in behavior tests like memory tests in maze paradigm [48].

Studies have reported that both D1 and D2 receptors are associated with intracranial self-stimulation behavior in the prefrontal cortex and nucleus accumbens of rats. D1 and D2 agonists stimulate this behavior, while antagonists inhibit it. Furthermore, D2-like receptors are reported to increase to seek further cocaine reinforcement in an animal model for cocaine seeking behavior. However, D1-like receptors decrease this behavior and thus agonists of these receptors may be a partner in the therapy of cocaine addiction. Both D1 and D2 receptors in the hippocampus of rat and prefrontal cortex in monkey have roles on learning and memory in pharmacological behavior experiments like performance measurement in working memory tasks [49].

D3 and D4 receptors are expressed mostly in the limbic and cortical regions but lesser amount in the dorsal striatum and may be useful in new antipsychotic drug discovery thanks to the lower incidence of extrapyramidal side effects [49].

2. Dopamine receptors and schizophrenia

The main reason of schizophrenia is the increase in dopaminergic neurotransmission in the brain. This increase may stem from either increased dopamine concentration in neurosynaptic junction between presynaptic and postsynaptic neurons or increased activity of the postsynaptic dopamine receptors like D2 [50]. Secretion of dopamine is changed abnormally and behavioral psychotic symptoms emerge in the patients with schizophrenia.

Schizophrenic patients are behaviorally more responsive to drugs such as amphetamine and methylphenidate increasing the amount of dopamine in neurosynaptic junction compared to healthy subjects. On used in these patients, these drugs trigger the psychotic symptoms. The main reason of this response is not only increased release of dopamine from presynaptic neuron, but also the increased amount of D2 receptors in the postsynaptic neurons. Both of these two main factors increase the dopaminergic neurotransmission and this neurotransmission is a basic source of delusion and hallucinations in schizophrenia. Even if presynaptic dopamine release is normal, D2 receptors are increased by an average of 5.8% in antipsychotic-free schizophrenia patients [50]. Increased psychotic response to psychostimulant drugs may stem from more D2 receptors in schizophrenia. It was reported that 75% of schizophrenia patients and 25% of healthy control subjects experienced new symptoms of psychosis after usage of the psychostimulants like amphetamine and methylphenidate [50].

2.1 Development and progression of schizophrenia

The consistency between acts and results provides the learning. Learning according to the amount of pleasure after act is an important way to learn. The mesolimbic dopaminergic pathways are related to motivation, providing a link between affect and action. These pathways provide connection between mood and act. Dopaminergic inputs to nucleus accumbens provide knowledge about importance and awareness of events occurring throughout the world. This knowledge contains rewarding and punisher stimuli and their foreseeability and novelty [51, 52].

The phasic firings in dopaminergic neurons, associated with the broad transient increase in synaptic dopamine release, stimulate postsynaptic signals encoding reward prediction or incentive awareness [53]. The abnormal functioning of this process in schizophrenia leads to abnormal perceptions of excessive novelty [54], awareness and thus to psychotic delusions [55].

In patients with schizophrenia, rate of habituation to the acoustic startle is decreased, and they exhibit higher scores of neuroticism compared to healthy control [56]. Attenuated acoustic startle response means to Prepulse Inhibition (PPI) is associated with central dopaminergic dysfunction. In PPI, startling stimulus is immediately preceded by a weaker, non-startling tone. Prepulse inhibition correlates with some schizophreniform cognitive dysfunctions like prolong maternal separations and variations in maternal care [57].

Recent studies indicate a significant increase in the levels of tyrosine hydroxylase, rate limiting enzyme involved in DA synthesis, suggesting increased production of DA in the midbrain. Studies using Positron Emission Tomography imaging (PET) showed abnormally high subcortical synaptic DA release after using DA stimulants like amphetamine, which induced psychotic symptoms in healthy individuals indicating that there is a presynaptic hyperdopaminergic abnormality in schizophrenia, and the antipsychotic drugs used to treat the disorder act by blocking DA receptors. However, it is also reported that glutamate, g-aminobutyric acid (GABA), acetylcholine and serotonin alterations, related to cognitive behavioral and social dysfunction, are involved in the pathophysiology of schizophrenia [58].

2.2 Psychosis and dopaminergic neurotransmission

Dopaminergic neurons in VTA and substantia nigra secret excess amount of the dopamine in patients with schizophrenia. These neurons provide the mesolimbic dopaminergic activity. This system projects into the medial and anterior portions of the limbic system composed of hippocampus, amygdala, prefrontal cortex and anterior caudate nucleus. These regions control the behavior. Increased phasic activity of subcortical dopaminergic neurotransmission on cortical regions results in behavioral impairments in patients with schizophrenia [59].

In the pathogenesis of schizophrenia, an abnormal dopaminergic neurotransmission occurs after genetic and environmental risk factors. Changes in the brain connections under the environmental effects like stress may lead to formation of psychosis, loss of brain mass and neurodegeneration in the formation of schizophrenia [60, 61]. The volume of the hippocampus in dominant hemisphere is decreased in patients with schizophrenia. However, an in vivo imaging study showed that main abnormality of the dopamine function in schizophrenia is also in the dorsal striatum related to the nigrostriatal pathway as well as the ventral (limbic) striatum related to the mesolimbic pathway [62].

During physiological conditions, sensation and explication of the novelty is provided by dopaminergic system. However, high activity in some brain regions of dopaminergic system results in an abnormal novelty sensation [63] and awareness [64]. These symptoms of schizophrenia can be reversed by antipsychotic drugs [63].

Main signs of the psychosis are delusions and hallucinations. Before the open psychosis, patients experience a prodromal period. During this period, dopaminergic neurons fire in a context independent manner. That condition results in a new novelty perception in patients. At this moment, perception is clearer and patients notice the things that they are not interested in before. Patients experience changed perceptions in the prodromal period.

Changes in mood and behavior, confusion and wonder increase day by day and transform to meaningful delusions. Abnormality of the dopaminergic system is the main source of the delusions. Personal and cultural history of the patient determine the basis of the delusion [55]. Decreased ability to use context information occurs in this late period [65]. After these pathological processes, delusions change abnormally the behavior of the patient. Patients or relatives of the patients request psychiatric examination in this active period. Usage of antipsychotics starts at this time.

Antipsychotics block the effect of the dopamine in CNS and decrease the abnormal perceptions. However, these drugs affect locomotor functions of the dopaminergic systems, as well. This effect emerges as disruption of the locomotor activity and prevents continuity of antipsychotic treatment [55].

3. Dopamine receptors and Parkinson's disease

PD is a common neurodegenerative disorder and affects 2–3% of the people, older than 65 years of age, throughout the world. Neuropathological markers of the PD are the aggregates of the α-synuclein as intracellular inclusion body and nigrostriatal dopaminergic neuronal loss [66].

Aging is an important risk factor for PD. While PD affects the 1% of the population older than 60 years, prevalence increases up to 5% in population older than 85 years [67].

The corticostriatal projections from the primary motor cortex, supplementary motor area, cingulate motor cortex and premotor cortex, which terminate on the dendrites of striatal medium spiny neurons, comprise the motor circuit of the dopaminergic system related to PD. Substantia nigra pars reticulata and globus pallidus internus are main dopaminergic output nuclei of the basal ganglia projecting into the ventrolateral thalamus and brainstem. Striatal projections on these output nuclei are composed of direct and indirect pathway. The direct pathway is between medium spiny neurons and GABAergic neurons in the globus pallidus internus and substantia nigra pars reticulata. This is a monosynaptic connection between these spiny neurons having D1 receptors and GABAergic neurons in these output nuclei. Projections from medium spiny neurons expressing D2 receptors to the globus pallidus externus constitute the indirect pathway. In a form of glutamatergic relay in the subthalamic nucleus, these projections arrive at globus pallidus internus, as well. Together with these two pathways, GABAergic output activity is regulated by dopaminergic projections from striatum. Changes in these relays result in PD.

Defect in the nigrostriatal dopaminergic activity results in different effects on direct and indirect pathways. In this condition, activity of direct pathway related to D1 receptor is reduced and activity of indirect pathway related to D2 receptor is increased. Hence firing rate of GABAergic neurons in basal ganglia strongly increases, inhibiting thalamocortical and brainstem areas [66].

3.1 Risk factors of Parkinson's disease

The number of the dopaminergic neurons in the substantia nigra decreases at a rate of 9.8% every 10 years during the aging process. Besides, the volume of these neurons decreases at a rate of 4.4% every 10 years [68]. The cognitive impairment of normal aging decreases the stimulation of the dopaminergic transmission from substantia nigra to other brain regions.

Family history of PD, family history of tremor, preceding constipation, prior mood disorder, exposure to pesticides, previous head injury, rural living, beta-blocker use and agricultural occupation were strongly and positively associated with PD. However, interestingly, smoking, coffee drinking, prior hypertension, use of NSAIDs, use of calcium channel blocker and alcohol consumption were associated negatively with PD [69]. Negative correlation between PD and smoking may result from the neuroprotective effect of nicotine [70, 71].

3.2 Physiopathology of Parkinson's disease

Dopaminergic dysfunction in basal ganglia is related to movement disorders such as PD, dystonia, chorea and tics [72]. PD is characterized with neurodegeneration in the dopamine producing neurons in the substantia nigra controlling motor functions of body. Dopaminergic degeneration mainly results from loss of the dopaminergic neurons in substantia nigra pars compacta. During neurodegeneration, some microscopic changes such as Lewy body and intracytoplasmic inclusion bodies composed of fibrillary α-synuclein occur [73]. After loss of dopaminergic neurons at a rate of 60–80%, symptoms can be detectable in patients with PD [74].

A part of the dopaminergic neuronal degeneration is the formation of the intracellular alpha-synuclein (SNCA) aggregates [75]. Involvement of miRNA is related to SNCA accumulation [76]. miRNAs control SNCA expression. miR-7 and miR-153 post-transcriptionally regulate SNCA and suppress SNCA expression. An advantage of the suppression of SNCA thanks to miR-7 and miR-153 is to protect cells from oxidative stress [77, 78].

Among pathologic reasons of the PD, there are mitochondrial dysfunction, oxidative stress, disruption of ubiquitin-proteasome system, neuro inflammation induced by microglia, excitotoxicity by glutamate receptor activation, iron deposition and familial PD [79].

Dysfunction of mitochondrial complex I has high importance in the formation of PD [80]. It was reported that dopaminergic neurons in substantia nigra died and PD occurred in genetically engineered mice lacking a gene (NDUFS2) encoding complex I subunit [81]. Mitochondrial complex I activity is significantly decreased in substantia nigra of patients with PD and mitochondrial DNA damage occurs in a high level [79]. Besides, excess amount of Reactive Oxygen Species (ROS) production, ATP consumption, mtDNA deletion, caspase secretion may occur in the table of mitochondrial dysfunction [82]. In a recent electrophysiological study, it was reported that lack of gene for mitochondrial transcription factor A in a Mitopark mice model resulted in loss of dopaminergic neurons of SN and provided a genetic model of PD. These neurons in SN exhibited age-dependent declines in electrophysiological parameters like disrupted pace maker firing regularity, decreased ion channel conductance and smaller D2 receptor-mediated outward currents [83]. These findings emphasize the importance of the mitochondrial dysfunction in the progression of PD.

Increased oxidative stress activates the Ubiquitin-Proteasome System (UPS). Hence, damaged and misfolded proteins are accumulated, leading to dopaminergic degeneration together with UPS [73]. Ubiquitin-proteasome system (UPS) is one of the degradation pathways for misfolded proteins in PD [79, 84]. Mutant Parkin, PINK1 and DJ-1 proteins disrupt the function of UPS and form an ubiquitin E3 ligase complex resulting in unfolded protein degradation [85]. The E3 ligase complex typically plays a vital role in controlling cell trafficking, DNA repair and signaling, which affect survival of dopaminergic neurons [86].

Neuroinflammation is among the specific compound of the PD [87]. Main actor of this inflammatory pattern is microglia [88]. After a genetic or environmental effect, α-synuclein protein is secreted from dying dopaminergic neurons and triggers the chemotaxis and activation of the microglia [89]. It was reported that the number of dopaminergic neurons of the substantia nigra is decreased in mice because of excess activation of the microglia in patients with PD [90]. Similarly, it was also reported that anti-inflammatory drugs decrease the loss of the dopaminergic neurons and symptoms of the disease in a mouse model of PD [91].

Excess stimulation of the ionotropic receptors of the glutamate results in the damage and death of the dopaminergic cells [92], resulted from the increase in the intracellular Ca^{+2} concentration, change in the mitochondrial membrane potential [93] and disorder of the production of the ROS and reactive nitrogen species [94]. After the hyperactivation of NMDA receptors, Ca^{+2} influx as a secondary messenger triggers dopaminergic neurodegeneration [95]. Effects of NMDA receptor activity in a dopaminergic neuron spread into other neighbor neurons by diffusion of Ca^{+2} through the gap junctions between dopaminergic neurons. If there are no gap junctions between cells, neurodegeneration is limited [96].

Iron accumulation is seen in patients with PD [97]. During aging, the concentration of the iron increases in the substantia nigra, putamen, globus pallidus and caudate nucleus that are basic dopamine synthesizing regions in the brain [79]. Accumulation of iron in the brain results from the increase in the permeability in Blood Brain Barrier (BBB) [98], increase in pro-inflammation [99] and gene mutations of the proteins related to iron transport, bind and metabolism [100].

Accumulation of α-synuclein is common in familial PD [101]. Parkin gene mutation is seen in familial autosomal recessive PD [102]. While prevalence of this mutation in all familial PD is 50%, it is seen at a rate of 20% in idiopathic PD [103].

3.3 Treatment of Parkinson's disease

In PD, dopamine synthesis is decreased in some specific brain regions like substantia nigra and striatum. DA receptor agonists are generally used to treat PD, which act by stimulating both presynaptic and postsynaptic dopaminergic receptors. DA deficiency in PD is substituted by a chemical precursor L-DOPA, which is the most effective drug to treat various symptoms. L-DOPA passes through the BBB and transforms to dopamine. L-DOPA has pivotal role in PD therapy strategy. However, changes in the concentration in body fluids of this drug result in some adverse effects like motor fluctuations. Intestinal gel infusions of L-DOPA provide continuous dopaminergic receptor stimulation thanks to more stable concentrations of drug and thus, prevents drug-induced dyskinesia [104].

The only drug used in the treatment of PD is not the L-DOPA. Dopaminomimetic drugs affect the striatal neurons via dopamine receptors. Dopaminomimetics directly activate the D2 receptor family. Ergot alkaloid bromocriptine and other dopaminomimetics have important role in PD therapy for motor symptoms [105, 106].

In terms of motor fluctuations and adverse effects of anti-Parkinson drugs, dopamine agonists are more attractive choices than L-DOPA [105, 107]. Dopamine agonists have less striatal dopamine receptor stimulation than L-DOPA and this provides reduced risk for motor complications during drug administration in initial PD monotherapy [106]. Besides, some dopaminomimetics like rotigotine are possible to be administrated as transdermal patch, providing constant drug concentration in cerebrospinal fluid [66].

However, dopamine agonists have some adverse effects including drowsiness and impulse dyscontrol resulted from D3 receptor activity in the ventral striatum causing to the stimulation of the brain reward system. Besides, dopamine agonists have more reduced effect size in PD compared to L-DOPA [108]. However, apomorphine has equal effect size to L-DOPA and affects both D1 and D2 receptors [109]. Continuous subcutaneous apomorphine administration prevents the motor response fluctuations and dyskinesia resulting from L-DOPA usage [110].

Current literature reports that metabolic stress could be the most important reason for the degeneration of DA neurons. A few selective voltage-gated ion channels, such as Ca^{+2} channels and ATP pumps under metabolic stress, fail to maintain membrane potential, thereby causing an imbalance in ion concentrations. These fluctuations in turn affect the neuronal network and cause dopaminergic neuron degeneration [111]. Because the symptoms cannot be identified at an earlier state of onset of disease, providing treatment on time is difficult for PD patients. To find early symptoms and protect dopaminergic neurons from degradation is the biggest challenge to date. Some studies show that supplementing PD patients with vitamin E or C at optimal doses is a potential treatment, because vitamin E and C produce large amounts of antioxidants, which can relieve a cell from metabolic stress by inhibiting the production of free radicals and reactive oxygen [112].

Dopamine receptor agonists are generally used to treat PD, which act by stimulating both presynaptic and postsynaptic dopaminergic receptors. DA deficiency in PD is substituted by a chemical precursor L-DOPA, which is the most effective drug to treat various symptoms.

4. Dopamine receptors and addiction

Dopamine is responsible for reward and addiction as well as control of coordinated movement, metabolism and hormonal secretion in CNS [113]. Addictive drugs generally largely and rapidly increase the extracellular concentration of dopamine in the nucleus accumbens [114]. Besides, addictive drug-evoked neurosynaptic plasticity results in behavioral responses in addicted patients [115]. Plasticity in the mesolimbic system triggers the compulsive behavior for seeking addictive matters after enough usage of addictive drugs [116]. These drugs trigger long-lasting synaptic adaptations in the mesolimbic reward system causing the additional pathological behaviors, as well [117].

Cannabinoids increase the dopamine levels in VTA through cannabinoid type 1 receptors. Cues related to cannabis smoking elicit phasic dopamine secretions and induce drug seeking behaviors like craving [118].

Cocaine controls the movement, cognition, motivation and reward in the CNS by blocking the reuptake of dopamine and thereby extracellular concentration of dopamine increases especially in the nucleus accumbens [119]. While psychostimulants like ecstasy, amphetamine and cocaine decrease dopamine reuptake, nicotine can directly increase the spike of dopaminergic neurons and thereby, the secretion of dopamine. Opioids, cannabinoids, γ-hydroxybutyrate and benzodiazepines inhibit the VTA GABAergic neurons [120]. This leads to a reduction in inhibition of dopaminergic neurons, resulting in increased dopamine secretion [120].

Cocaine shows its effects by phosphorylating ERK in the nucleus accumbens, providing D1 receptor-dependent synaptic potentiation [121] and behavioral adaptation [122] as well as increasing the mesolimbic dopamine level. ERK has important roles in gene regulation and drug addiction through chromatin remodeling and activation of gene transcription factors [121].

Addictive drugs elicit synaptic plasticity in dopaminergic neurons of VTA, leading to an increase in dopamine concentration in the mesolimbic reward system [122]. Cocaine provides insertion of GluA2-lacking AMPA receptors at glutamatergic synapse in dopaminergic neurons [122].

Addictive drugs cause a transient and significant increase in the extracellular concentration of dopamine in nucleus accumbens located in the ventral striatum in limbic system of the brain [123]. Increases in dopamine level in the ventral striatum triggered by addictive drugs like nicotine and alcohol provide euphoria during exposure [124].

After addicts notice the drug cues, mesolimbic projections on striatum are hyperresponsive to these cues and addicted patients desire to take drugs causing incentive salience and motivation for compulsive behaviors to take drugs. Hence these conditions result in relapse [125].

Reward and punishment stimuli bring search and avoidance responses, set by burst firing of dopaminergic neurons through long-term potentiation mechanism. Relationship between dopaminergic stimuli, glutamatergic inputs and GABAergic outputs enables learning and the ability to seek out rewarding behaviors and aversive ones [126]. Animals that lack of ability to synthesize dopamine cannot realize conditional reflexes or appetitive behavior. These animals have only unconditional and unlearned reflexes. To learn reward and punishment stimuli is mostly associated with phasic firing of dopaminergic neurons in the brain, establishing long-term memories. Independent firing of dopaminergic neurons motivates responses to reward and punishment cues. Interest in habitual rewards decreases because of reduction in the dopamine receptors resulted from habitual chronic usage of addictive drugs [127].

Decreased dopamine release from striatum to other brain regions within the reward circuitry may be a part of the deprivation neurophysiology in addicted chronic drug users. An altered feedback regulation of the reward circuit by prefrontal and amygdala pathways may also be responsible for disruption mechanism. Prefrontal regions and amygdala are involved in some behaviors related to addiction and deprivation like impulsivity, relapse and craving in chronic drug abusers that dopaminergic dysfunction occurs [123].

4.1 Treatment of addiction

Medications for addiction may be agonists, antagonists and anti-craving drugs. Methadone activates opiate receptors and prevents cravings for opiates and euphoria induced by usage of opiates [114, 128]. Naltrexone is a complete mu-receptor antagonist and it prevents relapse and euphoria resulted from abusing any opiate [129]. Buprenorphine is a partial mu-agonist and prevents cravings and euphoria because of usage of any opiate [114].

If D2 receptor activity in ventral striatum is increased in the reward system, self-administration of cocaine or alcohol can be reduced [130]. Similarly, impulsivity and compulsive pattern of self-administration in methamphetamine abuse is related to changed D2 receptor activity [131]. In addition, a potential strategy to address behavioral problems resulting from addiction and deprivation is to use transcranial magnetic stimulation or deep brain stimulation to eliminate cocaine-induced synaptic plasticity [132].

4.1.1 Dopamine and other neuropsychiatric diseases

Dopaminergic projections from VTA to hippocampus provide the formation of new memories. The ability to learn new information is lost when dopaminergic neurotransmission in this pathway is decreased. Hence, risk of dementia related diseases like Alzheimer's disease increases.

Pharmacological and imaging studies show that increase in dopamine neurotransmission, elevations in D2 and D3 receptors level in striatum and activation of reward circuit result in mania. However increased dopamine transporter level in striatum results in the decrease in the dopaminergic transmission and depressive attacks in bipolar affective disorder [133].

Attention Deficit Hyperactivity Disorder (ADHD) is diagnosed by lack of concentration, short attention span and physical restlessness. Patients with ADHD were reported at least one gene defect such as DRD2, DRD4 or dopamine transporter genes, resulting in decrease in the dopaminergic neurotransmission in the brain [134].

4.1.2 Future treatment strategies on drug design for neurodegenerative disorders

With the advent of computer-based technology, it is possible to find a solution and bring better treatment procedures for complex disorders. Computer-Aided Drug Design (CADD) may be useful to provide more rapidly the discovery of the drugs, more effective for neurodegenerative disorders such as PD and Alzheimer's disease [135]. CADD could emerge as an effective tool to minimize time and cost of the new lead molecules for extensively studying the DA receptors and other protein targets involved in dopaminergic signaling, and this gives a clear-cut idea of targets, which aids in designing New Chemical Entities (NCEs). After the discovery of NCE, it must be tested in terms of its safety and efficacy for humans as it is in the traditional drugs as well.

Dysfunctions of the dopamine neurotransmission in neuropsychiatric diseases are mostly related to presynaptic or postsynaptic dopamine receptors and can be reversed or stopped by targeting these receptors and their intracellular pathways. New researches must be focused on at this area to find more effective and cheaper solutions to treat these diseases.

Author details

Burak Yaman
Medical Faculty, Department of Physiology, Gaziantep University, Gaziantep, Turkey

*Address all correspondence to: burakyaman810@gmail.com

References

[1] Bhatia A, Lenchner JR, Saadabadi A. Biochemistry, Dopamine Receptors. StatPearls Publishing; 2022

[2] Beaulieu JM, Espinoza S, Gainetdinov RR. Dopamine receptors—IUPHAR Review 13. British Journal of Pharmacology. 2015;**172**(1):1-23

[3] Shimizu K, Stopfer M. Gap junctions. Current Biology. 2013;**23**(23)

[4] Grove JCR et al. Dopamine subsystems that track internal states. Nature. 2022;**608**(7922):374-380. DOI: 10.1038/s41586-022-04954-0

[5] Augustine V et al. Temporally and spatially distinct thirst satiation signals. Neuron. 2019;**103**(2):242-249.e4

[6] Fernandes AB et al. Postingestive modulation of food seeking depends on vagus-mediated dopamine neuron activity. Neuron. 2020;**106**(5):778-788.e6. DOI: 10.1016/J.NEURON.2020.03.009

[7] Beaulieu JM, Gainetdinov RR. The physiology, signaling, and pharmacology of dopamine receptors. Pharmacological Reviews. 2011;**63**(1):182-217. DOI: 10.1124/PR.110.002642

[8] Rehman S, Sharma S. Biochemistry, G Protein Coupled Receptors. StatPearls Publishing; 2018

[9] Sayın A. Dopamin reseptörleri ve sinyal iletim özellikleri. KlinPsikiyatri. 2008;**11**:125-134

[10] Yeragani V, Tancer M, Chokka P, Baker G. Arvid Carlsson, and the story of dopamine. Indian Journal of Psychiatry. 2010;**52**(1):87

[11] Xu TX et al. Hyperdopaminergic tone erodes prefrontal long-term potential via a D2 receptor-operated protein phosphatase gate. The Journal of Neuroscience. 2009;**29**(45):14086-14099. DOI: 10.1523/JNEUROSCI.0974-09.2009

[12] Sidhu A, Niznik HB. Coupling of dopamine receptor subtypes to multiple and diverse G proteins. International Journal of Developmental Neuroscience. 2000;**18**(7):669-677

[13] Witt KM, Harper DN, Ellenbroek BA. Dopamine D1 receptor and effort-based decision making in rats: The moderating effect of sex. Progress in Neuro-Psychopharmacology & Biological Psychiatry. 2023;**120**:110651

[14] Le Heron C et al. Dysfunctional effort-based decision-making underlies apathy in genetic cerebral small vessel disease. Brain. 2018;**141**(11):3193-3210

[15] Sun X et al. Accumbal adenosine A2A receptor inactivation biases for large and costly rewards in the effort- but not delay-based decision making. Neuropharmacology. 2023;**222**:109273

[16] Le Heron C et al. Distinct effects of apathy and dopamine on effort-based decision-making in Parkinson's disease. Brain. 2018;**141**(5):1455-1469. DOI: 10.1093/brain/awy110

[17] Brassard SL, Balodis IM. A review of effort-based decision-making in eating and weight disorders. Progress in Neuro-Psychopharmacology and Biological Psychiatry. 2021;**110**:110333

[18] Sung YK et al. The dopamine D2 receptor regulates the development of dopaminergic neurons via extracellular signal-regulated kinase and Nurr1 activation. The Journal of Neuroscience. 2006;**26**(17):4567-4576

[19] Mishra A, Singh S, Shukla S. Physiological and functional basis of dopamine receptors and their role in neurogenesis: Possible implication for Parkinson's disease. Journal of Experimental Neuroscience. 2018;**12**. DOI: 10.1177/1179069518779829

[20] Wrobel TM, Bartuzi D, Kaczor AA. Allosteric modulators of dopamine D2 receptors for fine-tuning of dopaminergic neurotransmission in CNS diseases: Overview, pharmacology, structural aspects and synthesis. Molecules. 2022;**28**(1):178

[21] Abi-dargham A, Moore H. Prefrontal DA transmission at D1 receptors and the pathology of schizophrenia. Neuroscientist. 2003;**9**(5):404-416. DOI: 10.1177/1073858403252674

[22] Seeman P et al. Dopamine supersensitivity correlates with D2 high states, implying many paths to psychosis. Proceedings of the National Academy of Sciences of the United States of America. 2005;**102**(9):3513-3518. DOI: 10.1073/PNAS.0409766102

[23] Seeman P, Ko F, Jack E, Greenstein R, Dean B. Consistent with dopamine supersensitivity, RGS9 expression is diminished in the amphetamine-treated animal model of schizophrenia and in postmortem schizophrenia brain. Synapse. 2007;**61**(5):303-309. DOI: 10.1002/SYN.20368

[24] Volkow ND, Fowler JS, Wang GJ, Baler R, Telang F. Imaging dopamine's role in drug abuse and addiction. Neuropharmacology. 2009;**56**(Suppl 1):3-8. DOI: 10.1016/J.NEUROPHARM.2008.05.022

[25] Nikolaus S, Antke C, Müller HW. In vivo imaging of synaptic function in the central nervous system: I. Movement disorders and dementia. Behavioural Brain Research. 2009;**204**(1, 1):-31. DOI: 10.1016/J.BBR.2009.06.008

[26] Rondou P, Haegeman G, Van Craenenbroeck K. The dopamine D4 receptor: Biochemical and signalling properties. Cellular and Molecular Life Sciences. 2010;**67**(12):1971-1986. DOI: 10.1007/S00018-010-0293-Y

[27] Parsons MJ et al. A dopamine D2 receptor gene-related polymorphism is associated with schizophrenia in a Spanish population isolate. Psychiatric Genetics. 2007;**17**(3):159-163. DOI: 10.1097/YPG.0B013E328017F8A4

[28] Bertram L. Genetic research in schizophrenia: New tools and future perspectives. Schizophrenia Bulletin. 2008;**34**(5):806-812

[29] Le Foll B, Gallo A, Le Strat Y, Lu L, Gorwood P. Genetics of dopamine receptors and drug addiction: A comprehensive review. Behavioural Pharmacology. 2009;**20**(1):1-17. DOI: 10.1097/FBP.0B013E3283242F05

[30] Roth BL, Sheffer DJ, Kroeze WK. Magic shotguns versus magic bullets: Selectively non-selective drugs for mood disorders and schizophrenia. Nature Reviews Drug Discovery. 2004;**3**(4):353-359. DOI: 10.1038/nrd1346

[31] Roth BL. Drugs and valvular heart disease. The New England Journal of Medicine. 2007;**356**(1):6-9. DOI: 10.1056/nejmp068265

[32] Namkung Y, Sibley DR. Protein kinase C mediates phosphorylation, desensitization, and trafficking of the D2 dopamine receptor. The Journal of Biological Chemistry. 2004;**279**(47):49533-49541. DOI: 10.1074/JBC.M408319200

[33] Cho EY, Cho DI, Park JH, Kurose H, Caron MG, Kim KM. Roles of protein

kinase C and actin-binding protein 280 in the regulation of intracellular trafficking of dopamine D3 receptor. Molecular Endocrinology. 2007;**21**(9):2242-2254. DOI: 10.1210/ME.2007-0202

[34] Morris SJ, Itzhaki Van-Ham I, Daigle M, Robillard L, Sajedi N, Albert PR. Differential desensitization of dopamine D2 receptor isoforms by protein kinase C: The importance of receptor phosphorylation and pseudosubstrate sites. European Journal of Pharmacology. 2007;**577**(1-3):44-53

[35] Rex EB, Rankin ML, Ariano MA, Sibley DR. Ethanol regulation of D1 dopamine receptor signaling is mediated by protein kinase C in an isozyme-specific manner. Neuropsychopharmacol. 2008;**33**(12):2900-2911. DOI: 10.1038/npp.2008.16

[36] Cokan KB et al. Critical impact of different conserved endoplasmic retention motifs and dopamine receptor interacting proteins (DRIPs) on intracellular localization and trafficking of the D2 dopamine receptor (D2-R) isoforms. Biomolecules. 2020;**10**:1355

[37] Duan J et al. "Synonymous mutations in the human dopamine receptor D2 (DRD2) affect mRNA stability and synthesis of the receptor". Human Molecular Genetics. Feb. 2003;**12**(3):205-216. DOI: 10.1093/ HMG/ DDG055

[38] Cutando L et al. Cerebellar dopamine D2 receptors regulate social behaviors. Nature Neuroscience. 2022;**25**(7):900-911

[39] Favier M, Carcenac C, Savasta M, Carnicella S. Dopamine D3 receptors: A potential target to treat motivational deficits in Parkinson's disease. Current Topics in Behavioral Neurosciences. 2023;**60**:109-132

[40] Gonda X, Tarazi FI. Dopamine D 3 receptors: From bench to bedside. Neuropsychopharmacologia Hungarica. 2021;**23**(2):272-280

[41] Bono F, Mutti V, Fiorentini C, Missale C. Dopamine D3 receptor heteromerization: Implications for neuroplasticity and neuroprotection. Biomolecules. 2020;**10**(7):1-15. DOI: 10.3390/biom10071016

[42] Kienast T, Heinz A. Dopamine and the diseased brain. CNS & Neurological Disorders Drug Targets. 2006;**5**(1):109-131

[43] Bonci A, Hopf FW. The dopamine D2 receptor: New surprises from an old friend. Neuron. 2005;**47**(3):335-338

[44] Kabbani N, Levenson R. A proteomic approach to receptor signaling: Molecular mechanisms and therapeutic implications derived from discovery of the dopamine D2 receptor signalplex. European Journal of Pharmacology. 2007;**572**(2-3):83-93. DOI: 10.1016/J.EJPHAR.2007.06.059

[45] Meisenzahl EM, Schmitt GJ, Scheuerecker J, Möller HJ. The role of dopamine for the pathophysiology of schizophrenia. International Review of Psychiatry. 2007;**19**(4):337-345

[46] Ciliax BJ et al. The dopamine transporter: Immunochemical characterization and localization in brain. Journal of Neuroscience. 1995;**15**(3):1714-1723

[47] Mercuri NB, Grillner P, Bernardi G. N-methyl-D-aspartate receptors mediate a slow excitatory postsynaptic potential in the rat midbrain dopaminergic neurons. Neuroscience. 1996;**74**(3):785-792

[48] Nieoullon A. Dopamine and the regulation of cognition and

attention. Progress in Neurobiology. 2002;**67**(1):53-83

[49] Missale C, Russel Nash S, Robinson SW, Jaber M, Caron MG. Dopamine receptors: From structure to function. Physiological Reviews. 1998;**78**(1):189-225

[50] Seeman P. Schizophrenia and dopamine receptors. European Neuropsychopharmacology. 2013;**23**(9):999-1009

[51] Salamone JD. The involvement of nucleus accumbens dopamine in appetitive and aversive motivation. Behavioural Brain Research. 1994;**61**(2):117-133

[52] Kelley AE. Ventral striatal control of appetitive motivation: Role in ingestive behavior and reward-related learning. Neuroscience and Biobehavioral Reviews. 2004;**27**(8):765-776. DOI: 10.1016/J.NEUBIOREV.2003.11.015

[53] Grace AA. Phasic versus tonic dopamine release and the modulation of dopamine system responsivity: A hypothesis for the etiology of schizophrenia. Neuroscience. 1991;**41**(1):1-24

[54] Martinelli C, Rigoli F, Averbeck B, Shergill SS. The value of novelty in schizophrenia. Schizophrenia Research. 2018;**192**:287-293

[55] Kapur S. How antipsychotics become anti-'psychotic'—From dopamine to salience to psychosis. Trends in Pharmacological Sciences. 2004;**25**(8):402-406

[56] Akdag SJ, Nestor PG, O'Donnell BF, Niznikiewicz MA, Shenton ME, McCarley RW. The startle reflex in schizophrenia: Habituation and personality correlates. Schizophrenia Research. 2003;**64**(2-3):165-173

[57] Zhang TY, Chrétien P, Meaney MJ, Gratton A. Influence of naturally occurring variations in maternal care on prepulse inhibition of acoustic startle and the medial prefrontal cortical dopamine response to stress in adult rats. The Journal of Neuroscience. 2005;**25**(6):1493-1502

[58] Yang AC, Tsai SJ. New targets for schizophrenia treatment beyond the dopamine hypothesis. International Journal of Molecular Sciences. 2017;**18**(8):03

[59] Dargham AA. Recent evidence for dopamine abnormalities in schizophrenia. European Psychiatry. 2002;**17**(Suppl. 4):341-347

[60] Sayin AI et al. Effects of the adverse life events and disrupted in schizophrenia-1 (DISC1) gene polymorphisms on acute symptoms of schizophrenia. DNA and Cell Biology. 2013;**32**(2):73-80. DOI: 10.1089/dna.2012.1894

[61] Tsuang M. Schizophrenia: Genes and environment. Biological Psychiatry. 2000;**47**(3):210-220. DOI: 10.1016/S0006-3223(99)00289-9

[62] McCutcheon RA, Abi-Dargham A, Howes OD. Schizophrenia, dopamine and the striatum: From biology to symptoms. Trends in Neurosciences. 2019;**42**(3):205. DOI: 10.1016/J.TINS.2018.12.004

[63] Tamminga CA et al. Hippocampal novelty activations in schizophrenia: Disease and medication effects. Schizophrenia Research. 2012;**138**(2-3):157-163

[64] Kapur S. Psychosis as a state of aberrant salience: A framework linking biology, phenomenology, and pharmacology in schizophrenia.

American Journal of Psychiatry. 2003;**160**(1):13-23. DOI: 10.1176/appi.ajp.160.1.13

[65] Bazin N, Perruchet P, Hardy-Bayle MC, Feline A. Context-dependent information processing in patients with schizophrenia. Schizophrenia Research. 2000;**45**(1-2):93-101. DOI: 10.1016/S0920-9964(99)00167-X

[66] Poewe W et al. Parkinson disease. Nature Reviews. Disease Primers. 2017;**3**:1-21

[67] Hipkiss AR. Aging risk factors and Parkinson's disease: Contrasting roles of common dietary constituents. Neurobiology of Aging. 2014;**35**(6):1469-1472. DOI: 10.1016/j.neurobiolaging.2013.11.032

[68] Ma SY, Yttä MR, Collan Y, Rinne JO, Röyttä M. Unbiased morphometrical measurements show loss of pigmented nigral neurones with ageing. Neuropathology and Applied Neurobiology. 1999;**25**:394-399

[69] Noyce AJ et al. Meta-analysis of early nonmotor features and risk factors for Parkinson disease. Annals of Neurology. 2012;**72**(6):893-901

[70] Tanner CM et al. Smoking and Parkinson's disease in twins. Neurology. 2002;**58**(4):581-588. DOI: 10.1212/WNL.58.4.581

[71] Carr LA, Rowell PP. Attenuation of 1-methyl-4-phenyl-1,2,3,6-tetrahydropyridine-induced neurotoxicity by tobacco smoke. Neuropharmacology. 1990;**29**(3):311-314

[72] Lanciego JL, Luquin N, Obeso JA. Functional neuroanatomy of the basal ganglia. Cold Spring Harbor Perspectives in Medicine. 2012;**2**(12)

[73] Abou-Sleiman PM, Muqit MMK, Wood NW. Expanding insights of mitochondrial dysfunction in Parkinson's disease. Nature Review Neuroscience. 2006;**7**(3):207-219. DOI: 10.1038/nrn1868

[74] Dauer W, Przedborski S. Parkinson's disease: Mechanisms and models. Neuron. 2003;**39**(6):889-909

[75] Pascale E, Divisato G, Palladino R, Auriemma M, Ngalya EF, Caiazzo M. Noncoding RNAs and midbrain DA neurons: Novel molecular mechanisms and therapeutic targets in health and disease. Biomolecule. 2020;**10**(9):1269. DOI: 10.3390/BIOM10091269

[76] Leggio L et al. microRNAs in Parkinson's disease: From pathogenesis to novel diagnostic and therapeutic approaches. International Journal of Molecular Sciences. 2017;**18**(12). DOI: 10.3390/IJMS18122698

[77] Doxakis E. Post-transcriptional regulation of α-synuclein expression by mir-7 and mir-153. The Journal of Biological Chemistry. 2010;**285**(17):12726

[78] Fragkouli A, Doxakis E. miR-7 and miR-153 protect neurons against MPP+-induced cell death via upregulation of mTOR pathway. Frontiers in Cellular Neuroscience. 2014;**8**:182

[79] Akbayır E, Şen M, Ay U, Şenyer S, Tüzün E, Küçükali Cİ. Parkinson HastalığınınEtyopatogenezi. Deneysel Tıp Araştırma Enstitüsü Dergisi. 2017;**7**(13):1-23

[80] Doric Z, Nakamura K. Mice with disrupted mitochondria used to model Parkinson's disease. Nature. 2021;**599**(7886):558-560. DOI: 10.1038/d41586-021-02955-z

[81] González-Rodríguez P et al. Disruption of mitochondrial complex

I induces progressive parkinsonism. Nature. 2021;**599**(7886):650-656

[82] Exner N, Lutz AK, Haass C, Winklhofer KF. Mitochondrial dysfunction in Parkinson's disease: Molecular mechanisms and pathophysiological consequences. The EMBO Journal. 2012;**31**(14):3038

[83] Branch SY, Chen C, Sharma R, Lechleiter JD, Li S, Beckstead MJ. Dopaminergic neurons exhibit an age-dependent decline in electrophysiological parameters in the MitoPark mouse model of Parkinson's disease. The Journal of Neuroscience. 2016;**36**(14):4026

[84] Nakamura T, Lipton SA. Cell death: Protein misfolding and neurodegenerative diseases. Apoptosis. 2009;**14**(4):455-468

[85] Xiong H et al. Parkin, PINK1, and DJ-1 form a ubiquitin E3 ligase complex promoting unfolded protein degradation. The Journal of Clinical Investigation. 2009;**119**(3):650-660. DOI: 10.1172/JCI37617

[86] Teixeira LK, Reed SI. Ubiquitin ligases and cell cycle control. Annual Review of Biochemistry. 2013;**82**:387-414. DOI: 10.1146/ANNUREV-BIOCHEM-060410-105307

[87] Nagatsu T, Sawada M. Inflammatory process in Parkinsons disease: Role for cytokines. Current Pharmaceutical Design. 2005;**11**(8):999-1016

[88] Hirsch EC, Hunot S. Neuroinflammation in Parkinson's disease: A target for neuroprotection? Lancet Neurology. 2009;**8**(4):382-397

[89] Kim C et al. Neuron-released oligomeric α-synuclein is an endogenous agonist of TLR2 for paracrine activation of microglia. Nature Communications. 2013;**4**:1562

[90] Cicchetti F, Brownell AL, Williams K, Chen YI, Livni E, Isacson O. Neuroinflammation of the nigrostriatal pathway during progressive 6-OHDA dopamine degeneration in rats monitored by immunohistochemistry and PET imaging. The European Journal of Neuroscience. 2002;**15**(6):991-998

[91] Kurkowska-Jastrzębska I et al. Dexamethasone protects against dopaminergic neurons damage in a mouse model of Parkinson's disease. International Immunopharmacology. 2004;**4**(10-11):1307-1318

[92] Mehta A, Prabhakar M, Kumar P, Deshmukh R, Sharma PL. Excitotoxicity: Bridge to various triggers in neurodegenerative disorders. European Journal of Pharmacology. 2013;**698**(1-3):6-18

[93] Abramov AY, Duchen MR. Mechanisms underlying the loss of mitochondrial membrane potential in glutamate excitotoxicity. Biochimica et Biophysica Acta, Bioenergetics. 2008;**1777**(7-8):953-964

[94] Dong XX, Wang Y, Qin ZH. Molecular mechanisms of excitotoxicity and their relevance to pathogenesis of neurodegenerative diseases. Acta Pharmacologica Sinica. 2009;**30**(4):379-387. DOI: 10.1038/APS.2009.24

[95] Van Laar VS et al. Glutamate excitotoxicity in neurons triggers mitochondrial and endoplasmic reticulum accumulation of Parkin, and, in the presence of N-acetyl cysteine, mitophagy. Neurobiology of Disease. 2015;**74**:180-193

[96] De Rivero Vaccari JC, Corriveau RA, Belousov AB. Gap junctions are required

for NMDA receptor-dependent cell death in developing neurons. Journal of Neurophysiology. 2007;**98**(5):2878-2886. DOI: 10.1152/jn.00362.2007

[97] Imai Y, Soda M, Inoue H, Hattori N, Mizuno Y, Takahashi R. An unfolded putative transmembrane polypeptide, which can lead to endoplasmic reticulum stress, is a substrate of Parkin. Cell. 2001;**105**(7):891-902

[98] Kortekaas R et al. Blood-brain barrier dysfunction in Parkinsonian midbrain in vivo. Annals of Neurology. 2005;**57**(2):176-179. DOI: 10.1002/ana.20369

[99] Gao HM, Hong JS. Why neurodegenerative diseases are progressive: Uncontrolled inflammation drives disease progression. Trends in Immunology. 2008;**29**(8):357-365. DOI: 10.1016/j.it.2008.05.002

[100] Borie C et al. Association study between iron-related genes polymorphisms and Parkinson's disease. Journal of Neurology. 2002;**249**(7):801-804

[101] Schiesling C et al. Review: Familial Parkinson's disease-genetics, clinical phenotype and neuropathology in relation to the common sporadic form of the disease. Neuropathology and Applied Neurobiology. 2008;**34**:255-271

[102] Klein C, Lohmann-Hedrich K, Rogaeva E, Schlossmacher MG, Lang AE. Deciphering the role of heterozygous mutations in genes associated with parkinsonism. Lancet Neurology. 2007;**6**(7):652-662

[103] Lücking CB et al. Association between early-onset Parkinson's disease and mutations in the Parkin gene. The New England Journal of Medicine. 2000;**342**(21):1560-1567. DOI: 10.1056/nejm200005253422103

[104] Antonini A et al. Effect of levodopa-carbidopa intestinal gel on dyskinesia in advanced Parkinson's disease patients. Movement Disorders. 2016;**31**(4):530-537. DOI: 10.1002/mds.26528

[105] Fox SH et al. The movement disorder society evidence-based medicine review update: Treatments for the motor symptoms of Parkinson's disease. Movement Disorders. 2011;**26**(S3). DOI: 10.1002/mds.23829

[106] Connolly BS, Lang AE. Pharmacological treatment of Parkinson disease: A review. JAMA. 2014;**311**(16):1670-1683. DOI: 10.1001/jama.2014.3654

[107] Jankovic J, Poewe W. Therapies in Parkinson's disease. Current Opinion in Neurology. 2012;**25**(4):433-447

[108] Voon V, Mehta AR, Hallett M. Impulse control disorders in Parkinson's disease: Recent advances. Current Opinion in Neurology. 2011;**24**(4):324-330. DOI: 10.1097/WCO.0b013e3283489687

[109] Frankel JP, Lees AJ, Kempster PA, Stern GM. Subcutaneous apomorphine in the treatment of Parkinson's disease. Journal of Neurology, Neurosurgery, and Psychiatry. 1990;**53**(2):96-101. DOI: 10.1136/jnnp.53.2.96

[110] Katzenschlager R et al. Continuous subcutaneous apomorphine therapy improves dyskinesias in Parkinson's disease: A prospective study using single-dose challenges. Movement Disorders. 2005;**20**(2):151-157

[111] Duda J, Pötschke C, Liss B. Converging roles of ion channels, calcium, metabolic stress, and activity

pattern of Substantia nigra dopaminergic neurons in health and Parkinson's disease. Journal of Neurochemistry. 2016;**139**(Suppl 1):156-178. DOI: 10.1111/jnc.13572

[112] Brown TM. Parkinsonism and vitamin C deficiency. Federal Practitioner. 2017;**34**(8):28

[113] Wang S, Che T, Levit A, Shoichet BK, Wacker D, Roth BL. Structure of the D2 dopamine receptor bound to the atypical antipsychotic drug risperidone. Nature. 2018;**555**(7695):269-273. DOI: 10.1038/nature25758

[114] Ndasauka Y, Wei Z, Zhang X. Received view of addiction, relapse and treatment. Advances in Experimental Medicine and Biology. 2017;**1010**:3-19

[115] Anderson SM et al. CaMKII: A biochemical bridge linking accumbens dopamine and glutamate systems in cocaine seeking. Nature Neuroscience. 2008;**11**(3):344-353. DOI: 10.1038/nn2054

[116] Simmler LD, Li Y, Hadjas LC, Hiver A, van Zessen R, Lüscher C. Dual action of ketamine confines addiction liability. Nature. 2022;**608**(7922):368-373. DOI: 10.1038/s41586-022-04993-7

[117] Tan KR et al. Neural bases for addictive properties of benzodiazepines. Nature. 2010;**463**(7282):769-774. DOI: 10.1038/nature08758

[118] Spanagel R. Cannabinoids and the endocannabinoid system in reward processing and addiction: From mechanisms to interventions. Dialogues in Clinical Neuroscience. 2020;**22**(3):241-250

[119] Volkow ND et al. Decreased striatal dopaminergic responsiveness in detoxified cocaine- dependent subjects. Nature. 1997;**386**(6627):830-833

[120] Bellone C, Loureiro M, Lüscher C. Drug-evoked synaptic plasticity of excitatory transmission in the ventral tegmental area. Cold Spring Harbor Perspectives in Medicine. 2021;**11**(4). DOI: 10.1101/cshperspect.a039701

[121] Brami-Cherrier K, Roze E, Girault JA, Betuing S, Caboche J. Role of the ERK/MSK1 signalling pathway in chromatin remodelling and brain responses to drugs of abuse. Journal of Neurochemistry. 2009;**108**(6):1323-1335. DOI: 10.1111/j.1471-4159.2009.05879.x

[122] Brown MTC et al. Drug-driven AMPA receptor redistribution mimicked by selective dopamine neuron stimulation. PLoS One. 2010;**5**(12)

[123] Volkow ND, Wang G-J, Fowler JS, Tomasi D, Telang F, Baler R. Addiction: Decreased reward sensitivity and increased expectation sensitivity conspire to overwhelm the brain's control circuit. BioEssays. 2010;**32**:748-755. DOI: 10.1002/bies.201000042

[124] Brody AL et al. Ventral striatal dopamine release in response to smoking a regular vs a denicotinized cigarette. Neuropsychopharmacology. 2009;**34**(2):282. DOI: 10.1038/NPP.2008.87

[125] Berridge KC, Robinson TE. Liking, wanting, and the incentive-sensitization theory of addiction. The American Psychologist. 2016;**71**(8):670-679. D OI: 10.1037/amp0000059

[126] Wise RA, Jordan CJ. Dopamine, behavior, and addiction. Journal of Biomedical Science. 2021;**28**(1). DOI: 10.1186/S12929-021-00779-7

[127] Wise RA, Robble MA. Dopamine and addiction. Annual

Review of Psychology. 2020;**71**:79-106. DOI: 10.1146/ANNUREV-PSYCH-010418-103337

[128] Substance Abuse and Mental Health Services Administration. Adult drug courts and medication-assisted treatment for opioid dependence. British. 2014;**8**(1):1-8

[129] Krupitsky E, Nunes EV, Ling W, Illeperuma A, Gastfriend DR, Silverman BL. Injectable extended-release naltrexone for opioid dependence: A double-blind, placebo-controlled, multicentre randomised trial. Lancet (London, England). 2011;**377**(9776):1506-1513

[130] Trifilieff P, Martinez D. Imaging addiction: D2 receptors and dopamine signaling in the striatum as biomarkers for impulsivity. Neuropharmacology. 2014;**76**:498-509. DOI: 10.1016/j.neuropharm.2013.06.031

[131] Lee B et al. Striatal dopamine D2/D3 receptor availability is reduced in methamphetamine dependence and is linked to impulsivity. The Journal of Neuroscience. 2009;**29**(47):14734-14740. DOI: 10.1523/JNEUROSCI.3765-09.2009

[132] Pascoli V, Turiault M, Lüscher C. Reversal of cocaine-evoked synaptic potentiation resets drug-induced adaptive behaviour. Nature. 2012;**481**(7379):71-76. DOI: 10.1038/nature10709

[133] Ashok AH et al. The dopamine hypothesis of bipolar affective disorder: The state of the art and implications for treatment. Molecular Psychiatry. 2017;**22**(5):666-679. DOI: 10.1038/mp.2017.16

[134] Blum K et al. Attention-deficit-hyperactivity disorder and reward deficiency syndrome. Neuropsychiatric Disease and Treatment. 2008;**4**(5):893-917. DOI: 10.2147/ndt.s2627

[135] Baig MH, Ahmad K, Rabbani G, Danishuddin M, Choi I. Computer aided drug design and its application to the development of potential drugs for neurodegenerative disorders. Current Neuropharmacology. 2017;**16**(6):740-748

Chapter 11

Oxygen Tissue Levels as an Effectively Modifiable Factor in Alzheimer's Disease Improvement

Arturo Solís Herrera

Abstract

Despite the advance in biochemistry, there are two substantial errors that have remained for at least two centuries. One is that oxygen from the atmosphere passes through the lungs and reaches the bloodstream, which distributes it throughout the body. Another major mistake is the belief that such oxygen is used by the cell to obtain energy, by combining it with glucose. Since the late nineteenth century, it began to be published that the gas exchange in the lungs cannot be explained by diffusion. Even Christian Bohr suggested that it looked like a cellular secretion. But despite experimental evidence to the contrary and based only on theoretical models, the dogma that our body takes the oxygen it contains inside from the air around it has been perpetuated to this day. The oxygen levels contained in the human body are high, close to 99%, and the atmosphere only contains between 19 and 21%. The hypothesis that there is a supposed oxygen concentrating mechanism has not been experimentally proven to date, after almost two centuries. The mistaken belief, even among neurologists, that our body takes oxygen from the atmosphere is widespread, even though there is no experimental basis to support it, just theoretical models. Our finding that the human body can take oxygen from the water it contains, not from the air around it, like plants, comes to mark a before and after in biology in general, and the CNS is no exception. Therefore, establishing the true origin of the oxygen present within our body and brain will allow us to better understand the physio pathogenesis of neurodegenerative diseases.

Keywords: oxygen, AD, water, ventricles, volume, CSF

1. Introduction

Current medicine is based in an important way on two wrong assumptions: (1) The oxygen present inside the body comes from the atmosphere because theoretically it can cross the thin alveolar membrane and reach the bloodstream, which distributes it to all the cells of the body [1]. (2) Oxygen from the atmosphere is used by cells to produce energy, by combining it with glucose or its intermediate metabolites, something like graduated combustion [2].

However, the passage from atmospheric oxygen to the blood circulation through the pulmonary alveoli has not been demonstrated so far in addition to going against

IntechOpen

the behavior of gases. Therefore, the first error gives rise to a second mistake: the combination of oxygen with glucose to produce energy.

Both concepts are entirely theoretical, and concepts so far-fetched and tangled that it is not possible to contrast them experimentally. Thereby, we do not have definitive and complete answers to important questions behind the simple picture that in mammals, oxygen is extracted from the atmospheric air in the lungs and carried by the bloodstream through the circulation to the tissue, where it is utilized mainly within the mitochondria [3].

The brain is an organ whose normal function depends critically on an uninterrupted delivery of oxygen. Unlike skeletal muscle that can survive for hours without oxygen, brain cells show irreversible damage within minutes from the onset of oxygen deficiency. Thus, theoretical studies (they cannot be otherwise) have special importance for understanding how oxygen is distributed in different structures of the brain under normal and hypoxic conditions [4].

Theoretical work on oxygen transport in the brain began with applications of the Krogh Equation [5] and the extension of the Krogh model to hexagonal space-filling tissue cylinders [6]. A systematic analysis of oxygen transport in the brain with the Krogh model was performed by Reneau and his coworkers [7]. Note that they all are theoretical in their entirety (**Figure 1**).

However, the architecture of the capillary network in the brain does not provide support for the Krogh model [8]. The oxygen consumption rate within the neuron is about ten times higher than in the glial cells, and that has a significant effect on oxygen distribution [9]. There is experimental evidence that significant precapillary loss of oxygen occurs in the cerebral circulation [10].

The problem of oxygen loading in the blood capillaries of the lung is, in a sense, inverse to the problem of oxygen unloading in other tissues. Therefore, for a better understanding of oxygen transport, simultaneous analysis of oxygen and carbon dioxide transport is necessary [11].

At present none of the models of oxygen transport (including Krogh's model) has been carefully tested against experimental data. The main reason appears to be the lack of accurate measurements of oxygen tension and hemoglobin saturation *in vivo* with the spatial resolution necessary for the validation of distributed transport models [12].

The mathematical and statistical models that are used to try to explain biological processes, such as gas exchange, usually do not work because, in biology, the variables

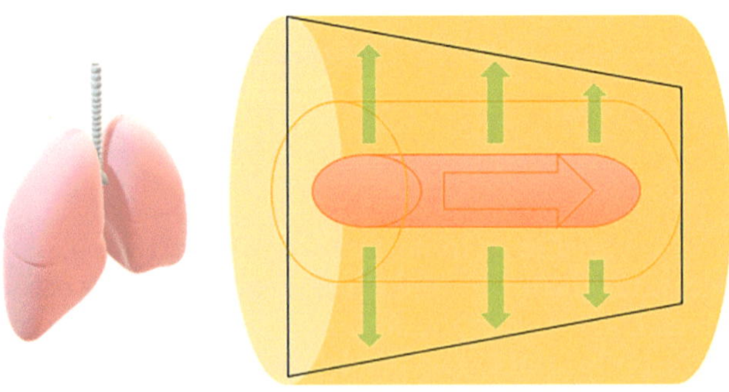

Figure 1.
Krogh Cylinder (simplified). The concepts handled by Krogh's models are so complex and far-fetched that they cannot even be experimentally contrasted. I quote few names: Anoxic lethal corner, O2 radial vectors, capillary radius, capillary X-section, cylinder radius, cylinder X-section, anoxic tissue, axial kick, augmented O2 radial vectors, OPF range, average ptO2, hypercapnic lethal corner, normal intracapillary blood flow velocity.

$$[O_2] = \alpha P \quad Hb{+}nO2 \rightleftarrows kk'Hb(O2)n \quad S{=}K[O2]n1{+}K[O2]n \quad S{=}(P/P50)n1{+}(P/P50)n$$

$$O2{+}Hb4(O2)i{-}1 \rightleftarrows kiki'Hb4(O2)i,i{=}1,2,3,4 \qquad S{=}(\sum i{=}14i[Hb4(O2)i])/(\sum i{=}14[Hb4(O2)i])$$

$$S{=}a1P{+}2a2P2{+}3a3P3{+}4a4P44(1{+}a1P{+}a2P2{+}a3P3{+}a4P4) \qquad a_i = \alpha^i K_1 K_2 \ldots K_i$$

$$S = (S_m - S_o)\exp[-(R/K)\exp(-KP)] + S_o \qquad P = \ln(R/K) - \ln(\ln[(S_m - S_o)/(S - S_o)])/K$$

$$O2{+}Hb \rightleftarrows kk'HbO2 \quad R = k'[O_2][Hb] - k[HbO_2] \quad ddt[O2]{=}{-}R,ddt[Hb]{=}{-}R,ddt[HbO2]{=}R$$

$$S{=}K[O2]1{+}K[O2] \quad k'{=}k1\alpha P(PP50)n \quad R{=}k[HbT](F(P)1{-}F(P)(1{-}S){-}S)$$

$$Ri{=}ki'[O2][Hb4(O2)i{-}1]{-}ki[Hb4(O2)i],i{=}1,2,3,4 \quad Mb{+}O2 \rightleftarrows kk'MbO2$$

$$S{=}[MbO2][Mb]{+}[MbO2]{=}K[O2]1{+}K[O2] \quad j{=}{-}D\partial c\partial n \quad j = -D\nabla c \quad \partial c\partial t{=}\nabla D\nabla c{+}R$$

$$j = D_o\nabla[O_2] + D_{Hb}\nabla[HbO_2] \quad j = D_o\nabla[O_2] + D_{Hb}[Hb_T]\nabla S \quad j{=}(Do{+}DHb[HbT]dSd[O2])\nabla[O2]$$

$$1{+}DHb\alpha Do[HbT]dSdP \quad \nabla[HbO2]{=}[HbT]\alpha{-}1dSdP\nabla P \quad \gamma{=}(LL\beta)2 \quad c = 1 \text{ at } r = R_L$$

$$Pe(u\partial c\partial x{+}v\partial c\partial r){=}\partial 2c\partial r2{+}1r\partial c\partial r{+}\partial 2c\partial x2 \quad c = 0 \text{ at } x = -1 \text{ and } x = 1$$

Figure 2.
A sample of the first 32 equations of already 120 described that have been implemented with the aim of building Krogh's acceptable theoretical (imaginary) model about oxygen transportation theory.

are continuous random (nonlinear behavior). When the phenomena to be studied are discrete variables (linear behavior), mathematical models work better, as is the case of predicting the production of a factory, the possibility that manufacturing processes produce wrong parts, etc. But this is not the case in biology, because the values that variables can take change from one moment to the next, and it is not understood why.

Hence, Krogh's equation of 1919, which is a mathematical (imaginary) model, has been added to other equations by different authors until reaching about 120 equations (**Figure 2**).

The result is a set of mathematical operations so far-fetched and tangled that it is impossible to contrast them in the laboratory. And we are talking about Krogh or Krogh–Erlang equation, which has been the basis of most physiological estimates for the last 70 years.

Some models assumed that tissue is spatially homogeneous. Tissue consists of cells and extracellular spaces. Further, there are intracellular heterogeneities, for example, those caused by discrete oxygen consumption by mitochondria. These heterogeneities may affect the distribution of oxygen in the tissue. Theoretically, inside the cell, oxygen is consumed almost exclusively within mitochondria [13].

It has been proposed that oxygen is transported from blood to mitochondria along channels of high solubility; the endoplasmic reticulum could serve to channel oxygen [14]. The cytosol is largely free of oxygen because of its low solubility. However, theoretical and experimental validation of this hypothesis (1980) remains to be done. It is frustrating that the bases of oxygen transport and gas exchange, which constitute the foundations of the clinic, cannot be experimentally contrasted because of how tangled they are.

2. Oxygen transportation (if any) and brain

Supposedly, the brain is an organ whose normal function depends critically on an uninterrupted delivery of oxygen. However, the element of real value for cell metabolism is hydrogen and it is produced at the same time than oxygen; both come from water dissociation. It is relatively simple to show that melanin dissociates the molecule from water, generating both molecular hydrogen and oxygen (**Figures 3** and **4**). It is difficult to measure the levels of molecular hydrogen inside the cells; it is more practical

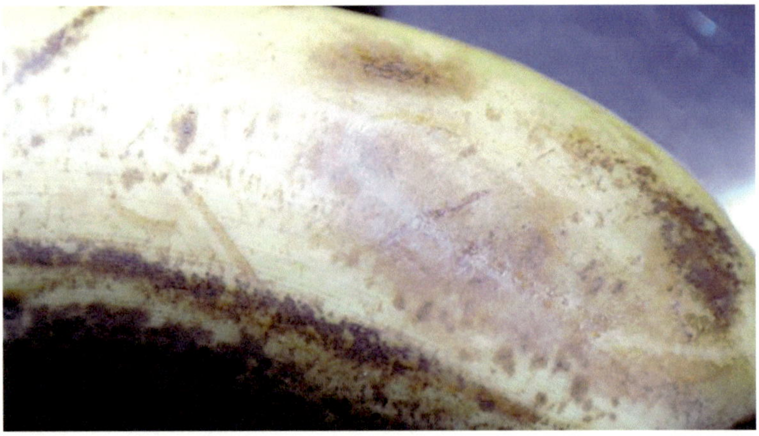

Figure 3.
The melanin in the banana peel, illuminated with polychromatic (white) light.

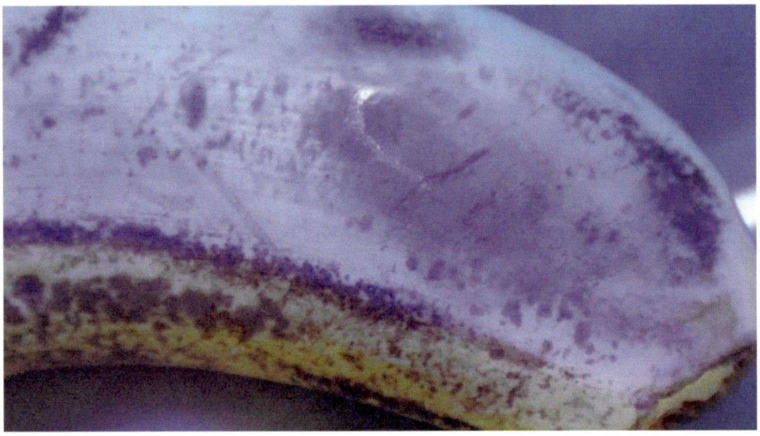

Figure 4.
*When the same specimen of **Figure 3** is illuminated with monochromatic light in the ultraviolet light range (10–400 nm), a distinctive fluorescence appears. Due to the presence of hydrogen that comes from the dissociation of water by melanin, oxygen does not fluoresce.*

to determine molecular oxygen levels. Thereby, oxygen levels are indirect markers of hydrogen levels because both elements come from the dissociation of water that occurs inside the cell, thanks to melanin and other pigments. It can be said that both hydrogen and oxygen are produced at the same time and in the same place.

Unlike skeletal muscle that can survive for hours without oxygen, brain cells show irreversible damage within minutes from the onset of oxygen deficiency that reflects low level of hydrogen by impairment of water dissociation mechanisms.

Theoretical work on oxygen transport in the brain began with applications of the Krogh Equation [5] and the extension of the Krogh model to hexagonal space-filling tissue cylinders [6]. A systematic analysis of oxygen transport in the brain with the Krogh model using the numerical finite-difference method to obtain solutions to steady and unsteady problems of physiological importance was performed in 1967 [15]. As expected, the architecture of the capillary network in the brain does not provide support for the Krogh model. Thereby, other models have been formulated trying to reflect the heterogeneity of capillary architecture and hemodynamics [8].

It is interesting that the oxygen consumption rate within the neuron is about ten times higher than in the glial cells [9], but this finding tells us that the intensity of water dissociation is 10 times more in glial cells than in neurons, because the neuron or any cells do not consume oxygen to produce energy, because the power requirements of the cells are based on the hydrogen that is released when water is dissociated, and molecular hydrogen (H_2) is the element that carries energy, not only in cells but throughout the universe. In AD patients, there is chronic hypoxia that, in turn, indicates a chronic lack of hydrogen, and therefore a generalized lack of energy. The source of the problem is that the brain tissues are not able to dissociate the water at the necessary rate, and then the liquid water accumulates characteristically in the ventricles.

In most studies of oxygen transport, the governing differential equations are solved numerically by a discretization method, either finite difference or finite element, which is typical of imaginary models and that can hardly become a representation of reality due, among other things, that biological processes are made up of continuous random variables.

There is experimental evidence that significant precapillary loss of oxygen occurs in the cerebral circulation [16], which for us means that water dissociation decreases in that region normally.

3. The role of oxygen in neurodegenerative diseases

So far, Alzheimer's disease (AD) is considered an incurable neurodegenerative disease [17]. Recent studies suggest that the neurobiology of AD pathology could not be explained solely by an increase in beta-amyloid levels. In fact, success with potential therapeutic drugs that inhibit the generation of beta amyloid has been low. Therefore, due to therapeutic failure in recent years, scientists are looking for alternative hypotheses to explain the causes of the disease and the cognitive loss. These early changes affect several key metabolic processes related to glucose uptake and insulin signaling, cellular energy homeostasis, mitochondrial biogenesis, and increased Tau phosphorylation by kinase molecules, such as mTOR and Cdk5 [18].

The condition involves a progressive deterioration in memory, cognition, and mobility. Numerous studies have demonstrated a critical role of dysregulated glucose metabolism in its pathogenesis. The already described metabolic alterations in the aging brain and AD-related metabolic deficits are associated with glucose metabolism dysregulation, glycolysis dysfunction, tricarboxylic acid (TCA) cycle, oxidative phosphorylation (OXPHOS) deficits, and pentose phosphate pathway impairment. There are numerous biochemical alterations that occur simultaneously.

AD pathophysiology is extremely complex and heterogeneous, entailing accumulation of senile plaques caused by abnormal amyloid β (Aβ) metabolism, and neurofibrillary tangles caused by tau hyperphosphorylation. The cerebrovascular system is seriously damaged, including the disturbance of the blood–brain barrier (BBB) and cerebral amyloid angiopathy [19]. Functional failures and anatomical changes are multiple and varied, as they do not follow a definite pattern, which is compatible with energy failure.

Supposedly, increased levels of reactive oxygen species (ROS) induce the transcription of pro-inflammatory genes and the release of cytokines (e.g., interleukin-1β [IL-1β], IL-6, and tumor necrosis factor-alpha [TNF-α]) and chemokines that cause neuroinflammation. Furthermore, reactive microglia and astrocytes and other pathological events also contribute to the dysfunction and deprivation of synapses and, ultimately, neuronal death [20]. It seems that the cells lose for some reason, the complex order that characterizes them even though neurons have done their job for millions of years, millions of times, every day.

It could be said that both functional and anatomical failure of the brain's human body is widespread. And in any system, when the faults are so extensive, one must first think about energy [21].

4. Oxygen as a biomarker of energy levels

The brain consumes the greatest amount of energy of all the organs in the body, except the retina photoreceptor layer [22]. There is an age-related decrease in glucose utilization in most human brains [23].

However, it is conflicting that oxygen consumption is studied by determining the levels of mitochondrial nitric oxide synthase when synthases are enzymes that do not use ATP as an energy source to carry out their function [24].

The pathological metabolic alterations in aging (e.g., cerebral glucose hypometabolism) are early and consistent events in the progression of AD. Glucose, the main transportation form of carbohydrate in our blood, is also the crucial and primary energy substrate for the brain under physiological conditions [25]. Glucose is the universal precursor of any organic molecule, but it cannot provide the energy that its own metabolism requires [26], thereby, the prevalent dogma about glucose as source of biomass and energy at the same time now is broken down into thousands of pieces after our discovery of the unexpected capacity of the human body to take oxygen from the water molecule, like plants.

Alternative substrates, such as glycogen, ketone bodies, and amino acids, are also important, but only as a source of carbon chains that our body uses to build up other organic molecules. Energy hypometabolism, particularly a decline in glucose metabolism, is one of the earliest and most common anomalies observed in patients with AD [27], but glucose should not be considered an energy substrate, but a metabolic intermediate that requires energy from the dissociation of water.

Statistically, our body begins to lose its capacity to take oxygen from water at 26 years old, at approximately 10% rate each decade; and after the fifties, goes into free fall. This is an important date because the decline in glucose use capacity by the cells observed with aging is congruous with the loss of capacity to take oxygen from water. Remember that glucose metabolism requires oxygen, this is: energy.

Despite those, the main intracellular energy metabolism pathways, (theoretical all of them) occurring in our brains are necessarily complicated and include anaerobic glycolysis and the pentose phosphate pathway (PPP) in the cytoplasm, as well as oxidative phosphorylation (OXPHOS) in mitochondria and the tricarboxylic acid (TCA) cycle (also known as the citric acid cycle and Krebs cycle) [28], these neuronal metabolic pathways are controversial in circa 98% like in other cells and tissues [29]. CNS biology is no exception to collective mistakes in regards to the wrong double role of glucose as a source of biomass and energy at the same time. No way.

Metabolic processes are regulated by a series of key enzymes. Indeed, a growing body of evidence suggests the presence of organic impairment of mitochondria [30] and damage to related metabolic enzymes [31]. In addition, oxygen and glucose metabolic rates are drastically changed in many neurodegenerative diseases, including AD due to marked alterations in the glycolytic pathway and TCA cycle [32]. Again, it seems like a generalized failure.

The picture is a metabolic dysregulation in many senses, it is a typical generalized fault. Traditionally, glucose is metabolized to ATP, an unstable high-energy compound. An entirely theoretical dogma. If we analyze the energy required by all the components that are described for glucose to end up in ATP, there would be nothing left for the cell.

Researchers are determined to explain the flow of energy where there is none, because it is not possible to obtain more energy than the molecule as is the case of glucose. They forget that the energy needs of the cell are constant, day and night. So, our discovery erases everything theoretically, because when the cell obtains oxygen from water, at the same time it obtains energy, which is transported by hydrogen, the main carrier of energy in the entire universe.

So, oxygen is important for life, it is fundamental; but not in the role that had been assigned to it —combustion of glucose—but to form the cellular scaffolding, of tissues, organs, and systems, which optimizes the use of energy that comes from the sun, but not through food as had been believed to date, but our body is able to capture it directly, like plants.

5. The oxygen inside our body (and brain) does not come from the atmosphere

There is a deeply rooted dogma that oxygen from the atmosphere passes through lung tissues by simple diffusion and reaches the bloodstream, which distributes them to all cells of the body. But from the mid-nineteenth and early twentieth centuries, intense controversy was generated due to the works of Carl Ludwig, Christian Bohr, Haldane, and others, who sought experimentally, both in man and other lung animals, the mechanism by which the %SpO2 rises to more than 95%. And not only did they not find it, but they realized that diffusion alone (the theory in vogue) could not explain the gas exchange in the lungs [33].

So, if the source of oxygen in the body is the water it contains, then the water of the cerebral-spinal fluid (CSF) acquires unusual importance. Well, it is the source of oxygen and hydrogen in the CNS.

Our finding that the human body has several molecules capable of transforming light power into chemical energy, through the dissociation of water [34], like plants, is a disruptive discovery.

6. Conclusion

It is not known if oxygen is transported in blood mainly by pure convection. The roles of diffusion and chemical kinetics are not defined yet. The importance of the resistances to oxygen transport by various membranes is unknown. It is uncertain that oxygen cross cell membranes (red blood cells, endothelial cell, and parenchymal cell) by pure diffusion or if it is facilitated by a carrier. The mechanisms of oxygen transport inside the cells are not known. It is not possible, so far, to identify active transport in oxygen delivery. It is unknown the supposed main site of oxygen exchange between the blood and tissue (arterioles, capillaries, or venules). Sadly, we do not have definitive and conclusive answers to these fundamental questions due to the experiments that are required to do so, in regards to Krogh's model technically are not possible to date. A clear understanding of the physical mechanisms of oxygen transport throughout the pathway is a way beyond, starting because oxygen does not come from the atmosphere, and therefore is not transported.

Krogh laid the wrong foundation for the theory of oxygen transport to the tissue [35]. He proposed, without experimental foundations and based only on theoretical (imaginary) models, that oxygen is transported in the tissue by passive diffusion driven by gradients of oxygen tension (PO_2). Krogh tissue cylinder or simply Krogh's model is a simple geometrical model of the elementary tissue unit supplied by a single capillary. Krogh formulated a differential equation governing oxygen diffusion and uptake in the tissue cylinder assisted by Erlang, a mathematician.

The solution to this equation theoretically expresses oxygen tension in the tissue as a function of spatial position within the tissue cylinder. This simple assumption so-called Krogh equation, known as the Krogh or Krogh–Erlang equation, has been the basis of most physiological estimates for the last 70 years, but now it breaks into a thousand pieces thanks to the discovery of the unsuspected ability of the human body to take oxygen from the water it contains [36], just as plants do.

Only a decade ago, the picture of oxygen delivery from cells to the sites of oxygen consumption, even though it became unnecessarily complex, had not differed qualitatively from that described by Krogh in 1919. In the past 10 years, theoretical Krogh's concept of radial PO_2 gradients in the tissue from the capillary has undergone drastic changes and has all but reversed. Indeed, it is now proposed, in yet another attempt to explain to exploit with mathematical models a theory that cannot be tested experimentally, that the dominant PO_2 gradients on the pathway from hemoglobin to mitochondria occur not in the tissue but inside the vessels. These new concepts, also entirely theoretical; require further and highly complex experimental validation and new theoretical developments. However, if they are valid, then much of our understanding of oxygen transport to tissue will have to be reassessed.

In any case, the models based on the Krogh theorems and the recent trend of non-Krogh models will continue to be futile, as they try to explain how oxygen from the atmosphere passes through the lungs and reaches the bloodstream to be distributed throughout the body.

The discovery of the human body's unsuspected ability to take oxygen from the water contained within cells, such as plants, constitutes the beginning of a new era in the study and treatment of neurodegenerative diseases such as Alzheimer's.

Acknowledgements

This work was supported by Human Photosynthesis™ Research Centre. Aguascalientes 20000, México.

Author details

Arturo Solís Herrera
Human Photosynthesis™ Study Center, Aguascalientes, México

*Address all correspondence to: comagua2000@yahoo.com

References

[1] Nova Z, Skovierova H, Calkovska A. Alveolar-capillary membrane-related pulmonary cells as a target in endotoxin-induced acute lung injury. International Journal of Molecular Sciences. 2019;**20**(4):831. DOI: 10.3390/ijms20040831 PMID: 30769918; PMCID: PMC6412348

[2] Popel AS. Theory of oxygen transport to tissue. Critical Reviews in Biomedical Engineering. 1989;**17**(3):257-321

[3] Traystman RJ. Microcirculation of the brain. In: Mortillaro NA, editor. The Physiology and Pharmacology of the Microcirculation. Vol. 1. New York: Academic Press; 1984. p. 237

[4] Reneau DD Jr, Bruley DF, Knisely MH. A digital simulation of transient oxygen transport in capillary-tissue systems (cerebral gray matter). Development of a numerical method for solution of transport equations describing coupled convection-diffusion systems. AIChE Journal. 1969;**15**:916

[5] Opitz E, Schneider M. Uber die Sauerstoffversorgung des Gehirns und den mechanismus von mangelwirkungen. Electroretinograms of Physiology. 1950;**46**:126

[6] Thews G. Die sauerstoffdiffusion im gehirn. Ein beitrag lur frage der sauerstroffversorgung der organe. Pflügers Archive. 1960;**271**:197

[7] Knisely MH, Reneau DD Jr, Bruley DF. The development and use of equations for predicting the limits on the rates of oxygen supply to the cells of living tissues and organs. A contribution to the biophysics of health and disease. Angiology Journal of Vase Diseases. 1969;**20**:S1

[8] Metzger H. The influence of space-distributed parameters on the calculation of substrate and gas exchange in microvascular units. Mathematical Biosciences. 1976;**30**:31

[9] Ivanov KP, Kislyakov YY, Samoilov MO. Microcirculation and transport of oxygen to neurons of the brain. Microvascular Research. 1979;**18**:434

[10] Sharan M, Jones MD Jr, Koehler RC, Traystman RJ, Popel AS. A compartmental model for oxygen transport in brain microcirculation. Annals of Biomedical Engineering. 1989;**17**:13

[11] Weibel ER. The Pathway for Oxygen Structure and Function in the Mammalian Respiratory System. Cambridge, MA: Harvard University Press; 1984

[12] Lomen DO, Gross JF. A mathematical model of the effect of oxygen consumption on the resistance to flow of sickle cell blood in capillaries. Mathematical Biosciences. 1977;**37**:63

[13] Clark A Jr, Clark PAA, Connett RJ, Gayeski TEJ, Honig CR. How large is the drop in PO2 between cytosol and mitochondrion? The American Journal of Physiology. 1987;**252**:C583

[14] Longmuir IS. Channels of oxygen transport from blood to mitochondria. Advances in Physiology Science. 1980;**25**:19

[15] Reneau DD Jr, Bruley DF, Knisely MH. A mathematical simulation of oxygen release, diffusion, and consumption in the capillaries and tissue of the human brain. In: Hershey D,

editor. Chemical Engineering in Medicine and Biology. New York: Plenum Press; 1967. p. 135

[16] Popel AS, Gross JF. Analysis of oxygen diffusion from arteriolar networks. The American Journal of Physiology. 1979;**237**:H681

[17] Yan X, Hu Y, Wang B, Wang S, Zhang X. Metabolic dysregulation contributes to the progression of Alzheimer's disease. Frontiers in Neuroscience. 2020;**14**:530219. DOI: 10.3389/fnins.2020.530219

[18] Pedros I, Patraca I, Martinez N, Petrov D, Sureda FX, Auladell C, et al. Molecular links between early energy metabolism alterations and Alzheimer's disease. Frontiers in Bioscience (Landmark Edition). 2016;**21**(1):8-19. DOI: 10.2741/4372 PMID: 26709757

[19] Viswanathan A, Greenberg SM. Cerebral amyloid angiopathy in the elderly. Annals of Neurology. 2011;**70**:871-880

[20] Martins RN, Villemagne V, Sohrabi HR, Chatterjee P, Shah TM, Verdile G, et al. Alzheimer's disease: A journey from amyloid peptides and oxidative stress, to biomarker technologies and disease prevention strategiesgains from AIBL and DIAN cohort studies. Journal of Alzheimer's Disease. 2018;**62**:965-992. DOI: 10.3233/jad-171145

[21] Harrison CG, Williams PR. A systems approach to natural disaster resilience. Simulation Modelling Practice and Theory. 2016;**65**:11-31. DOI: 10.1016/j.simpat.2016.02.008

[22] Herrera AS, Esparza DCAM, Ashraf MG, Zamyatnin AA, Aliev G. Beyond mitochondria, what would be the energy source of the cell? Central Nervous System Agents in Medicinal Chemistry. 2015;**15**(1):32-41. DOI: 10.2174/1871524915666150203093656 PMID: 25645910

[23] Petit-Taboué MC, Landeau B, Desson JF, Desgranges B, Baron JC. Effects of healthy aging on the regional cerebral metabolic rate of glucose assessed with statistical parametric mapping. NeuroImage. 1998;**7**:176-184. DOI: 10.1006/nimg.1997.0318

[24] Alvarez S, Valdez LB, Zaobornyj T, Boveris A. Oxygen dependence of mitochondrial nitric oxide synthase activity. Biochemical and Biophysical Research Communications. 2003;**305**(3):771-775. ISSN 0006-291X. DOI: 10.1016/S0006-291X(03)00818-0

[25] Bouzier-Sore AK, Voisin P, Bouchaud V, Bezancon E, Franconi JM, Pellerin L. Competition between glucose and lactate as oxidative energy substrates in both neurons and astrocytes: A comparative NMR study. The European Journal of Neuroscience. 2006;**24**:1687-1694. DOI: 10.1111/j.1460-9568.2006.05056.x

[26] Solís-Herrera A, Ashraf GM, Esparza d CAM, Arias RI, Bachurin SO, Barreto GE, et al. Biological activities of QIAPI 1 as a melanin precursor and its therapeutic effects in wistar rats exposed to arsenic poisoning. Central Nervous System Agents in Medicinal Chemistry. 2015;**15**(2):99-108. DOI: 10.2174/1871524915666150424113831 PMID: 25909193

[27] Small GW, Kepe V, Barrio JR. Seeing is believing: Neuroimaging adds to our understanding of cerebral pathology. Current Opinion in Psychiatry. 2006;**19**:564-569. DOI: 10.1097/01.yco.0000245747.53008.e2

[28] Dienel GA. Brain glucose metabolism: Integration of energetics

with function. Physiological Reviews. 2019;**99**:949-1045. DOI: 10.1152/physrev.00062.2017

[29] Stobbe, Miranda D. 2012. The Road to Knowledge: From Biology to Databases and Back Again. University of Amsterdam, UvA-DARE (Digital Academic Repository). Available from: https://hdl.handle.net/11245/1.385827 [Accessed: May 16, 2022]

[30] Macdonald R, Barnes K, Hastings C, Mortiboys H. Mitochondrial abnormalities in Parkinson's disease and Alzheimer's disease: Can mitochondria be targeted therapeutically? Biochemical Society Transactions. 2018;**46**:891-909. DOI: 10.1042/bst20170501

[31] Bubber P, Haroutunian V, Fisch G, Blass JP, Gibson GE. Mitochondrial abnormalities in Alzheimer brain: Mechanistic implications. Annals of Neurology. 2005;**57**:695-703. DOI: 10.1002/ana.20474

[32] van Gijsel-Bonnello M, Baranger K, Benech P, Rivera S, Khrestchatisky M, de Reggi M, et al. Metabolic changes and inflammation in cultured astrocytes from the 5xFAD mouse model of Alzheimer's disease: Alleviation by pantethine. PLoS One. 2017;**12**:e0175369. DOI: 10.1371/journal.pone.0175369

[33] Gjedde A. Diffusive insights: On the disagreement of christian bohr and august krogh at the centennial of the seven little devils. Advances in Physiology Education. 2010;**34**(4):174-185

[34] Herrera AS. The biological pigments in plants physiology. Agricultural Sciences. 2015;**6**:1262-1271. DOI: 10.4236/as.2015.610121

[35] Krogh A. The number and distribution of capillaries in muscles with calculations of the oxygen pressure head necessary for supplying the tissue. Journal of Physiology (London). 1919;52:409. PubMed: 16993405]

[36] Herrera AS. The unsuspected intrinsic property of melanin to transform light into chemical energy and the seed growth. In: Rigobelo EC, editor. Plant Growth. London: IntechOpen; 2016 [cited June 6, 2022]. DOI: 10.5772/64542 Available from: https://www.intechopen.com/chapters/51547

Chapter 12

Diffusion Magnetic Resonance Imaging (MRI)-Biomarkers for Diagnosis of Parkinson's Disease

Gloria Cruz, Shengdong Nie and Juan Ramírez

Abstract

Parkinson's disease (PD) is a degenerative neurological disorder, the origin of which remains unclear. The efficacy of treatments is limited due to the small number of remaining neurons. Diffusion magnetic resonance imaging (MRI) has revolutionized clinical neuroimaging. This noninvasive and quantitative method gathers *in vivo* microstructural information to characterize pathological processes that modify nervous tissue integrity. The changes in signal intensity result from the motion of the water molecules; they can be quantified by diffusivity measures. Diffusion MRI has revealed "biomarkers" in several brain regions that could be useful for PD diagnosis. These regions include the olfactory tracts, putamen, white matter, superior cerebellar peduncles, middle cerebellar peduncle, pons, cerebellum, and substantia nigra. There are encouraging preliminary data that differentiate PD from atypical parkinsonian diseases based on these microstructural changes.

Keywords: brain imaging, Parkinson's disease, diffusion MRI, atypical parkinsonian diseases, neuroimaging

1. Introduction

Parkinson's disease (PD) was first described in 1817 by James Parkinson and is characterized by the selective loss of dopaminergic neurons in the substantia nigra pars compacta (SNpc) [1–3]. Although PD has been known for more than two centuries, its origin remains unclear. The motor symptoms in patients with PD appear when at least 50–80% of dopaminergic neurons have been lost in the substantia nigra (SN). For this reason the quantity of remaining neurons limits the efficacy of treatments. PD begins with a reduction in dopamine signaling from the SN to the basal ganglia, which causes a decrease in the neuronal excitation localized in the thalamus. This abnormal condition is reflected by the symptoms of bradykinesia (slow or difficult movements), rigidity, postural instability, resting tremor, and non-motor symptoms in conjunction with fatigue, reduced facial expressions, sleep and smell disturbances, depression, and cognitive decline [4].

Conventional magnetic resonance imaging (MRI) does not provide adequate contrast to study changes in the brain of patients with PD. Indeed, conventional

 IntechOpen

1.5 T T1- and T2-weighted sequences do not collect information for the SNpc. Hence, conventional MRI cannot detect structural lesions that cause PD and cannot differentiate PD from characteristic alterations of atypical parkinsonism diseases (APD), such as multiple system atrophy (MSA) and progressive supranuclear palsy (PSP). Conventional MRI neuroimaging is not specifically recommended for routine diagnosis in clinical practice of the difficulty in PD [5].

Diffusion MRI is an evolution of conventional MRI and has the potential to differentiate between PD and APD. This ability includes identifying the principal changes in the SN and the lower part of the putamen/caudate complex, the location of most nigrostriatal dopaminergic neurons. Changes in these areas in patients with PD could provide valuable information to aid in the diagnosis and assess disease progression. Diffusion MRI involves two techniques: (1) diffusion-weighted imaging (DWI) shows the change in a particular water molecule diffusing from one location to another over a given period of time estimated by the apparent diffusion coefficient (ADC). (2) Diffusion tensor imaging (DTI) is a useful method to measure the directionality of water inside living systems, which is estimated by fractional anisotropy (FA). The fundamental aims of the use of diffusion MRI in PD are: (1) to contribute to the differential clinical diagnosis between PD and APD; (2) to determine biomarkers of disease progression and, therefore, to demonstrate the usefulness of potential therapies that delay or improve disease progression; (3) to allow presymptomatic diagnosis in people with PD; and (4) to identify in advance the motor and non-motor complications.

This chapter reviews the available data on the use of diffusion MRI to determine the pathophysiological mechanisms responsible for PD and APD. This technique could be used to identify microstructural changes earlier and thus initiate treatment more quickly after PD onset. It also offers the potential to differentiate between PD and APD.

2. Basic of diffusion

Diffusion is the physical property that describes the Brownian (random) movement of water molecules in biological tissue in response to thermal energy [5]. The human body is composed of 75% water, which is located in three compartments: intravascular, intracellular, and extracellular (**Figure 1**). The movement of water molecules at the microscopic level of these compartments is sensitive to the diffusion sequence. Of note, it is the movement of water molecules in the extracellular space that is most useful to identify quantifiable markers that reflect tissue alterations. Microscopic displacement of water molecules occurs within brain tissue by following diffusion [7, 8]. Identifying these alterations in these movements could be useful to characterize neurodegenerative diseases, such as PD.

In 1965, Stejskal and Tanner [9] were the first to apply the property of diffusion to MR sequences. In 1980, researchers reported the first biological tissues imaged based on the principles of nuclear magnetic resonance established by Carr et al. [10]. In 1986, Le Bihan et al. developed the first diffusion image from a brain MRI [11]. In 1992, Warach et al. [12] first applied this technique to study cerebral infarction. An advantage of this technique is its noninvasive nature and it does not require ionizing radiation and paramagnetic contrast. There is a great interest in MRI use to measure water diffusion. This application could provide maps of the diffusion coefficients in tissues, particularly *in vivo* [7]. Identifying areas of interest could be useful in defining biomarkers that could improve the diagnosis or traceability of a specific pathology.

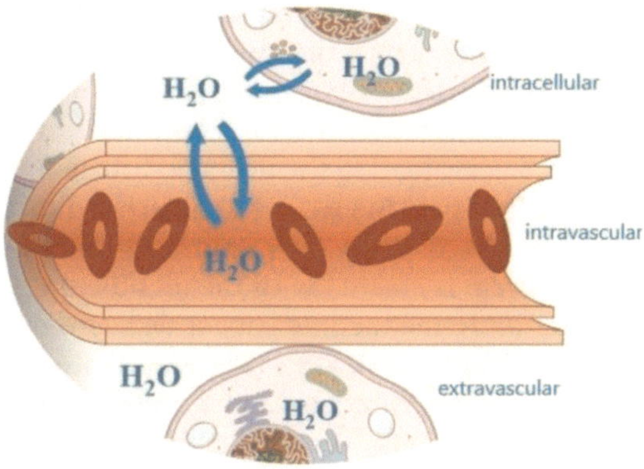

Figure 1.
A model of biological tissue described by three compartments: extravascular, intravascular, and intracellular. In healthy brain, water (H_2O, which forms the basis for the magnetic resonance signal) is present and exchanged among all three compartments. This figure is based on the model from Anderson et al. [6].

2.1 Brief background of diffusion MRI

Diffusion MRI, also known as DWI, is a procedure of MRI based upon measuring the motion of water molecules within a voxel of biological tissue. Diffusion MRI detected the Brownian motion that is observed in the random or uncontrolled movement of particles in a fluid as they constantly collide with other molecules [13]. The pulsed gradient spin echo sequence, shown in **Figure 2**, is the most used acquisition scheme to generate diffusion weighting in an MRI image. It is also widely used to measure the displacement of water molecules in tissue. It consists of two radiofrequency (RF) pulses, one at 90° and the second at 180°, and two magnetic gradients with intensity G and pulse duration δ, before and after the 180° RF pulse.

In the MRI literature, the sequence parameters (see **Figure 2**) are commonly represented by a single diffusion parameter, b. It can be calculated according to Eq. (1):

$$b = \gamma^2 G^2 \delta^2 \left(\Delta - \frac{\delta}{3} \right). \tag{1}$$

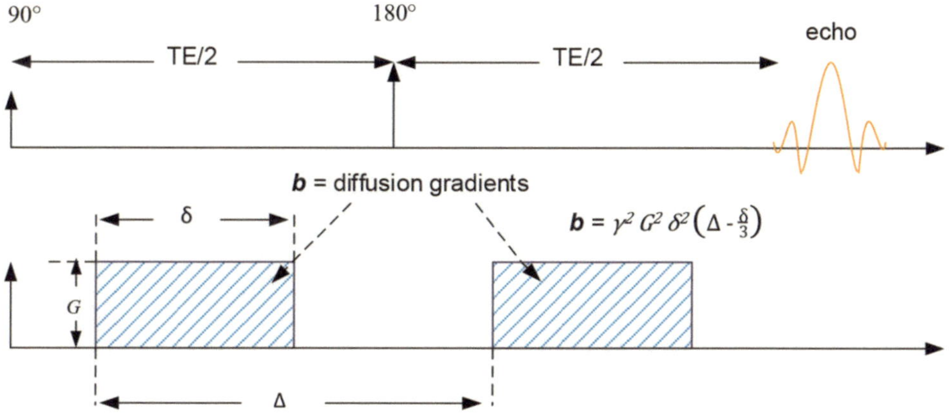

Figure 2.
The Stejskal-Tanner pulsed-gradient spin echo (PGSE) sequence [9]. δ is the pulse duration, G is the pulse gradient, Δ is the diffusion time and echo time (TE) is the time to echo [14, 15].

Diffusion MRI quantifies the motion of water molecules (see **Table 1**). Microstructural changes in neuronal tissue are determined by quantifying the diffusion coefficients, measured by applying a diffusion-sensitizing gradient using the isotropic signal decay formulated by Stejskal-Tanner, which is called the apparent diffusion coefficient (ADC). This measure allows for evaluating the average diffusion in the area of interest of a tissue. Isotropic diffusion refers to the lack of a preferred direction for diffusion. An example is cerebrospinal fluid in which the diffusion rate of molecules is equal in all directions [16, 17]. The ADC map is created with the mono-exponential model by applying a square noise filter to define the intensity scale based on b-values (**Figure 3**).

DTI was first described by Basser et al. [18]. It provides information about the local tissue when diffusion depends on the direction and is restricted by the normal architecture of the brain and the neuronal tracts, a condition known as anisotropy. Hence, DTI allows for calculating fractional anisotropy (FA) [19]. Anisotropic diffusion is not equal in all directions. An example is diffusion in neural tracts, where water molecules diffuse more longitudinally along the tract than to the sides. This directionality is largely determined by the cellularity and cell integrity in the tissues [16, 17]. FA is an important measure to detect any structural change with respect to a direction defined by the neuronal tissue. DTI is a sensitive, noninvasive method to detect the early stages of PD [20]. It even differentiates microstructural changes in PD (**Figures 4** and **5**) [21].

Diffusion imaging	Measures	Details
Diffusion-weighted imaging	Apparent diffusion coefficient (ADC), or trace (D) diffusion coefficient is a measure of the strength (velocity) of diffusion in tissue.	Isotropic diffusion are called the distance to travel by the water molecules in the tissue, without barriers that restrictand the move nor the direction.
Diffusion tensor imaging	Fractional anisotropy	The molecules are limited to a determined direction of the tissue, generating a tensor that has three diffusion components on each axis (x, y, and z).

Table 1.
Diffusion MRI techniques.

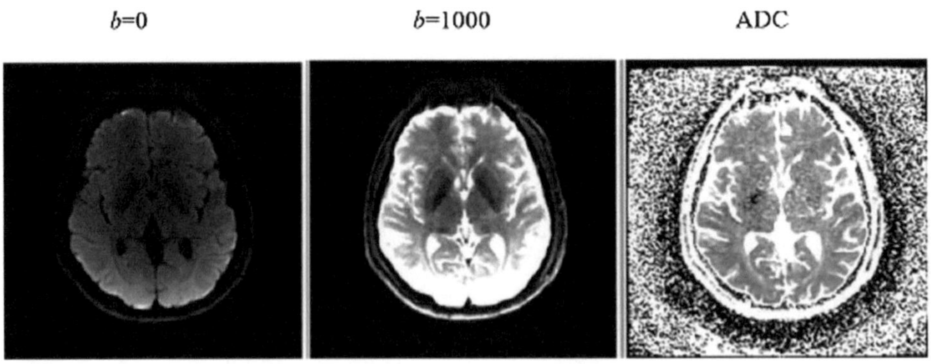

Figure 3.
PD-DWI images use two different b*-values, 43-year-old patient PD, male. Apparent diffusion coefficient (ADC) maps created from the linear representation of the mono-exponential model in patients with Parkinson's disease. The signal obtained with the* b*-value provides information about the diffusion constant (made by the authors).*

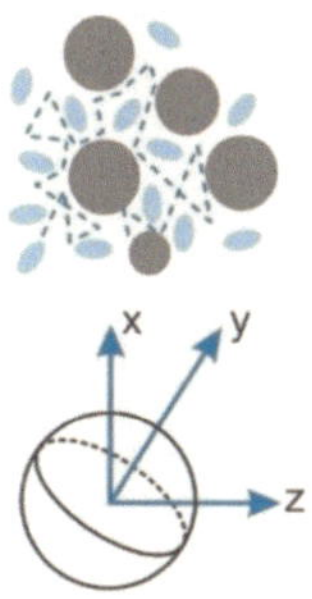

Figure 4.
Random barriers are present. Information on the microscopic motion of water protons (made by the authors).

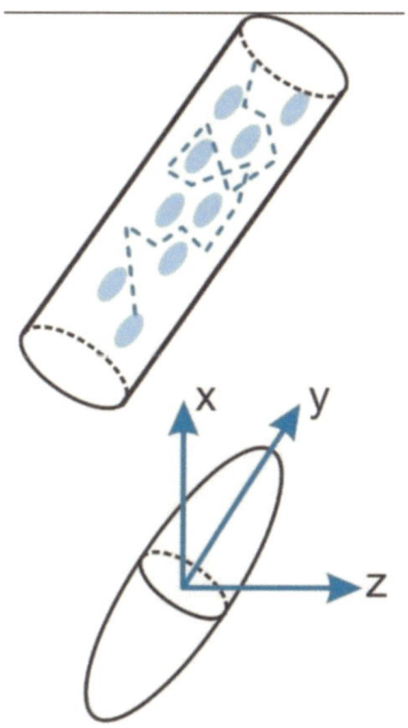

Figure 5.
Coherent axonal bundle. Information on diffusion directionality, for example, it is possible to reconstruct axonal or muscle fiber images (made by the authors).

3. Diagnosis of PD and APD

PD and APD are characterized by progressive dopaminergic dysfunction. Diagnosis and treatment of diseases in their early stages can be complicated [20]. While conventional MRI has provided information on these diseases (**Table 2**), diffusion MRI can help to provide additional information and specific biomarkers to help distinguish among them (**Figures 6–8**) [29].

3.1 Diffusional MRI findings in PD

DWI and DTI provide quantifiable information to detect microstructural changes in PD. Neuronal loss alters the structural architecture of the central nervous system, producing potential biomarkers that could be assessed with imaging to diagnose PD (**Table 3**) (**Figures 9–20**) [28, 29, 32, 51–53].

Definition	Affected areas	Typical imaging findings
MSA including MSA-P and MSA-C [22]	The putamen and cerebellum are both affected in MSA, and nigral dopaminergic neuronal loss is observed in both MSA and PD [23]. Increased putaminal diffusivity in a patients with MSA. ADC is increased in the area of the lenticular nucleus in the patient with MSA [24].	
PSP is characterized by postural instability and supranuclear gaze palsy; it is sometimes called Richardson's syndrome [25]	Pathological changes in the SCP and dentate nucleus. Extensive atrophy in the brain stem, particularly in the midbrain, and also in the basal ganglia and cortex [24]	
CBS includes apraxia, the alien-limb phenomenon, and disturbed epicritic sensitivity [26]	The most common motor feature in CBS is asymmetrical parkinsonism affecting a limb, typically an arm.	

Abbreviations: ADC: apparent diffusion coefficient; CBS: corticobasal syndrome; FLAIR: fluid-attenuated inversion recovery; MSA: multiple system atrophy; MSA-C: multiple system atrophy with predominant cerebellar dysfunction; MSA-P: multiple system atrophy with predominant parkinsonian features; PD: Parkinson's disease; PSP: Progressive supranuclear palsy; SCP: superior cerebellar peduncle.

Table 2.
The main diagnosis of parkinsonian diseases.

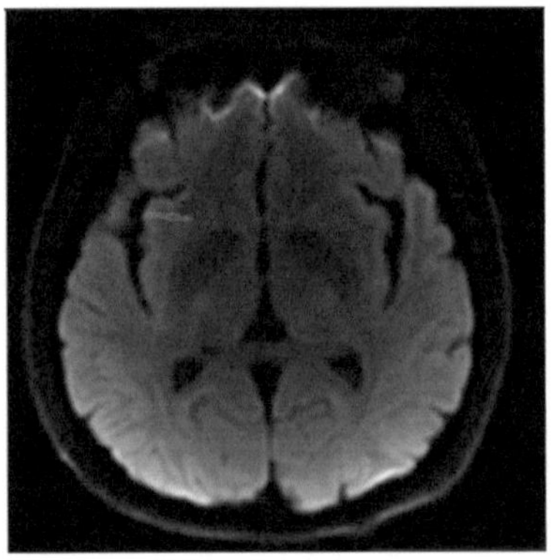

Figure 6.
The area of the lenticular nucleus 43-year-old patient PD, male (made by the authors).

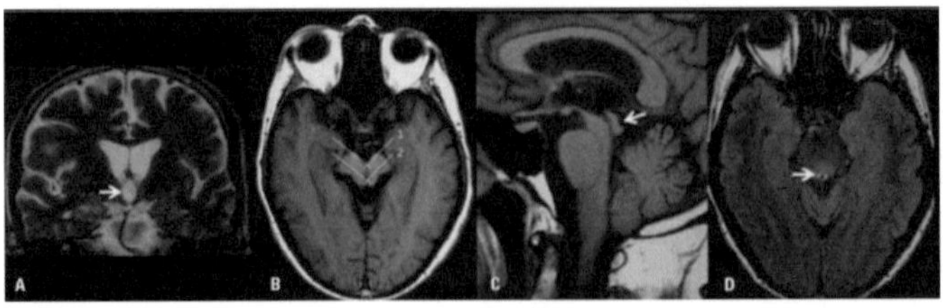

Figure 7.
DWI images of a patient with PSP. (A) Enlargement of the third ventricle (B). Internal-1 and external-2 interpeduncular angles show midbrain atrophy. (C) Quadrigeminal thickness showing atrophy. (D) Periaqueductal hypersignal. Adapted from Barsottini et al. [27].

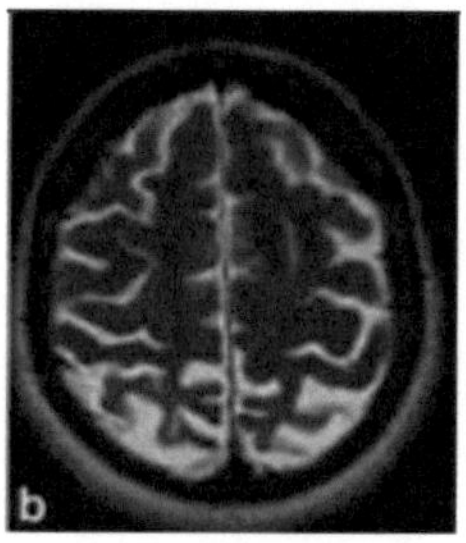

Figure 8.
Corticobasal degeneration. T2-weighted spin echo (b) demonstrates thinning of the sulci in the parietal cortex combined with subtle hyperintensity of the subcortical white matter. Adapted from Mascalchi et al. [28].

Technique and region	Diffusion MRI findings	Key diffusion measures	Reference
DWI in olfactory tracts	Patients with PD showed significant increases in trace of diffusion (D) values in both olfactory tracts in a cohort of patients with PD versus healthy controls. Adapted from Ref. [30].	**Patients with PD** Trace (D) $>0.78 \times 10^{-3}$ mm^2/s **Healthy controls** Trace (D) $<0.78 \times 10^{-3}$ mm^2/s	[30]
DTI to show olfactory dysfunction	Understanding the neurological substrates of olfactory dysfunction in early PD could be used in combination with clinical markers. Identify evidence of white matter areas with increased/ decreased connectivity in patients with PD with complete or severe loss of olfaction.		[31]
DWI of the putamen	PD, MSA-P, and healthy controls marked differences in putaminal ADC maps among patients. Putaminal ROIs denote descending regional ADC values. Adapted from Ref. [32].	**Putaminal regional ADC** **Patients with MSA-P** ADC median = 0.791×10^{-3} mm^2/s **Patients with PD** ADC median = 0.698×10^{-3} mm^2/s **Healthy controls** ADC median = 0.727×10^{-3} mm^2/s	[32]
DTI of the putamen	Schocke et al. [33] provided trace (D) imaging, which appears to be more accurate to separate patients with MSA-P from patients with PD, as rADC values in one direction are dependent on the slice orientation relative to the directions of fiber tracts. The ADC maps in the y-direction and z-direction clearly show the bilateral putaminal hyperintensity in	**Putamen** Increased putaminal diffusivity: rADC in the y- and z-direction as well as trace (D) clearly show bilateral putaminal hyperintensity. **Patients with MSA-P** rADC in the y-direction = $1.011 \pm 0.196 \times 10^{-3}$ mm^2/s rADC in the x-direction = $0.750 \pm 0.180 \times 10^{-3}$ mm^2/s Trace (D) = $0.926 \pm 0.208 \times 10^{-3}$ mm^2/s **Patients with PD** rADC in the y-direction = $0.766 \pm 0.036 \times 10^{-3}$ mm^2/s	[33]

Technique and region	Diffusion MRI findings	Key diffusion measures	Reference
	a patient with MSA, indicating increased putaminal rADCs and rTrace (D) values. The putaminal hyperintensity is poorly demarcated on the ADC map in the x-direction.	rADC in the x-direction = $0.591 \pm 0.0058 \times 10^{-3}$ mm^2/s Trace (D) = $0.718 \pm 0.030 \times 10^{-3}$ mm^2/s **Healthy controls** rADC in the y-direction = $0.769 \pm 0.025 \times 10^{-3}$ mm^2/s rADC in the x-direction = $0.637 \pm 0.071 \times 10^{-3}$ mm^2/s Trace (D) = $0.745 \pm 0.024 \times 10^{-3}$ mm^2/s	
DTI of white matter	Significant differences between patients with MSA-P and patients with PD.	**White matter** **Patients with MSA-P** rADC in the y-direction = $0.833 \pm 0.067 \times 10^{-3}$ mm^2/s ($P = 0.004$) **Patients with PD** rADC in the y-direction = $0.769 \pm 0.052 \times 10^{-3}$ mm^2/s ($P = 0.004$) **Healthy controls** rADC in the y-direction = $0.733 \pm 0.039 \times 10^{-3}$ mm^2/s ($P = 0.004$)	[33]
DTI of the caudate nucleus	Significant differences in trace (D) of the caudate nucleus between patients with MSA-P and patients with PD. The caudate nucleus also shows significant differences in the rADC in the y-direction between patients with MSA-P or PD and healthy controls.	**Caudate nucleus** **Patients with PD** Trace (D) = 0.725 $\pm 0.035 \times 10^{-3}$ mm^2/s **Patients with MSA-P** Trace (D) = 0.802 $\pm 0.125 \times 10^{-3}$ mm^2/s **Patients with PD** rADC in y-direction = 0.808 $\pm 0.043 \times 10^{-3}$ mm^2/s **Patients with MSA-P** rADC in y-direction = 0.914 $\pm 0.120 \times 10^{-3}$ mm^2/s **Healthy controls** rADC in y-direction = 0.823 $\pm 0.051 \times 10^{-3}$ mm^2/s	[33]
DTI of the globus pallidus	Significant differences: 1. rADC between patients with MSA-P or PD patients and healthy controls for the z- and x-directions. 2. Trace (D) between patients with MSA-P or PD and healthy controls.	**Globus pallidus** **Patients with MSA-P** rADC in the z-direction = 0.829 $\pm 0.109 \times 10^{-3}$ mm^2/s **Patients with PD** rADC in the z-direction = 0.737 $\pm 0.049 \times 10^{-3}$ mm^2/s **Healthy controls** rADC in the z-direction = 0.798 $\pm 0.068 \times 10^{-3}$ mm^2/s **Patients with MSA-P** rADC in the x-direction = 0.879 $\pm 0.120 \times 10^{-3}$ mm^2/s **Patients with PD** rADC in the x-direction = 0.736 $\pm 0.108 \times 10^{-3}$ mm^2/s	[33]

Technique and region	Diffusion MRI findings	Key diffusion measures	Reference
		Healthy controls rADC in the x-direction = 0.721 $\pm$ 0.092$\times$ 10^{-3} mm^2/s **Patients with MSA-P** Trace (D) = 0.802 $\pm$ 0.125$\times$ 10^{-3} mm^2/s **Patients with PD** Trace (D) = 0.725 $\pm$ 0.035$\times$ 10^{-3} mm^2/s **Healthy controls** Trace (D) = 0.747 $\pm$ 0.034$\times$ 10^{-3} mm^2/s	
DWI of the SCP ADC differentiates between patients with PSP and patients with PD		**SCP** **Patients with PSP** Median rADC = 0.98 $\times$ 10^{-3} mm^2/s **Patients with MSA-P** Median rADC = 0.79 $\times$ 10^{-3} mm^2/s ($P < 0.001$) **Patients with PD** Median rADC = 0.79 $\times$ 10^{-3} mm^2/s ($P < 0.001$) **Healthy controls** Median rADC = 0.80 $\times$ 10^{-3} mm^2/s ($P < 0.001$)	[34, 35]
DTI of the putamen in patients with MSA-P	Putaminal trace (D) in patients with MSA-P has been mapped at the level of the mid-striatum. The diffuse hyperintensity corresponding to increased trace (D) in the putaminal region of the patient with MSA [36].	**The patient with MSA** **Putamen** Trace (D) >0.80 $\times$ 10^{-3} mm^2/s **Posterior putamen** Trace (D) >0.80 $\times$ 10^{-3} mm^2/s	[37]
DWI of the middle cerebellar peduncle to differentiate between patients with MSA-P, PSP or PD	Increased middle cerebellar peduncle rADC. The images show patients with MSA without cruciform hyperintensity and patients with MSA with cruciform hyperintensity [37].	Increased middle cerebellar peduncle rADC differentiates patients with MSA-P from patients with PSP and PD. **Patients with MSA-P** Median rADC = 0.93 $\times$ 10^{-3} mm^2/s ($P < 0.001$) **Patients with PSP** Median rADC = 0.82 $\times$ 10^{-3} mm^2/s **Patients with PD** Median rADC = 0.79 $\times$ 10^{-3} mm^2/s ($P < 0.001$) **Healthy controls** Median rADC = 0.81 $\times$ 10^{-3} mm^2/s ($P < 0.001$)	[38]
DWI of the middle cerebellar peduncle and rostral pons to differentiate between patients with MSA-P, PSP,	The optimal cut-off level to discriminate patients with MSA-P from patients with PSP was a middle cerebellar peduncle rADC of $\geq$0.733 $\times$ 10^{-3} mm^2/s (sensitivity = 91%,	Increased rADC in the middle cerebellar peduncle and rostral pons in patients with MSA-P compared with patients with PSP or PD. **Pons (caudal):** **Patients with PSP** rADC = 0.785 $\pm$ 0.090 $\times$ 10^{-3} mm^2/s	[39]

Technique and region	Diffusion MRI findings	Key diffusion measures	Reference
or PD (caudal and rostral)	specificity = 84%). ADC measurements may have been utilized as surrogate markers in trials of disease-modifying medications [38].	**Patients with MSA** rADC = $0.845 \pm 0.133 \times 10^{-3}$ mm²/s **Patients with PD** rADC = $0.771 \pm 0.101 \times 10^{-3}$ mm²/s **Healthy controls** rADC = $0.763 \pm 0.079 \times 10^{-3}$ mm²/s **Pons (rostral):** **Patients with PSP** rADC = $0.745 \pm 0.110 \times 10^{-3}$ mm²/s	
DWI of the putamen and SCP	Significantly higher SCP ADC in patients with PSP compared with patients with CBS or PD and healthy controls. The median ADC in the higher-valued hemisphere was significantly increased in patients with CBS. The hemispheric symmetry ratio in patients with CBS was lower than in patients with RS or PD and healthy controls.	Putaminal ADC provides good discrimination between patients with PD and patients with APD (RS and CBS). **Patients with CBS** 0.77 (0.75–0.79) $\times 10^{-3}$ mm²/s **Patients with RS** 0.75 (0.74–0.79) $\times 10^{-3}$ mm²/s **Patients with PD** 0.72 (0.71–0.73) $\times 10^{-3}$ mm²/s **Healthy controls** 0.70 (0.69–0.71) $\times 10^{-3}$ mm²/s	[35]
DTI of the pons, cerebellum, and putamen to differentiate between patients with MSA-P and patients with PD.	FA and ADC detected early pathological involvement prior to magnetic resonance signal changes in patients with MSA-P. Early FA reduction and ADC increase are likely to be associated with subtle early degenerative processes in patients with MSA-P.	Increased ADC in the pons, cerebellum, and putamen, and reduced FA in patients with MSA compared with patients with PD and healthy controls. **FA** Pons = 0.38 Cerebellum = 0.30 Putamen = 0.35 **ADC** Pons = 0.98×10^{-3} mm²/s Cerebellum = 0.96×10^{-3} mm²/s Putamen = 0.83×10^{-3} mm²/s **Sensitivity and specificity of FA:** 70.0% and 100.0% in the pons; 70.0% and 63.6% in the cerebellum; and 70.0% and 87.5% in the putamen.	[40]
DTI in patients with an implanted deep brain stimulation (DBS) device.	DTI is safe and delineation of the white matter pathway is feasible for patients with PD and an implanted DBS device.	The FA of the left SN was significantly lower than that of the right SN ($P < 0.05$ in both DBS-on and DBS-off states)	[41]
Dopamine transporter imaging	The neuromelanin value was significantly lower and the diffusion tensor values except FA were significantly higher in the RBD and PD groups than in the healthy group. Diffusion MRI detects nigrostriatal changes in RBD and early PD.	Neuromelanin/mean diffusivity value. **Patients with RBD** SNpc = 0.76/0.82 **Patients with PD** SNpc = 0.83/0.80	[42]

Technique and region	Diffusion MRI findings	Key diffusion measures	Reference
Conventional MRI DTI of the SN		The reduced volume of the SN in the patient with PD is attributable to iron deposition. FA was lower in the patient with PD than in the patient without PD (0.425 vs. 0.581), indicating a loss of neuronal integrity.	[43]
DTI of the SN and middle cerebellar peduncle.	FA was increased in all three subareas of the SN.	FA was increased in the three nigral subareas in patients with PD ($P < 0.01$). The right SN had higher FA than the left in all subareas ($P < 0.01$). The left middle cerebellar peduncle had increased FA ($P < 0.001$).	[44]
DWI of the putamen.	Putaminal diffusivity measurements to distinguish MSA-P from PD.	Prominent neuronal loss in the putamen; structural damage in the putamen would lead to enhanced diffusivity. Meta-analysis showed an overall sensitivity of 90% and specificity of 93%.	[29]
DTI of the rostral, middle and caudal SN and cerebral peduncle	Assessment of FA in the rostral, middle, and caudal regions of the SN. SN distinguishes early-stage *de novo* patients with PD from healthy controls.	Decreased FA in the caudal part of the substantial nigra with increased sensitivity and specificity even between individual subjects. **Rostral region** t = 1.5; P = 0.12 **Middle region** t = 3.7; P = 0.001 **Caudal region** t = 11.9; P = 0.00001	[20]
DTI of the SN	The FA is decreased in the nigrostriatal projection in parkinsonian patients, even during the early clinical stages	Decreased FA in the ROI along a line between the SN and the lower part of the putamen/caudate complex in patients with PD, even during the early clinical stages of the disease. FA in patients with PSP was decreased in most of the ROIs except for those in the neostriatum of parkinsonian patients showed a significant decrease in FA of the subthalamic ROI beside the SN. FA in the white matter of the premotor cortices was significantly smaller in patients with PSP or advanced PD compared with healthy controls.	[45]
DTI of the SN, red nucleus, and cerebral peduncle		FA was reduced in the rostral SN of subjects with early-stage PD.	[46]
DWI of the SN with increased iron (R2)		Reduction of FA inside the SN in patients with PD demonstrated a high correlation with an increase in iron.	[47]
DTI of the SN with increased iron (R2)	Differences between patients with PD and controls from voxel-based analysis of R2, mean	Reduction of FA inside the SN demonstrated a high correlation with an increase in iron in patients with PD.	[48]

Technique and region	Diffusion MRI findings	Key diffusion measures	Reference
	diffusivity, and FA maps [48].		
DTI of the SN		FA in the SN based on DTI was lower in patients with PD compared with healthy controls.	[49]
DTI of the SN		Decreased FA in the SN is associated with the increased motor in patients with PD.	[50]
DTI of the SN		Decreased FA in the SN is associated with the increase of motor symptoms in patients with PD.	[21]

Abbreviations: ADC: apparent diffusion coefficient; APD: atypical parkinsonism diseases; CBS: corticobasal syndrome; DBS: deep brain stimulation; DTI: diffusion tensor imaging; DWI: diffusion-weighted imaging; FA: fractional anisotropy; MSA: multiple system atrophy; MSA-P: multiple system atrophy with predominant parkinsonian features; PD: Parkinson's disease; PSP: progressive supranuclear palsy; rADC: regional apparent diffusion coefficient; RBD: rapid eye movement sleep behavior disorder; ROI: region of interest; RS: Richardson's syndrome; rTrace (D): regional trace (D); SCP: superior cerebellar peduncles; SN: substantial nigra; Unified Parkinson's Disease Rating Scale (UPDRS). AC: anterior commissure; CN: caudate nucleus; Ctr: age matched normal subjects as control; GP: globus pallidus; GPe: globus pallidus lateral segment; GPi: globus pallidus medial segment; PC: posterior commissure; PD12: Parkinson's disease in the early-stage group; PD345: Parkinson's disease in the advanced stage group. ROI: region of interest; SN: substantia nigra; SNc: substantia nigra pars compacta; SNr: substantia nigra pars reticulate; STN: subthalamic nucleus; VL: nucleus ventralis lateralis.

Table 3.
Biomarkers in the diagnosis of PD and APD.

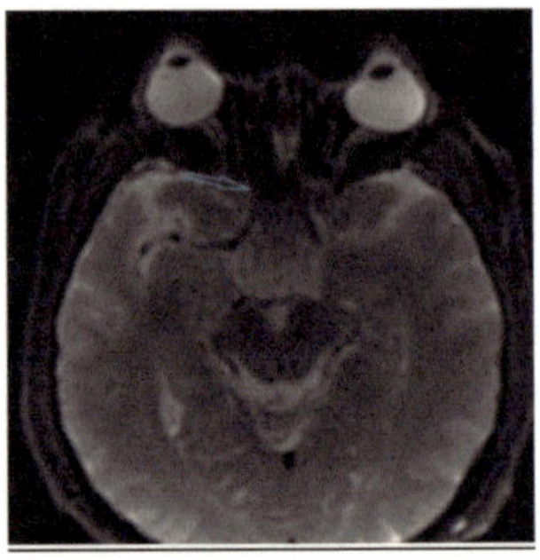

Figure 9.
DWI, 43-year-old patient PD, male (made by the authors).

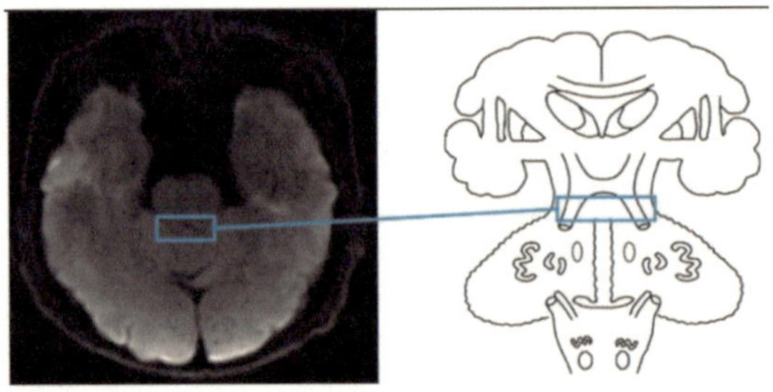

Figure 10.
Superior cerebellar peduncles (SCP) on the ROI map from 43-year-old patient PD, male. Adapted from results with interesting ROI (made by the authors).

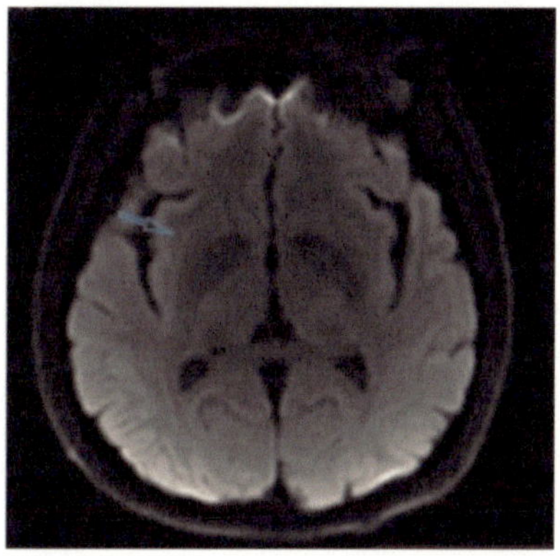

Figure 11.
Adapted from results with putaminal ROI from 43-year-old patient PD (made by the authors).

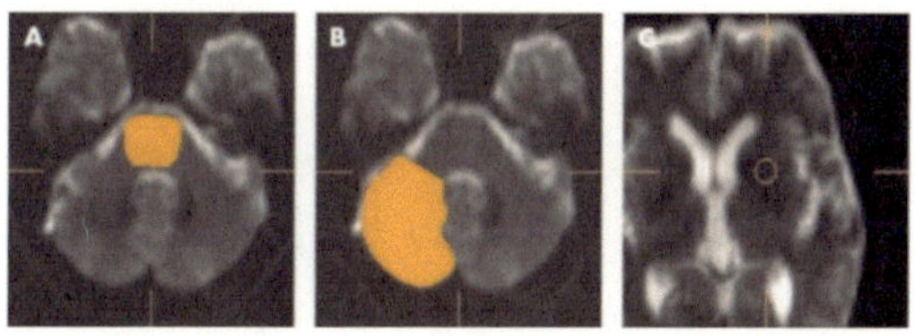

Figure 12.
ROIs in the pons (A), cerebellum (B), and putamen (C). Adapted from Ito et al. [40].

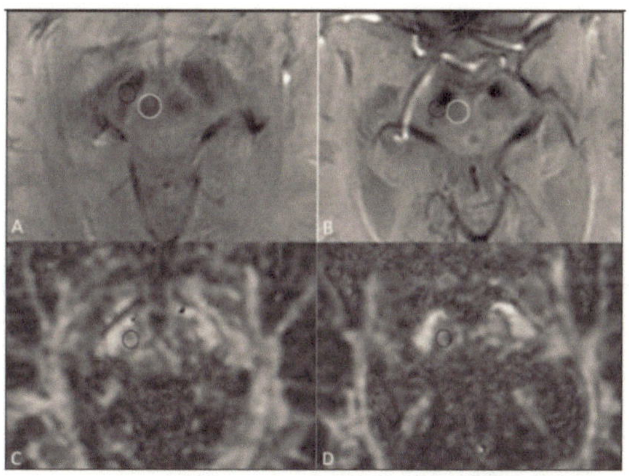

Figure 13.
DWI image in a 66-year-old-patient without PD (A), an axial slice of the midbrain shows a delineated SN (black circle), showing well-defined cleavage with the red nucleus (white circle). In a 68-year-old patient with PD (B), an axial slice of the midbrain on susceptibility-DWI shows a poorly delineated. Adapted from Oliveira et al. [43].

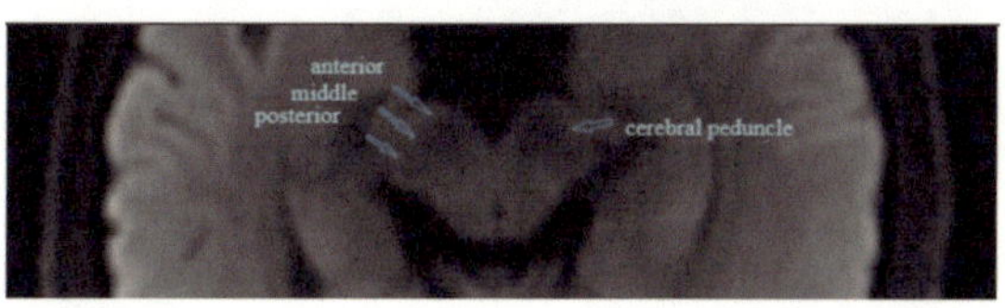

Figure 14.
Anterior, middle, and posterior SN in a 43-year-old patient PD (Adapted from results by the authors).

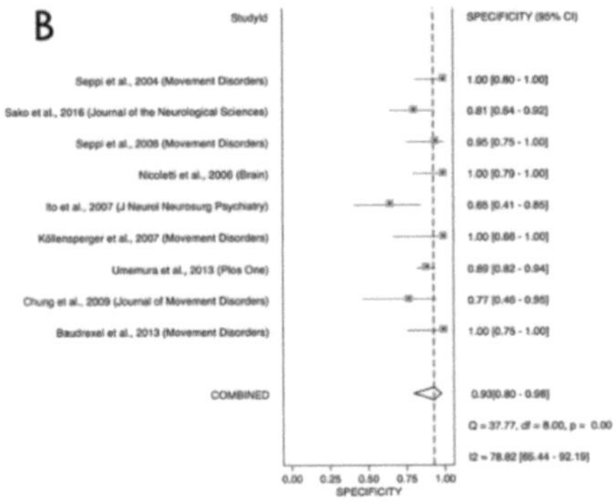

Figure 15.
The overall specificity of putaminal diffusivity to discriminate MSA-P from PD. Adapted from Bajaj et al. [29].

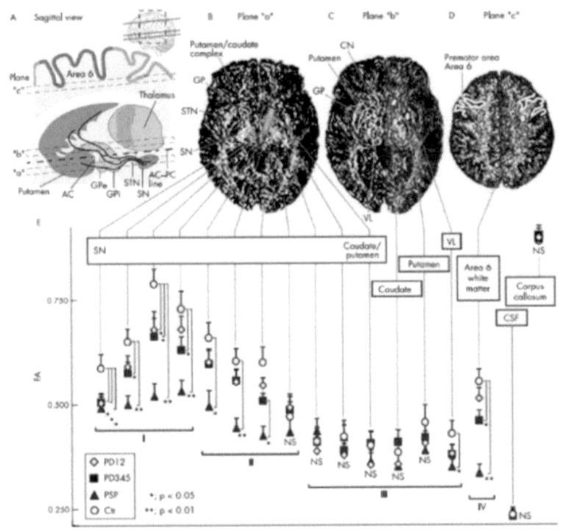

Figure 16.
Anatomy of the extrapyramidal system in the paramedian sagittal view (A). Fibers of nigro-neostriatal projection, which are selectively lost in PD, are illustrated by black lines originating from the SN. FA images are derived from diffusion tensor images (B–D). FA in the extrapyramidal system of normal subjects and patients (E). Adapted from Ref. [45].

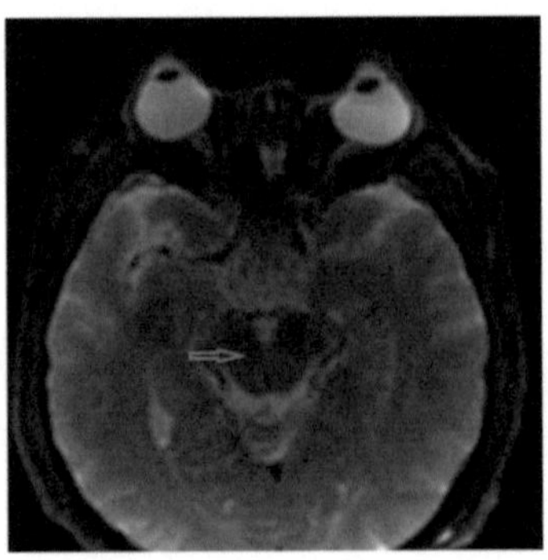

Figure 17.
Axial sequences depicting the SN and red nucleus (blue arrow) from a 43-year-old patient PD (adapted by the authors).

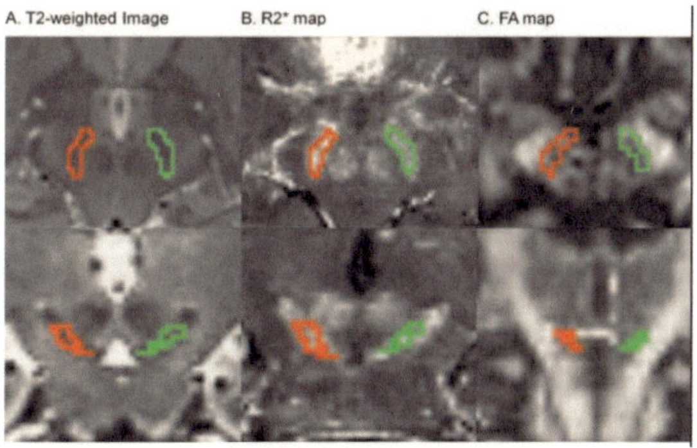

Figure 18.
Image illustrating the location of the SN in T2-weighted images (A) and the co-registered ROIs on the R2 (B) and FA (C) maps on both axial (top row) and coronal (bottom row) sections. Adapted from Du et al. [47].*

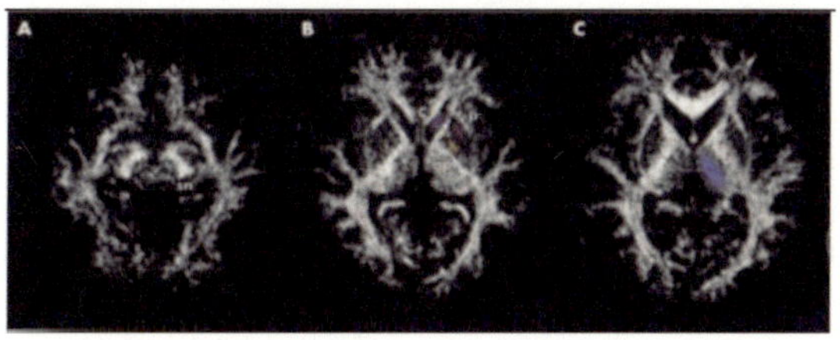

Figure 19.
ROIs of gray matter structures: (A) substantia nigra (sn), (B) caudate (c), putamen (p), globus pallidus (gp), and (C) thalamus (t), drawn on axial diffusion tensor DTI images on the FA map. Adapted from Chan et al. [49].

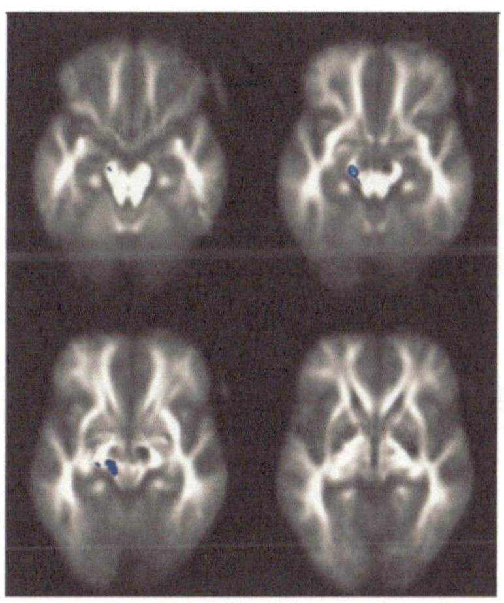

Figure 20.
Significant voxel-wise correlations ($P < 0.05$, corrected) between decreased FA and increased total UPDRS scores were detected in the white matter at the level of the SN. Adapted from Zhan et al. [21].

4. Conclusion

Diffusion MRI, including isotropic and anisotropic techniques, has become increasingly important in the evaluation and diagnosis of patients with PD, and even in other neurodegenerative diseases. The most common quantitative biomarkers are ADC and FA. Moreover, diffusion MRI has the advantages of being noninvasive, repeatable, and quantifiable, and has the ability to localize damage. It is likely that neuroimaging methods will become important research techniques in the area of biomarkers in future. In conclusion, the parameters estimated with diffusion MRI in patients with moderate-stage PD can distinguish between patients with PD or APD and healthy controls.

Acknowledgements

Greatly appreciated to the authors who allowed the use of the images as part of the construction of the chapter and to the Chinese Academy of Sciences for supporting this publication. It is necessary to clarify that the main author was affiliated with the Universidad Manuela Beltran and the Universidad ECCI as a research professor, but it is published with the authors' own resources without any financial interest.

Conflict of interest

The authors declare no conflict of interest.

Author details

Gloria Cruz[1]*, Shengdong Nie[2] and Juan Ramírez[3]

1 Faculty of Engineering, Department of Biomedical Engineering, Universidad ECCI, Bogotá, Colombia

2 Institute of Medical Imaging and Engineering School of Medical Instrument and Food Engineering, University of Shanghai for Science and Technology USST, Shanghai, China

3 Faculty of Engineering, Universidad Distrital Francisco José de Caldas, Bogotá, Colombia

*Address all correspondence to: g_milena@yahoo.com

References

[1] Braak H, Rüb U, Gai W, et al. Idiopathic Parkinson's disease: Possible routes by which vulnerable neuronal types may be subject to neuroinvasion by an unknown pathogen. Journal of Neural Transmission. 2003;**110**:517-536

[2] Hodaie M, Neimat J, Lozano A. The dopaminergic nigrostriatal system and Parkinson's disease: Molecular events in development, disease, and cell death, and new therapeutic strategies. Neurosurgery. 2007;**60**:17-28

[3] Braak H, Del Tredici K, Rüb U, et al. Staging of brain pathology related to sporadic Parkinson's disease. Neurobiology of Aging. 2003;**24**:197-211

[4] Deutschlander AB, Konno T, Soto-Beasley AI, et al. Association of MAPT subhaplotypes with clinical and demographic features in Parkinson's disease. Annals of Clinical Translational Neurology. 2020;**7**:1557-1563

[5] Politis M. Neuroimaging in Parkinson disease: From research setting to clinical practice. Nature Reviews. Neurology. 2014;**10**:708-722

[6] Anderson VC, Lenar DP, Quinn JF, et al. The blood-brain barrier and microvascular water exchange in alzheimer's disease. Cardiovascular Psychiatry Neurology. 2011;**2011**. DOI: 10.1155/2011/615829. [Epub ahead of print]

[7] Dietrich O, Biffar A, Baur-Melnyk A, et al. Technical aspects of MR diffusion imaging of the body. European Journal of Radiology. 2010;**76**:314-322

[8] Le Bihan D, Johansen-Berg H. Diffusion MRI at 25: Exploring brain tissue structure and function. NeuroImage. 2012;**61**:324-341

[9] Stejskal EO, Tanner JE. Spin diffusion measurements: Spin echoes in the presence of a time-dependent field gradient. The Journal of Chemical Physics. 1965;**42**:288

[10] Carr H, Purcell E. Effects of diffusion on free precession in nuclear magnetic resonance experiments. Physics Review. 1954;**94**:630-638

[11] LeBihan D, Breton E, Lallemand D, et al. MR imaging of intravoxel incoherent motions: Application to diffusion and perfusion in neurologic disorders. Radiology. 1986;**161**:401-407

[12] Warach S, Chien D, Li W, et al. Fast magnetic resonance diffusion-weighted imaging of acute human stroke. Neurology. 1992;**42**:1717-1723

[13] Mitchell JG, Kogure K. Bacterial motility: Links to the environment and a driving force for microbial physics. FEMS Microbiology Ecology. 2006;**55**:3-16

[14] Mori S. Introduction to Diffusion Tensor Imaging. Elsevier; 2007. DOI: 10.1016/B978-044452828-5/50017-X

[15] Kon T, Mori F, Tanji K, et al. An autopsy case of preclinical multiple system atrophy (MSA-C). Neuropathology. 2013;**33**:667-672

[16] Jones DK. Diffusion MRI: Theory, Methods, and Applications. DOI: 10.1093/med/9780195369779.001.0001

[17] Chilla GS, Tan CH, Xu C, et al. Diffusion weighted magnetic resonance imaging and its recent trend-a survey. Quantitative Imaging in Medicine and Surgery. 2015;**5**:407-422

[18] Basser PJ, Mattiello J, Lebihan D. Estimation of the effective self-diffusion tensor from the NMR spin Echo. Journal of Magnetic Resonance - Series B. 1994; **103**:247-254

[19] Hagmann P, Jonasson L, Maeder P, et al. Understanding diffusion MR imaging techniques: From scalar diffusion-weighted imaging to diffusion tensor imaging and beyond. Radiographics. Oct 2006;**26**. DOI: 10.1148/rg.26si065510. [Epub ahead of print]

[20] Vaillancourt D, Spraker M, Prodoehl J, et al. High-resolution diffusion tensor imaging in the substantia nigra of de novo Parkinson disease. Neurology. 2009;**72**:1378-1384

[21] Zhan W, Kang GA, Glass GA, et al. Regional alterations of brain microstructure in Parkinson's disease using diffusion tensor imaging. Movement Disorders. 2012;**27**:90-97

[22] Niethammer M, Eidelberg D. Chapter five—Network imaging in parkinsonian and other movement disorders: Network dysfunction and clinical correlates. In: Politis M, editor. Imaging in Movement Disorders: Imaging in Non-Parkinsonian Movement Disorders and Dementias, Part 2. Academic Press; 2019. pp. 143-184

[23] Sako W, Murakami N, Izumi Y, et al. The difference in putamen volume between MSA and PD: Evidence from a meta-analysis. Parkinsonism & Related Disorders. 2014;**20**:873-877

[24] Lehericy S, Bensimon G, Vidailhet M. Parkinsonian Syndromes. Elsevier Inc; 2015. DOI: 10.1016/B978-0-12-397025-1.00088-9

[25] Williams DR, de Silva R, Paviour DC, et al. Characteristics of two distinct clinical phenotypes in pathologically proven progressive supranuclear palsy: Richardson's syndrome and PSP-parkinsonism. Brain. 2005;**128**:1247-1258

[26] Boelmans K, Bodammer NC, Suchorska B, et al. Diffusion tensor imaging of the corpus callosum differentiates corticobasal syndrome from Parkinson's disease. Parkinson Related Disorders. 2010;**16**:498-502

[27] Barsottini OGP, Felício AC, de Aquino CC, et al. Progressive supranuclear palsy: New concepts. Arquivos de Neuro-Psiquiatria. 2010;**68**:938-946

[28] Mascalchi M, Vella A, Ceravolo R. Movement disorders: Role of imaging in diagnosis. Journal of Magnetic Resonance Imaging. 2012;**35**:239-256

[29] Bajaj S, Krismer F, Palma J-A, et al. Diffusion-weighted MRI distinguishes Parkinson disease from the parkinsonian variant of multiple system atrophy: A systematic review and meta-analysis. PLoS One. 2017;**12**:e0189897

[30] Scherfler C, Schocke MF, Seppi K, et al. Voxel-wise analysis of diffusion weighted imaging reveals disruption of the olfactory tract in Parkinson's disease. Brain. 2006;**129**:538-542

[31] Sobhani S, Rahmani F, Aarabi MH, et al. Exploring white matter microstructure and olfaction dysfunction in early Parkinson disease: Diffusion MRI reveals new insight. Brain Imaging and Behavior. 2019;**13**:210-219

[32] Schocke M, Seppi K, Esterhammer R, et al. Diffusion-weighted MRI differentiates the Parkinson variant of multiple system atrophy from PD. Neurology. 2002;**58**:575-580

[33] Schocke M, Seppi K, Esterhammer R, et al. Trace of diffusion tensor differentiates the Parkinson variant of

multiple system atrophy and Parkinson's disease. NeuroImage. 2004;**21**:1443-1451

[34] Nicoletti G, Tonon C, Lodi R, et al. Apparent diffusion coefficient of the superior cerebellar peduncle differentiates progressive supranuclear palsy from Parkinson's disease. Movement Disorders. 2008;**23**:2370-2376

[35] Rizzo G, Martinelli P, Manners D, et al. Diffusion-weighted brain imaging study of patients with clinical diagnosis of corticobasal degeneration, progressive supranuclear palsy and Parkinson's disease. Brain. 2008;**131**:2690-2700

[36] Seppi K, Schocke M, Mair KJ, et al. Progression of putaminal degeneration in multiple system atrophy: A serial diffusion MR study. NeuroImage. 2006; **31**:240-245

[37] Nicoletti G, Fera F, Condino F, et al. Imaging of middle cerebellar peduncle width: Differentiation of multiple system atrophy from purpose: Methods: Results: Conclusion. Radiology. 2006;**239**:825-830

[38] Paviour D, Thornton J, Lees A, et al. Diffusion-weighted magnetic resonance imaging differentiates parkinsonian variant of multiple-system atrophy from progressive supranuclear palsy. Movement Disorders. 2007;**22**:68-74

[39] Seppi K, Schocke MF, Prennschuetz-Schuetzenau K, Mair K, et al. Topography of putaminal degeneration in multiple system atrophy: A diffusion magnetic resonance study. Movement Disorders. 2006;**21**:847-865

[40] Ito M, Watanabe H, Kawai Y, et al. Usefulness of combined fractional anisotropy and apparent diffusion coefficient values for detection of involvement in multiple system atrophy. Journal of Neurology, Neurosurgery, and Psychiatry. 2007;**78**:722-728

[41] Li Y, He N, Zhang C, et al. Mapping motor pathways in Parkinson's disease patients with subthalamic deep brain stimulator: A diffusion MRI Tractography study. Neurological Theraphy. 2022:659-677

[42] Takahashi H, Kashiwagi N, Arisawa A, et al. Imaging of the nigrostriatal system for evaluating the preclinical phase of Parkinson's disease development: The utility of neuromelanin, diffusion MRI, and DAT-SPECT. The British Journal of Radiology. 2022;**95**:40-41

[43] de Oliveira RV, Pereira JS. The role of diffusion magnetic resonance imaging in Parkinson's disease and in the differential diagnosis with atypical parkinsonism. Radiologia Brasileira. 2017;**50**:250-257

[44] Lenfeldt N, Larsson A, Nyberg L, et al. Fractional anisotropy in the substantia nigra in Parkinson's disease: A complex picture. European Journal of Neurology. 2015;**22**:1408-1414

[45] Yoshikawa K. Early pathological changes in the parkinsonian brain demonstrated by diffusion tensor MRI. Journal of Neurology, Neurosurgery, and Psychiatry. 2004;**75**:481-484

[46] Modrego PJ, Fayed N, Artal J, et al. Correlation of findings in advanced MRI techniques with global severity scales in patients with Parkinson disease. Academic Radiology. 2011;**18**:235-241

[47] Du G, Lewis MM, Styner M, et al. Combined R2* and diffusion tensor imaging changes in the substantia Nigra in Parkinson's disease. Movement Disorders. 2011;**26**:1627-1632

[48] Péran P, Cherubini A, Assogna F, et al. Magnetic resonance imaging markers

of Parkinson's disease nigrostriatal signature. Brain. 2010;**133**:3423-3433

[49] Chan L-L, Rumpel H, Yap K, et al. Case control study of diffusion tensor imaging in Parkinson's disease. Journal of Neurology, Neurosurgery, and Psychiatry. 2007;**78**:1383-1386

[50] Prakash BD, Sitoh Y-Y, Tan LCS, et al. Asymmetrical diffusion tensor imaging indices of the rostral substantia nigra in Parkinson's disease. Parkinsonism & Related Disorders. 2012; **18**:1029-1033

[51] Seppi K, Schocke MFH, Donnemiller E, Esterhammer R, Kremser C, Scherfler C, et al. Comparison of diffusion-weighted imaging and [123I]IBZM-SPECT for the differentiation of patients with the Parkinson variant of multiple system atrophy from those with Parkinson's disease. Movement Disorders. 2004;**19**:1438-1445

[52] Paviour D, Price S, Stevens J, et al. Quantitative MRI measurement of superior cerebellar peduncle in progressive supranuclear palsy. Neurology. 2005;**64**:675-679

[53] Nicoletti G, Fera F, Condino F, et al. MR imaging of middle cerebellar peduncle width: Differentiation of multiple system atrophy from Parkinson disease. Radiology. 2006;**239**:825-830